Iatrogenic Conditions of the Chest, Abdomen, and Pelvis

Editors

GABRIELA GAYER
DOUGLAS S. KATZ

RADIOLOGIC CLINICS OF NORTH AMERICA

www.radiologic.theclinics.com

Consulting Editor
FRANK H. MILLER

September 2014 • Volume 52 • Number 5

ELSEVIER

1600 John F. Kennedy Boulevard • Suite 1800 • Philadelphia, Pennsylvania, 19103-2899

http://www.theclinics.com

RADIOLOGIC CLINICS OF NORTH AMERICA Volume 52, Number 5
September 2014 ISSN 0033-8389, ISBN 13: 978-0-323-32343-7

Editor: John Vassallo (j.vassallo@elsevier.com)
Developmental Editor: Donald Mumford

Radiologic Clinics of North America (ISSN 0033-8389) is published bimonthly by Elsevier Inc., 360 Park Avenue South, New York, NY 10010-1710. Months of issue are January, March, May, July, September, and November. Periodicals postage paid at New York, NY and additional mailing offices. Subscription prices are USD 460 per year for US individuals, USD 709 per year for US institutions, USD 220 per year for US students and residents, USD 535 per year for Canadian individuals, USD 905 per year for Canadian institutions, USD 660 per year for international individuals, USD 905 per year for international institutions, and USD 315 per year for Canadian and foreign students/residents. To receive student and resident rate, orders must be accompanied by name of affiliated institution, date of term and the signature of program/residency coordinatior on institution letterhead. Orders will be billed at individual rate until proof of status is received. Foreign air speed delivery is included in all *Clinics* subscription prices. All prices are subject to change without notice. **POSTMASTER:** Send address changes to *Radiologic Clinics of North America*, Elsevier Health Sciences Division, Subscription Customer Service, 3251 Riverport Lane, Maryland Heights, MO63043. **Customer Service: Telephone: 1-800-654-2452** (U.S. and Canada); **1-314-447-8871** (outside U.S. and Canada). **Fax: 1-314-447-8029. E-mail: journalscustomerservice-usa@ elsevier.com** (for print support); **journalsonlinesupport-usa@elsevier.com** (for online support).

Reprints. For copies of 100 or more of articles in this publication, please contact the Commercial Reprints Department, Elsevier Inc., 360 Park Avenue South, New York, New York 10010-1710. Tel.: +1-212-633-3874; Fax: +1-212-633-3820; E-mail: reprints@elsevier.com.

Radiologic Clinics of North America also published in Greek Paschalidis Medical Publications, Athens, Greece.

Radiologic Clinics of North America is covered in *MEDLINE/PubMed (Index Medicus), EMBASE/Excerpta Medica, Current Contents/Life Sciences, Current Contents/Clinical Medicine, RSNA Index to Imaging Literature, BIOSIS, Science Citation Index,* and *ISI/BIOMED*.

Printed in the United States of America.

Contributors

CONSULTING EDITOR

FRANK H. MILLER, MD
Chief, Body Imaging Section and Fellowship
Program and GI Radiology; Medical Director
MRI; Professor, Department of Radiology,
Northwestern University, Feinberg School of
Medicine, Northwestern Memorial Hospital,
Chicago, Illinois

EDITORS

GABRIELA GAYER, MD
Clinical Professor, Division of Abdominal
Imaging, Department of Radiology, Stanford
University Medical Center, Stanford, California;
Department of Radiology, Sheba Medical
Center, Sackler School of Medicine, Tel Aviv
University, Ramat-Gan, Israel

DOUGLAS S. KATZ, MD, FACR
Vice Chair for Clinical Research and
Education; Director of Body Imaging;
Professor, Department of Radiology,
Winthrop-University Hospital, Mineola,
New York; Professor of Clinical Radiology,
State University of New York at Stony Brook,
Stony Brook, New York

AUTHORS

MAHER A. ABBAS, MD, FACS, FASCRS
Digestive Disease Institute, Cleveland Clinic,
Al Maryah Island, Abu Dhabi, United Arab
Emirates

LAURA L. AVERY, MD
Division of Emergency Radiology, Department
of Diagnostic Radiology, Massachusetts
General Hospital, Boston, Massachusetts

SPENCER C. BEHR, MD
Assistant Professor, Department of Radiology
and Biomedical Imaging, University of
California, San Francisco, San Francisco,
California

SANJEEV BHALLA, MD
Professor of Radiology, Mallinckrodt Institute
of Radiology, Washington University School of
Medicine, St Louis, Missouri

PUNEET BHARGAVA, MD
Associate Professor, Department of
Radiology, University of Washington School
of Medicine; Department of Radiology,
VA Puget Sound Health Care System,
Seattle, Washington

PRIYA BHOSALE, MD
Associate Professor, Department of Diagnostic
Radiology, UT MD Anderson Cancer Center,
Houston, Texas

JARED D. CHRISTENSEN, MD
Division Chief; Assistant Professor,
Department of Radiology, Duke University
Medical Center, Durham, North Carolina

FERGUS V. COAKLEY, MD
Chair, Department of Radiology, Oregon
Health and Science University, Portland,
Oregon

BARRY DALY, MD, FRCR
Professor, Department of Diagnostic
Radiology, University of Maryland School of
Medicine, Baltimore, Maryland

JOSEPH DAVIES, MD
Department of Radiology, Royal London
Hospital, Barts and The London NHS Trust,
London, United Kingdom

SAEED ELOJEIMY, MD
Resident, Department of Radiology, University
of Washington School of Medicine, Seattle,
Washington

NAVEEN GARG, MD
Assistant Professor, Department of Diagnostic
Radiology, UT MD Anderson Cancer Center,
Houston, Texas

GABRIELA GAYER, MD
Clinical Professor, Division of Abdominal
Imaging, Department of Radiology, Stanford
University Medical Center, Stanford, California;
Department of Radiology, Sheba Medical
Center, Sackler School of Medicine, Tel Aviv
University, Ramat-Gan, Israel

DOUGLAS S. KATZ, MD, FACR
Vice Chair for Clinical Research and Education;
Director of Body Imaging; Professor,
Department of Radiology, Winthrop-University
Hospital, Mineola, New York; Professor of
Clinical Radiology, State University of New
York at Stony Brook, Stony Brook, New York

SAURABH KHANDELWAL, MD
Assistant Professor; Director of Bariatric
Surgery, Department of Surgery, University of
Washington School of Medicine, Seattle,
Washington

BRUCE LEHNERT, MD
Assistant Professor, Department of Radiology,
University of Washington School of Medicine,
Seattle, Washington

MINH LU, MD
Department of Diagnostic Radiology,
University of Maryland School of Medicine,
Baltimore, Maryland

MEGHAN G. LUBNER, MD
Assistant Professor of Radiology, Department
of Radiology, University of Wisconsin School of
Medicine and Public Health, Madison,
Wisconsin

SURESH MAXIMIN, MD
Assistant Professor, Department of Radiology,
University of Washington School of Medicine;
Department of Radiology, VA Puget Sound
Health Care System, Seattle, Washington

CHRISTINE O. MENIAS, MD
Professor of Radiology, Mayo Clinic; Mayo
Clinic Hospital; Mayo Clinic LL Radiology,
Scottsdale, Arizona

NANDINI M. MEYERSOHN, MD
Department of Diagnostic Radiology,
Massachusetts General Hospital, Boston,
Massachusetts

MARIAM MOSHIRI, MD
Associate Professor, Department of Radiology,
University of Washington School of Medicine,
Seattle, Washington

SHERIF OSMAN, MD
Fellow, Emergency Radiology, Department of
Radiology, University of Washington School of
Medicine, Seattle, Washington

BHAVIK N. PATEL, MD
Assistant Professor, Division of Abdominal
Imaging, Department of Radiology, Duke
University Medical Center, Durham, North
Carolina

CHRISTINE M. PETERSON, MD
Department of Radiology, Penn State Hershey,
Hershey, Pennsylvania

PERRY J. PICKHARDT, MD
Chief, Gastrointestinal Imaging; Professor of
Radiology, Department of Radiology,
University of Wisconsin School of Medicine
and Public Health, Madison, Wisconsin

ANTONIO PINTO, MD, PhD
Department of Diagnostic Imaging, Section
of General and Emergency Radiology,
"A. Cardarelli" Hospital, Naples, Italy

GAETANO REA, MD
Department of Diagnostic Imaging, Section of
General Radiology, Azienda Ospedali dei Colli,
P.O. Monaldi, Naples, Italy

TRACY J. ROBINSON, MD
Seattle Radiologists P.S., Seattle, Washington

LUIGIA ROMANO, MD
Department of Diagnostic Imaging, Section of General and Emergency Radiology, "A. Cardarelli" Hospital, Naples, Italy

GIOVANNI ROSSI, MD
Department of Diagnostic Imaging, Section of General Radiology, Azienda Ospedali dei Colli, P.O. Monaldi, Naples, Italy

TARA SAGEBIEL, MD
Assistant Professor, Department of Diagnostic Radiology, UT MD Anderson Cancer Center, Houston, Texas

MARIANO SCAGLIONE, MD
Locum Consultant Radiologist, Department of Radiology, Royal London Hospital, Barts and The London NHS Trust, London, United Kingdom; Department of Diagnostic Imaging, Pineta Grande Medical Center, Castel Volturno, Caserta, Italy

DANIELLE M. SEAMAN, MD
Assistant Professor, Department of Radiology, Duke University Medical Center, Durham, North Carolina

MYLENE TRUONG, MD
Professor, Department of Diagnostic Radiology, UT MD Anderson Cancer Center, Houston, Texas

TULLIO VALENTE, MD
Department of Diagnostic Imaging, Section of General Radiology, Azienda Ospedali dei Colli, P.O. Monaldi, Naples, Italy

DAVID M. VALENZUELA, MD
Department of Radiology and Biomedical Imaging, University of California, San Francisco, San Francisco, California

CHITRA VISWANATHAN, MD
Associate Professor, Department of Diagnostic Radiology, UT MD Anderson Cancer Center, Houston, Texas

Z. JANE WANG, MD
Associate Professor, Department of Radiology and Biomedical Imaging, University of California, San Francisco, San Francisco, California

LACEY WASHINGTON, MD
Associate Professor, Department of Radiology, Duke University Medical Center, Durham, North Carolina

EMILY M. WEBB, MD
Associate Professor, Department of Radiology and Biomedical Imaging, University of California, San Francisco, San Francisco, California

BENJAMIN M. YEH, MD
Professor, Department of Radiology and Biomedical Imaging, University of California, San Francisco, San Francisco, California

Contents

Common medical interventions performed by cardiologists, radiologists, surgeons, dentists, and alternative practitioners can result in complications within the thorax that lead to significant patient morbidity. Prompt radiologic identification of iatrogenic complications of medical procedures in the thorax is essential to guide patient triage and treatment. Understanding the approach to common thoracic interventions and the placement of thoracic medical devices can aid radiologists in the evaluation of iatrogenic complications.

Iatrogenic complications of thoracic and cardiovascular surgery are relatively uncommon, but contribute to potentially significant patient morbidity and mortality. The incidence of iatrogenic disease reflects the complexity of surgical procedures, including lung resection, esophagectomy, coronary artery bypass grafting, thoracic aorta repair, and cardiac valve replacement. Some iatrogenic complications are minor and common to all procedures, whereas others can be potentially devastating and are associated with precise technical components of specific surgeries. Multimodality imaging plays an important role in the diagnosis and management of operative thoracic and cardiovascular iatrogenic disease.

Aortic aneurysms remain a significant problem in the population, and there is a concerted effort to identify, define, image, and treat these conditions to ultimately improve outcomes. The rapid development of diagnostic modalities, operative strategies, and endovascular techniques within the realm of this aortic disease has transformed the field and broadened the spectrum of patients that can be treated with minimally invasive techniques. This investigation has a broad spectrum of normal expected findings that must be differentiated from early or late complications in which intervention is required. In this article, normal and abnormal postoperative and post-TEVAR/EVAR MDCT findings are described.

Every form of medical and surgical treatment, even the most trivial one, carries with it some chance of complications. This risk is usually small, and the benefit of the treatment should clearly outweigh the risk. Treatment-related complications may occur, however, presenting either soon after the intervention or remote from it. In this review, the focus is on imaging findings of surgical materials used in abdominal surgery, and of a wide array of implanted abdominal devices. The pertinent complications of these devices and of retained surgical objects are highlighted and illustrated.

Oncologic therapy is constantly evolving to improve patient outcomes, especially with regard to chemotherapy. The use of combination therapies and development and implementation of molecular targeted therapy lead to iatrogenic conditions that the radiologist must be aware of in interpreting studies of and caring for the oncologic patient. Knowledge of the chemotherapeutic agents and the imaging appearances of associated toxicities can impact patient management and decrease patient morbidity and mortality.

Radiation injuries often occur during or after radiation therapy in the abdomen or pelvis. Although any organ in the abdomen or pelvis may be exposed to and injured by radiation therapy directed to a nearby organ, this article focuses on more frequently encountered imaging findings of inadvertent radiation damage. It is important for the radiologist to be familiar with the imaging appearances of inadvertent radiation damage to abdominopelvic viscera in order to sustain clinical relevance and not mistake radiation injuries for other entities.

Intraluminal procedures for the gastrointestinal tract range from simple intubation for feeding or bowel decompression to endoscopic procedures including stenting and pancreatobiliary ductal catheterization. Each of these procedures and interventions carries a risk of iatrogenic injury, including bleeding, perforation, infection, adhesions, and obstruction. An understanding of how anatomy and function may predispose to injury, and the distinct patterns of injury, can help the radiologist identify and characterize iatrogenic injury rapidly at computed tomography (CT) imaging. Furthermore, selective use of intravenous or oral CT contrast material can help reveal injury and triage clinical management.

Several techniques for the surgical management of obesity are available to bariatric surgeons. These interventions are performed more frequently with worsening of the obesity epidemic. Radiologists should be familiar with the surgical techniques, normal postoperative appearances, and potential complications for which imaging may be employed to establish a diagnosis to optimize patient care.

PROGRAM OBJECTIVE

The objective of the *Radiologic Clinics of North America* is to keep practicing radiologists and radiology residents up to date with current clinical practice in radiology by providing timely articles reviewing the state of the art in patient care.

TARGET AUDIENCE

Practicing radiologists, radiology residents, and other health care professionals who provide patient care utilizing radiologic findings.

LEARNING OBJECTIVES

Upon completion of this activity, participants will be able to:

1. Discuss imaging of abdominal, pelvic surgical and post-procedural foreign bodies.
2. Review imaging of complications of thoracic and cardiovascular surgery.
3. Discuss CT findings of complications of surgical and endovascular treatment of aortic aneurysms.

ACCREDITATION

The Elsevier Office of Continuing Medical Education (EOCME) is accredited by the Accreditation Council for Continuing Medical Education (ACCME) to provide continuing medical education for physicians.

The EOCME designates this enduring material for a maximum of 15 *AMA PRA Category 1 Credit*(s)™. Physicians should claim only the credit commensurate with the extent of their participation in the activity.

All other health care professionals requesting continuing education credit for this enduring material will be issued a certificate of participation.

DISCLOSURE OF CONFLICTS OF INTEREST

The EOCME assesses conflict of interest with its instructors, faculty, planners, and other individuals who are in a position to control the content of CME activities. All relevant conflicts of interest that are identified are thoroughly vetted by EOCME for fair balance, scientific objectivity, and patient care recommendations. EOCME is committed to providing its learners with CME activities that promote improvements or quality in healthcare and not a specific proprietary business or a commercial interest.

The planning committee, staff, authors and editors listed below have identified no financial relationships or relationships to products or devices they or their spouse/life partner have with commercial interest related to the content of this CME activity:

Maher A. Abbas, MD, FACS, FASCRS; Laura L. Avery, MD; MD; Sanjeev Bhalla, MD; Priya Bhosale, MD; Jared D. Christensen, MD; Fergus V. Coakley, MD; Barry Daly, MD, FRCR; Joseph Davies, MD; Saeed Elojeimy, MD, PhD; Naveen Garg, MD; Gabriela Gayer, MD; Kristen Helm; Brynne Hunter; Douglas S. Katz, MD, FACR; Saurabh Khandelwal, MD; Sandy Lavery; Bruce Lehnert, MD; Minh Lu, MD; Suresh T. Maximin, MD; Jill McNair; Christine O. Menias, MD; Nandini M. Meyersohn, MD; Frank H. Miller, MD; Sherif Osman, MD; Bhavik N. Patel, MD; Christine M. Peterson, MD; Perry J. Pickhardt, MD; Antonio Pinto, MD, PhD; Gaetano Rea, MD; Tracy J. Robinson, MD, MS; Luigia Romano, MD; Giovanni Rossi, MD; Tara Sagebiel, MD; Mariano Scaglione, MD; Danielle M. Seaman, MD; Karthikeyan Subramaniam; Mylene Truong, MD; Tullio Valente, MD; David M. Valenzuela, MD; John Vassallo; Chitra Viswanathan, MD; Z. Jane Wang, MD; Lacey Washington, MD; Emily M. Webb, MD.

The planning committee, staff, authors and editors listed below have identified financial relationships or relationships to products or devices they or their spouse/life partner have with commercial interest related to the content of this CME activity:

Spencer C. Behr, MD has a research grant from General Electric Healthcare; has royalties/patents with OTC Foundation; and is a consultant/advisor for Grand Rounds Health.
Puneet Bhargava, MD, MBB, DNB; S has an employment affiliation with Elsevier.
Meghan G. Lubner, MD has a research grant from GE Medical.
Mariam Moshiri, MD is a consultant/advisor for Amirsys.
Benjamin M. Yeh, MD is a consultant/advisor for and has a research grant with General Electric Healthcare; also, both he and his spouse/partner are consultants/advisors for Nextrast, Inc.

UNAPPROVED/OFF-LABEL USE DISCLOSURE

The EOCME requires CME faculty to disclose to the participants:

1. When products or procedures being discussed are off-label, unlabelled, experimental, and/or investigational (not US Food and Drug Administration (FDA) approved); and
2. Any limitations on the information presented, such as data that are preliminary or that represent ongoing research, interim analyses, and/or unsupported opinions. Faculty may discuss information about pharmaceutical agents that is outside of FDA-approved labelling. This information is intended solely for CME and is not intended to promote off-label use of these medications. If you have any questions, contact the medical affairs department of the manufacturer for the most recent prescribing information.

TO ENROLL

To enroll in the *Radiologic Clinics of North America* Continuing Medical Education program, call customer service at 1-800-654-2452 or sign up online at http://www.theclinics.com/home/cme. The CME program is available to subscribers for an additional annual fee of USD $315.

METHOD OF PARTICIPATION

In order to claim credit, participants must complete the following:

1. Complete enrolment as indicated above.
2. Read the activity.
3. Complete the CME Test and Evaluation. Participants must achieve a score of 70% on the test. All CME Tests and Evaluations must be completed online.

CME INQUIRIES/SPECIAL NEEDS

For all CME inquiries or special needs, please contact elsevierCME@elsevier.com.

RADIOLOGIC CLINICS OF NORTH AMERICA

ISSUE OF RELATED INTEREST

Neuroimaging Clinics of North America, May 2014 (Vol. 24, No. 2)
Imaging of the Postoperative Spine
A. Orlando Ortiz, *Editor*

DOWNLOAD
Free App!

Review Articles
THE CLINICS

NOW AVAILABLE FOR YOUR iPhone and iPad

Preface

Imaging of Iatrogenic Conditions of the Chest, Abdomen, and Pelvis

 CrossMark

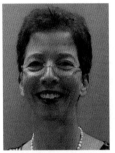 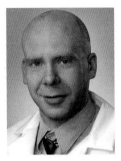

Gabriela Gayer, MD   Douglas S. Katz, MD, FACR
Editors

The "definitive source" of all information at present, the Web site Wikipedia.org, defines an iatrogenic effect or injury/complication as "a potentially preventable harm resulting from medical treatment (or advice to patients)." The term "iatrogenic" derives from the Greek meaning "originating from a physician." Ultimately, therefore, all complications in medicine are iatrogenic, whether from physicians or from their associated health care practitioners, if one is to use the original definition of this word. Some of these iatrogenic effects are clearly defined, such as direct complications of a surgical or other procedure, whereas others are potentially less obvious, for example, the negative interaction of medications, or the negative outcome from not undergoing a specific surgery or other treatment path. Per Wikipedia, the term iatrogenic can be used to refer to complications of chance, medical errors, negligence, and the adverse effects of other types of therapies. The term can also be used without negative connotation to describe the results of treatment.

As has been well-known since the start of modern medicine and before, the prime directive of medical care is to "first do no harm" (ie, *primum non nocere*). Everything we do in medicine—every prescribed medication, every treatment ordered, every surgery, every procedure, and every test (nonimaging or imaging)—has the potential to have an adverse effect, whether direct or indirect,

and to potentially harm patients. Managing risk-benefit ratios, and then managing subsequent complications if and when they arise, whether they were potentially preventable or not, remains a mainstay of modern medical therapy, regardless of the specific field of practice.

This issue of the *Radiologic Clinics of North America* is devoted to the imaging of iatrogenic conditions of the chest, abdomen, and pelvis. Eleven articles review a wide variety of complications arising from many different types of invasive and noninvasive treatments, including surgery, endoscopy, and radiation. Treatment-related complications may present either soon after the intervention or remote from it. The radiologist often plays a critical role in recognizing and assessing such complications, particularly when the presentation is remote from the treatment/intervention and the clinical suspicion of a treatment-related problem is low. The correct diagnosis may be reached when the clinical information is available and the imaging findings are carefully analyzed. Referring physicians, however, tend to provide only scant pertinent information regarding prior procedures or surgery that the patient had undergone. With the increasing use of electronic medical records, radiologists may have access to important information that will shed light on relevant details in a patient's history and account for the imaging findings. However, the key to recognizing iatrogenic complications is in particular

Radiol Clin N Am 52 (2014) xiii–xiv
http://dx.doi.org/10.1016/j.rcl.2014.05.007
0033-8389/14/$ – see front matter © 2014 Published by Elsevier Inc.

familiarity with the scope of imaging appearances related to treatment. This issue aims to familiarize radiologists with the broad spectrum of imaging findings pertaining to various complications arising from a variety of treatments.

We especially appreciate the efforts of our teams of contributing authors from multiple institutions who have participated in this issue. It is not particularly easy, for a variety of reasons, to prepare articles on this topic, especially given the sensitive nature of this endeavor. It is not pleasant to review the complications from one's own institution(s) in particular, and to demonstrate, how and when "drugs, scopes, probes, and robots have gone bad."[a] It is hoped that the honesty of the authors, and that of those authors who have reported their complications cited in the many references included in this issue, will be to the benefit of our current and future patients, and to the current and future practice of medical care.

Gabriela Gayer, MD
Department of Radiology
Sheba Medical Center
Derech Sheba 2, Tel-Hashomer
Ramat-Gan 52621, Israel

Department of Radiology
Stanford University Medical Center
300 Pasteur Drive
Stanford, CA 94304, USA

Douglas S. Katz, MD, FACR
Department of Radiology
Winthrop-University Hospital
Mineola, NY 11501, USA

State University of New York at Stony Brook
Stony Brook, NY 11794, USA

E-mail addresses:
ggayer@stanford.edu (G. Gayer)
dkatz@winthrop.org (D.S. Katz)

---

[a] Title of a recent Radiological Society of North America exhibit, co-authored by the two co-editors and several other contributors to this issue.

Imaging of Iatrogenic Conditions of the Thorax

Nandini M. Meyersohn, MD[a], Laura L. Avery, MD[b],*

KEYWORDS

- Iatrogenic • Thoracic complications • Device lead fracture • Catheter placement
- Medical procedures

KEY POINTS

- Common medical interventions performed by cardiologists, radiologists, surgeons, dentists, and alternative practitioners can result in complications within the thorax that lead to significant patient morbidity.
- Prompt radiologic identification of iatrogenic complications of medical procedures in the thorax is essential to guide patient triage and treatment.
- Understanding the approach to common thoracic interventions and the placement of thoracic medical devices can aid radiologists in the evaluation of iatrogenic complications.

INTRODUCTION

Iatrogenic thoracic conditions resulting from the placement of medical devices, access catheters, cardiovascular procedures, and interventional radiology procedures can be a significant source of patient morbidity. Radiologists play an essential role in identifying iatrogenic thoracic conditions that may result from these common procedures in a timely fashion so that patients receive appropriate management.

The objectives of this article are to review the expected radiographic findings after common interventions and to guide radiologists in identifying iatrogenic complications within the thorax. The subtypes of interventions and procedures discussed include cardiac conduction devices, vascular catheters, cardiothoracic endovascular procedures, diagnostic and interventional radiology procedures, dental procedures, and alternative/complementary medicine procedures.

IMAGING FINDINGS/PATHOLOGY
Cardiology Interventions

Cardiac conduction devices
The placement of cardiac pacemakers and implantable cardioverter defibrillators has become a common procedure in the United States and is performed by cardiologists trained in cardiac electrophysiology. The 3 most common types of cardiac conduction devices seen on radiographs are single-chamber, dual-chamber, and biventricular devices.[1,2]

A single-chamber device lead is typically placed in the right ventricle (RV) with the tip at the ventricular apex projecting to the left of the spine on an anteroposterior (AP) chest radiograph. Dual-chamber devices typically have a similar RV lead, with a second lead in the right atrium (RA), usually with its tip in the right atrial appendage, leading to an upward curvature of the lead tip on a lateral chest radiograph (**Fig. 1**). Biventricular pacing

a Department of Diagnostic Radiology, Massachusetts General Hospital, 55 Fruit Street, FND 2-216, Boston, MA 02114, USA; b Division of Emergency Radiology, Department of Diagnostic Radiology, Massachusetts General Hospital, 55 Fruit Street, FND 2-210, Boston, MA 02114, USA
* Corresponding author.
E-mail address: Lavery@partners.org

Radiol Clin N Am 52 (2014) 913–928
http://dx.doi.org/10.1016/j.rcl.2014.05.005
0033-8389/14/$ – see front matter © 2014 Elsevier Inc. All rights reserved.

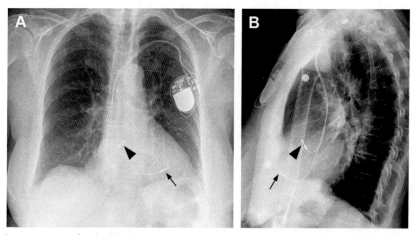

Fig. 1. Normal appearance of a dual-lead pacemaker. (A, B) PA and lateral radiographs demonstrate a dual-lead pacemaker with pulse generator overlying the left chest wall. Pacemaker wires descend over the expected location of the SVC into the RA and RV. The atrial lead (*arrowheads*) typically curves upward in a "J" configuration to reside in the right atrial appendage. The ventricular lead (*arrows*) ideally terminates in the ventricular apex to the left of the spine.

includes an RV lead and an additional lead placed through the RA into the coronary sinus and terminating in a cardiac vein along the free wall of the left ventricle (LV). The LV is thus paced in an epicardial fashion.[1,2] An RA lead may also be present in biventricular pacing. All of these leads are typically placed transvenously via the axillary or subclavian vein. Common minor immediate postprocedural complications include pneumothorax and hematoma.

A potential major complication is inadvertent intraarterial lead placement via the subclavian artery into the aorta. This diagnosis is suggested when leads follow a course medial to the expected position of the superior vena cava (SVC), suggesting that they are within the aorta (Fig. 2). Intraarterial leads are associated with a high thromboembolic risk, whereas leads extending into the coronary arteries may result in cardiac ischemia. Immediate CT imaging and echocardiography should be used to exclude coronary artery or ventricular perforation to allow for anticoagulation. Pacemaker lead removal requires multidisciplinary intervention.

Ventricular leads are fixed into the myocardium either actively via a screw tip or passively via radiolucent tines at the tip of the lead that are caught within trabeculated myocardium.[2] Another potential major complication is myocardial perforation, which can be symptomatic or asymptomatic (Figs. 3 and 4). On radiographs, the only clue to this diagnosis may be abnormally lateral or superior positioning of the RV lead tip. An important finding suggesting this diagnosis on CT is

hemopericardium, although the absence of a pericardial effusion does not exclude the possibility of perforation (see Fig. 4). Myocardial perforation can also occur with atrial leads, which in unusual situations can be symptomatic due to irritation of the chest wall or diaphragm (Fig. 5).

Cardiac conduction leads can also become dislodged over time (Fig. 6). It is important when interpreting routine chest radiographs to compare lead tip position with prior examinations to ensure that lead position has not changed. Dislodged RA or RV leads can migrate into other areas of the right heart, the SVC, or inferior vena cava (IVC), which can result in insufficient or inappropriate pacing (see Fig. 6). Perhaps the most commonly detected abnormality on radiographs is lead fracture. A common location for failure is near the generator on the chest wall; this location should be carefully examined for lead fracture or disconnection. Additionally, a region of friction exists where the wires extend between the first rib and clavicle prior to entering the subclavian vein, known as subclavian crush. These fractured leads can result in noncapture and lack of cardiac pacing in addition to stimulation and contraction of chest wall muscles. Uncommonly, lead fragments can migrate into the RV outflow tract or even into the liver via the IVC (Fig. 7).

Pulmonary vein ablation
Pulmonary vein radiofrequency ablation or pulmonary vein isolation (PVI) is a common procedure performed by cardiologists to treat symptomatic atrial fibrillation.[3] PVI is performed via an

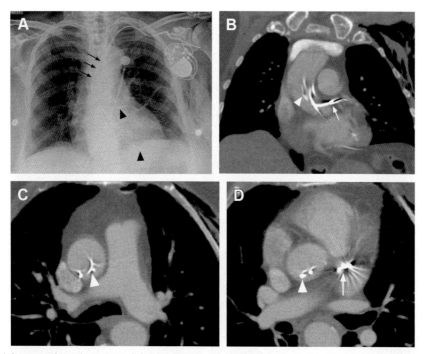

Fig. 2. Arterial pacemaker placement. (*A*) Portable chest radiograph demonstrates a dual-lead pacemaker with the course of the leads medial to the SVC within the aorta (*arrows*). The tips of the atrial and ventricular leads cross to the left of the spine (*arrowheads*). A chest tube is visualized in the left hemithorax related to procedurally induced pneumothorax. (*B–D*) Coronal and axial CT images demonstrate the arterial course of the pacemaker within the aorta (*arrowheads*) with atrial lead tip extending into the ostium of the left main coronary artery (*arrows*). The patient was heparinized and a multidisciplinary approach was undertaken for pacemaker removal. Cardiology extracted the pacemaker leads percutaneously, with catheters seated in the proximal aorta prepared for the possibility of coronal artery rupture. Removal occurred without rupture; however, a procedurally-induced thrombus was identified and retrieved via suction thrombectomy. Subsequently, a covered stent was used to repair the arteriotomy of the subclavian artery.

endovascular approach, and ablation lesions are placed around the pulmonary vein ostia to isolate arrhythmogenic foci from the remainder of the left atrium. A transseptal approach is used in which the transvenous catheter is advanced centrally to the RA, then subsequently through the atrial septum into the left atrium. In a minority of patients, this septal perforation results in an ongoing iatrogenic atrial septal defect (**Fig. 8**). Patients with preprocedural increased pulmonary arterial pressure are at increased risk of a persistent interatrial septal defect, which can potentially become hemodynamically significant.[3]

The posterior left atrial wall lies in close approximation to the esophagus, and high temperatures are achieved during the radiofrequency ablation. This can lead to inadvertent thermal injury to the esophagus and result in ulceration secondary to thermal and ischemic causes (**Fig. 9**).[4] Esophageal ulceration can progress transmurally and result in an esophageal–left atrial fistula with a

poor prognosis secondary to embolic phenomena (**Fig. 10**).[4]

After pulmonary vein ablation, up to 38% of patients have been reported to develop at least some degree of pulmonary vein stenosis secondary to circumferential ablation zones around the vein ostia.[5,6] Pulmonary vein stenosis can often be clinically misdiagnosed, because the presenting symptoms of dyspnea and cough can be mistaken for respiratory disease or even lung malignancy.[7] Radiographically, pulmonary stenosis can result in isolated lobar edema that can be misdiagnosed as pneumonia. ECG-gated CT is a useful imaging modality for detection of this condition (**Fig. 11**).

Vascular Procedures

Pulmonary arterial catheters

Pulmonary arterial catheters, commonly known as Swan-Ganz catheters, have been in use for several decades as a means of providing important

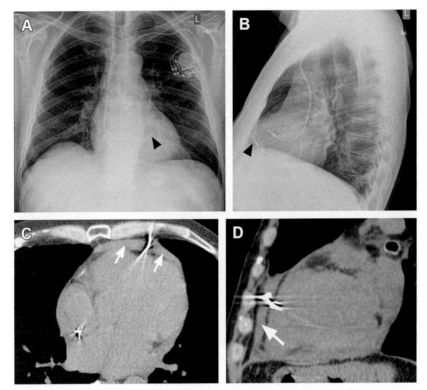

Fig. 3. Symptomatic ventricular lead perforation. Patient complained of chest pain after recent pacemaker place-ment. Bedside ultrasound was positive for pericardial effusion. (*A, B*) PA and lateral radiographs of the chest demonstrate a dual-lead pacemaker. The PA view demonstrates the ventricular lead to be more superior than ex-pected (*arrowhead*). On the lateral view, the ventricular lead is slightly anterior to the expected position (*arrow-head*). (*C, D*) Noncontrast axial and sagittal CT images demonstrate ventricular perforation of the ventricular lead with a small volume of hemopericardium (*arrows*).

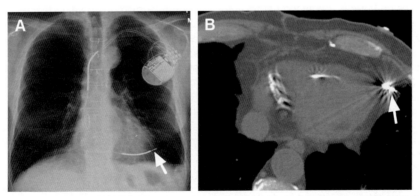

Fig. 4. Asymptomatic ventricular lead perforation. Patient with a remote history of pacemaker placement. (*A*) Frontal chest radiograph shows a more lateral position of the RV pacemaker lead than expected (*arrow*). (*B*) Axial noncontrast CT image demonstrates the lead extending into the pericardial fat (*arrow*) without pericardial effu-sion, a finding consistent with chronic myocardial perforation. This was left untreated without consequence.

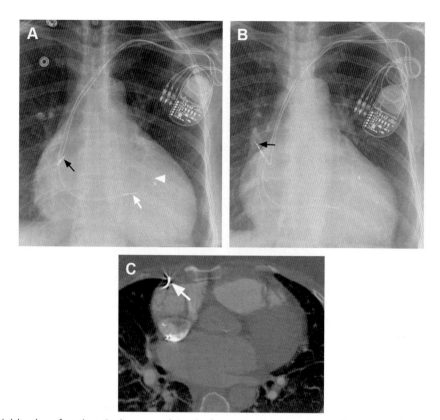

Fig. 5. Atrial lead perforation. Patient complained of peculiar chest wall sensations 1 month after pacemaker placement. (*A*) Initial PA radiograph demonstrates a biventricular pacemaker in position. Leads within the RA (*black arrow*), RV (*white arrow*), and coronary sinus (*arrowhead*) are identified in normal position. (*B*) Subsequent PA chest radiograph 1 month later demonstrates a change in the trajectory of the atrial lead (*black arrow*). The lead now resides beyond the cardiac silhouette. (*C*) Axial CT scan confirms atrial perforation with the pacemaker lead abutting the chest wall musculature causing the patient's symptoms.

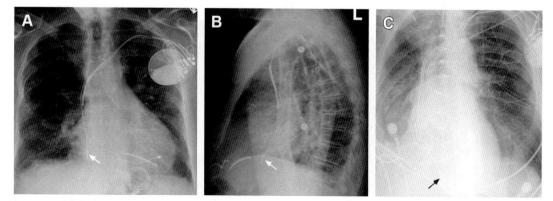

Fig. 6. Lead dislodgement in 2 patients. (*A, B*) The right atrial lead is suspended vertically in the RA (*white arrows*) rather than positioned in the atrial appendage. (*C*) The RV lead extends into the IVC in a different patient (*black arrow*).

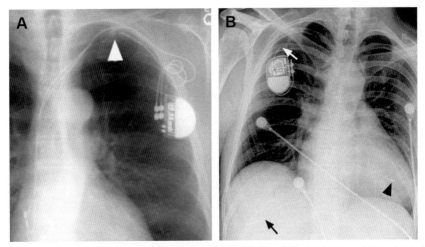

Fig. 7. Pacemaker lead fracture and migration in 2 patients. (*A*) Magnified AP view of the chest demonstrates lead fracture between the clavicle and first rib (*white arrowhead*), a region subject to crush injury in this patient who had recently taken up weightlifting. (*B*) AP chest radiograph demonstrates a fracture of the proximal lead near the generator (*white arrow*). There has been subsequent migration of the lead to the IVC and hepatic vein (*black arrow*). Note the tip remains adherent to the RV wall (*black arrowhead*).

hemodynamic measurements in patients in the critical care setting.[8] A balloon on the distal catheter is inflated while in a large main pulmonary artery (PA) and then advanced until wedged into a more distal PA branch. A major complication of this procedure is damage to the vessel wall, resulting in rupture with pseudoaneurysm formation (**Fig. 12**), which can present in the short term within 24 to 48 hours but in some cases may not be detected until months after catheter removal.[8] Patients who have been in a critical care setting and subsequently present with hemoptysis should raise a radiologist's suspicion for PA pseudoaneurysm, which can be demonstrated by CT or conventional angiography and treated with endovascular coiling.

Central venous access catheters

Central venous access catheters are routinely placed in inpatient and outpatient settings by physicians from many specialties. For radiologists, the preferred approach is via the right internal jugular (IJ) vein and the right brachiocephalic vein into the SVC and RA. Other access sites, including the left IJ, subclavian, or femoral veins, may be necessary in patients with extenuating circumstances, such

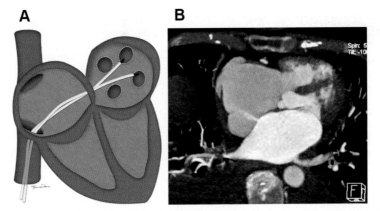

Fig. 8. Pulmonary vein ablation for paroxysmal atrial fibrillation. (*A*) Illustration demonstrating the endovascular approach for pulmonary vein ablation. Note the transseptal course of the ablation catheters. (*B*) Axial CT image demonstrates contrast flowing through an iatrogenic atrial septal defect after pulmonary vein ablation.

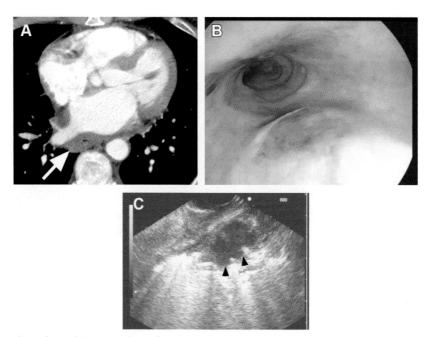

Fig. 9. Thermal esophageal injury without fistula. The patient developed hemoptysis immediately after pulmonary vein ablation. (*A*) Axial CT image demonstrates circumferential esophageal thickening (*arrow*). (*B*) Endoscopic image of the esophagus demonstrates mucosal ulceration. (*C*) Endoscopic ultrasound of the esophagus demonstrates submucosal fluid and air consistent with thermal injury leading to necrosis (*arrowheads*).

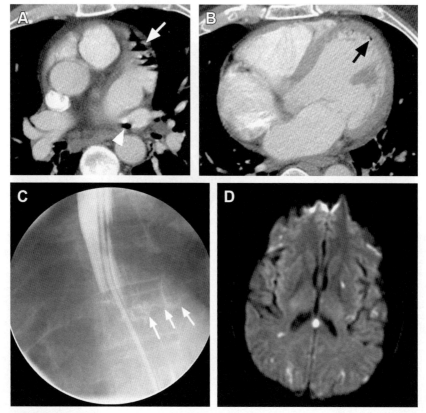

Fig. 10. Esophageal-to-left atrial fistula after pulmonary vein ablation. Patient complained of progressive weakness 1 month after pulmonary vein ablation. (*A*) Axial CT image demonstrates multiple foci of air within the left atrial appendage (*white arrow*). An additional focus of air is seen in the left pulmonary vein (*arrowhead*). (*B*) Additional air seen in the LV (*black arrow*). (*C*) Image from a gastrografin swallow demonstrates extravasation of contrast from the midesophagus (*white arrows*). The contrast rapidly washed away. (*D*) Diffusion-weighted axial MR image of the brain demonstrating multiple embolic infarcts with restricted diffusion.

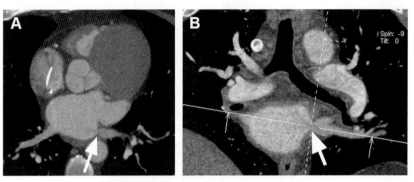

Fig. 11. Pulmonary vein stenosis after pulmonary vein ablation. (*A, B*) Axial and coronal contrast-enhanced CT images demonstrate stenosis of the left inferior pulmonary vein with orifice narrowing and turbulent blood flow (*arrows*). A pacemaker lead is partially visualized in the RA. (*Courtesy of* Brian Ghoshhajra, MD, Division of Cardiac Imaging, Department of Radiology, Massachusetts General Hospital, Boston, MA.)

as previous fibrotic or thrombotic disease. An uncommon but highly morbid complication of central venous access catheter placement is rupture of the central veins or the SVC, a complication to which patients with multiple prior transvenous interventions are predisposed due to prior vessel wall injury.[9] The presence of a cardiac conduction device with transvenous leads can also increase the likelihood of such a complication (**Fig. 13**). Suspicion for central vein or SVC rupture should be raised in the presence of a new pleural effusion or change in the mediastinal contour on radiography

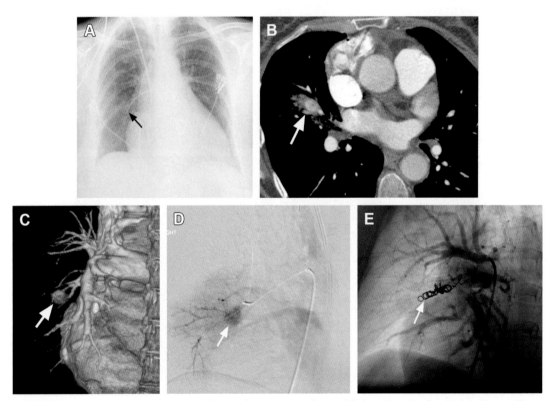

Fig. 12. PA pseudoaneurysm after PA catheter placement. Patient with hemoptysis after Swan-Ganz catheter placement. (*A*) A Swan-Ganz catheter is visualized with distal tip in the interlobar PA (*black arrow*). (*B*) Axial CT image demonstrates contrast opacifying a pseudoaneurysm caused by distal catheter balloon inflation (*white arrow*). Note surrounding pulmonary hemorrhage. Volumetric CT reformat (*C*) demonstrates the pseudoaneurysm, which was subsequently coiled via endovascular access (*white arrows* in *D, E*).

after catheter placement (**Fig. 14**). In a stable patient, contrast-enhanced thoracic CT with injection of contrast from the contralateral side is an appropriate next step for evaluation of pseudoaneurysm or suspected central venous rupture.

Cardiovascular Surgery Complications

Coronary artery bypass procedures

Coronary artery bypass grafting (CABG) has become a staple in the treatment of coronary artery disease. Intraoperatively, the ascending aorta is cannulated to provide extracorporeal circulation while the coronary arteries grafts are performed (**Fig. 15D**).[10] Delayed pseudoaneurysms can form at the aortic cannulation site (see **Fig. 15**) as well as within the bypass grafts themselves or at graft anastomotic sites. The mediastinal contours on radiographs of post-CABG patients should be carefully evaluated for focal abnormalities that may reflect aortic cannulation site or graft pseudoaneurysm, which can be well characterized using ECG-gated contrast-enhanced CT.

Aortic stent graft procedures

Radiographs are an important imaging modality for the surveillance of endovascular aortic stent grafts now used routinely for aneurysm repair or the treatment of aortic dissection via a surgical and/or endoscopic approach.[11] It is important for radiologists to note both the position and the morphology of the stent graft as well as the contours of the aneurysm sac and to compare with prior radiographs for changes over time. A change in morphology, distortion, or separation of the stent graft elements on radiography can indicate failure of the graft material (**Fig. 16**), which can eventually result in aneurysm rupture if not revised.[11]

A potential complication of thoracic aortic stent graft placement with high morbidity and mortality is the formation of an aortoesophageal fistula (**Fig. 17**). A periaortic collection containing air in the region of a stent graft should raise suspicion for this complication. The presumed mechanism of fistula formation is infection of the stent graft with resulting erosion through the thoracic aortic

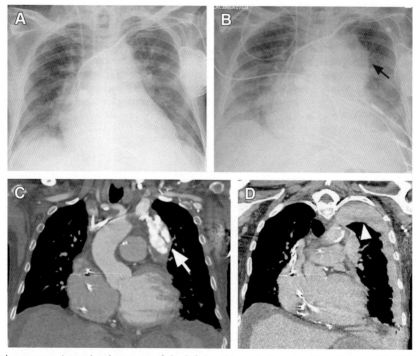

Fig. 13. Pseudoaneurysm/contained rupture of the left brachiocephalic vein after attempted left subclavian catheter placement. (*A*) Radiograph of the chest prior to left subclavian catheter placement; note left-sided automatic implantable cardioverter defibrillator (AICD). (*B*) Radiograph obtained after attempted catheter placement demonstrates development of an opacity adjacent to the aortic knob (*black arrow*). (*C*) Coronal CT image demonstrates pseudoaneurysm from the left brachiocephalic vein with dense contrast opacification from a left-sided venous injection (*white arrow*). (*D*) Immediate delay coronal image demonstrates pseudoaneurysm rupture and contrast/hemorrhage in the left pleural space (*arrowhead*).

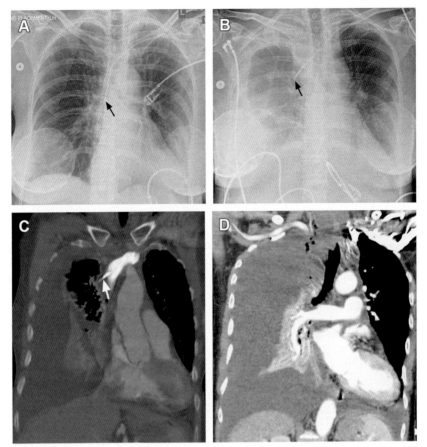

Fig. 14. Subclavian catheter perforation through SVC with rapidly developing right pleural effusion resulting from saline infusion through the catheter. (*A*) Precatheter repositioning radiograph with catheter curving into the SVC (*black arrow*). (*B*) Postrepositioning radiograph demonstrates the catheter tip abutting and possibly extending beyond the lateral margin of the SVC (*black arrow*). A large right pleural effusion has developed. (*C, D*) Coronal CT images demonstrate catheter tip penetrating the SVC (*white arrow*) with a large volume of right pleural fluid, associated with signs of tension, including mediastinal shift and diaphragm depression.

wall into the mediastinum and esophagus.[12] Although attempted repair via a surgical and/or endoscopic approach can at times be successful in the treatment of aortoesophageal fistulas, the rate of mediastinitis remains high.[12]

Additional detailed information regarding complications of aortic stent grafts is presented in another article in this issue.[11]

Radiology Procedural Complications

Vertebroplasty
Percutaneous vertebroplasty with polymethylmethacrylate (PMMA) is a common procedure performed by interventional radiologists for the treatment of vertebral collapse. Leakage of PMMA outside of the vertebral body has been reported to recur in 30% to 72% of procedures and

is normally well tolerated.[13] An uncommon complication of cement leakage is pulmonary embolism of PMMA due to venous migration of the cement material during the procedure (**Fig. 18**), which when present in large volumes can be symptomatic. Early detection of venous migration of PMMA during the procedure can help avert further complications, particularly pulmonary embolism.[13]

Fluoroscopic barium studies
Fluoroscopic examinations using orally administered barium solutions are a routine part of diagnostic radiology. Barium solutions have traditionally been used for their rare incidence of pneumonitis after aspiration compared with other contrast agents.[14] In more severe cases (**Fig. 19**), however, with significant extension of barium into the distal airways, morbidity related to rapidly

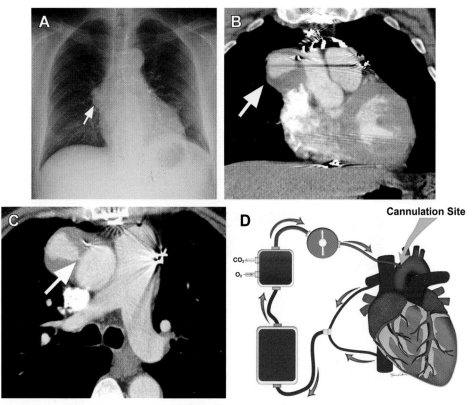

Fig. 15. Pseudoaneurysm at aortic cannulation site after cardiopulmonary bypass during CABG. (*A*) Chest radiograph demonstrates the patient to be status poststernotomy and CABG. An abnormal opacity at the right hilum in continuity with the mediastinum was noted (*arrow*). (*B*) Coronal contrast-enhanced image demonstrates a contrast-opacified pseudoaneurysm from the aorta (*arrow*). (*C*) Axial CT image better demonstrates the pseudoaneurysm, with a narrow neck from prior needle cannulation site (*arrow*). (*D*) Illustration of cardiac bypass; note cannulation site on aorta.

developing pneumonitis and impaired oxygenation can result and in rare instances even be fatal.[14,15] Fluoroscopic examinations involving oral barium solutions should be carefully monitored for penetration of contrast into the airway to minimize the extent of aspiration. High-density (thick) barium has also been linked with an increased incidence of pneumonitis after aspiration.[15]

Dental Procedures

The use of devices, such as high-speed, compressed air–driven turbine drills in dental surgical procedures has been associated with postprocedural subcutaneous emphysema, which is readily detectable clinically.[16] The swelling related to subcutaneous emphysema may be misdiagnosed by a dentist as an allergic reaction to local anesthetics. Because the roots of the mandibular molars directly communicate with the sublingual and submandibular spaces, compressed air may dissect into the retropharyngeal spaces and mediastinum. Hence, pneumomediastinum may be detected by radiographs (**Fig. 20**). A young patient with a history of recent dental procedures and chest pain should raise suspicion for this diagnosis and lead to careful scrutiny of the mediastinum on radiographs. CT is usually not necessary, because the source of pneumomediastium is well established.

Aspiration or ingestion of dental prostheses or tooth fragments can also be seen after dental procedures. Although ingestion into the digestive tract is more common, aspiration into the tracheobronchial system is a more severe complication.[17,18] Prompt detection of aspirated foreign bodies of dental origin after dental procedures or, in some cases, traumatic endotracheal intubation is essential to avoid delaying bronchoscopic retrieval (**Fig. 21**).[17,18]

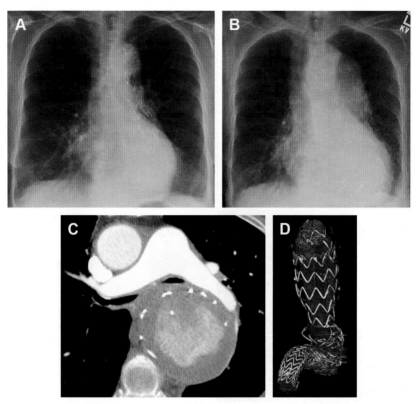

Fig. 16. Failure of a thoracic endovascular aortic stent graft. Patient with 2 weeks of back pain. (*A*) Prefailure chest radiograph demonstrating normal appearance of a thoracic aortic stent graft. Note tight metallic struts. (*B*) Postfailure chest radiograph demonstrating widening of the metallic struts. (*C*) Axial CT image demonstrating substantial dilatation of the aorta, with fractured and recoiled graft located along the anterior wall, and lack of graft covering of the posterior wall. (*D*) Volumetric reformation demonstrates the fractured superior component with widely spaced uncoiled struts and the intact inferior component with normally spaced struts.

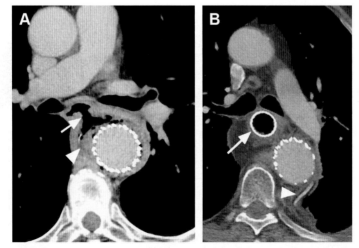

Fig. 17. Aortoesophageal fistula after aortic stent graft repair. The patient presented with back pain 2 months after aortic stent grafting. (*A*) Axial CT image demonstrates a fistulous tract visualized from the esophagus to the aortic stent graft (*arrow*). A periaortic fluid/air collection is visualized (*arrowhead*). (*B*) Axial CT image after primary repair with intercostal muscle flap and endoluminal esophageal stenting (*arrow*). Note characteristic appearance of an intercostal muscle flap with soft tissue and fat and enhancing intercostal artery (*arrowhead*).

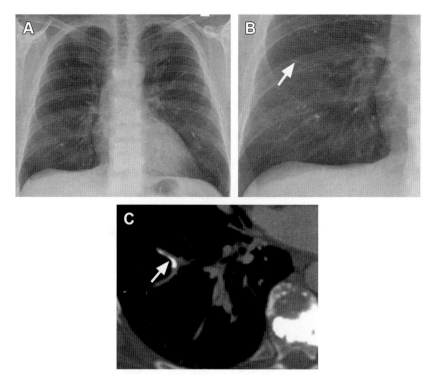

Fig. 18. PMMA pulmonary embolism after vertebroplasty. A patient with a history of osteoporosis secondary to seizure medication use requiring multiple vertebroplasties. (*A, B*) Chest radiograph and magnification view of the right lower lung demonstrates linear high-density foci within the lungs in a lower lobe predominant distribution (*arrow*). High-density material is identified within the vertebral bodies from the vertebroplasties. (*C*) Axial noncontrast CT scan demonstrates high-density material with a PA branch (*arrows*), representing PMMA pulmonary embolism.

Alternative/Cosmetic Medical Procedures

Cosmetic silicone injection

The injection of free silicone directly into subcutaneous tissue for cosmetic augmentation of the breasts and/or buttocks has been associated with a clinical syndrome of subacute pneumonitis. Silicone pneumonitis appears radiographically as patchy peripheral opacities often but not always wedge-shaped and similar in appearance to eosinophilic pneumonia and cryptogenic organizing pneumonia.[19] Although it is not clear what

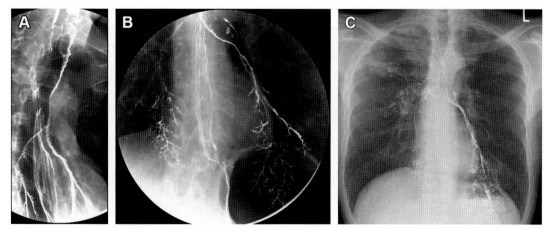

Fig. 19. Barium aspiration. (*A, B*) Selected images from a fluoroscopic barium swallow demonstrate extensive penetration of barium into the trachea and lower lobe airways. (*C*) Follow-up radiograph immediately following the swallow examination shows the extensive nature of aspiration into both lower lobes and into the right upper lobe.

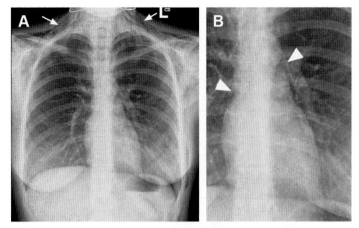

Fig. 20. Pneumomediastinum from dental extraction. The patient presented with chest pain after wisdom tooth extraction. (A) PA chest radiograph demonstrates air dissecting into the soft tissues of the neck (arrows). (B) Enlargement image demonstrates pneumomediastinum with air lifting the mediastinal pleura (arrowheads) seen as a linear opacity parallel to heart extending above the normal pericardial reflection.

the mechanism of pulmonary injury is, the observation that most documented cases have resolved after the administration of steroids implies that there is an immune-mediated component.[19] The observation of the characteristic appearance of subcutaneous silicone nodules (Fig. 22) should prompt a careful evaluation of the lungs for evidence of silicone pneumonitis.

Acupuncture

A specific form of acupuncture, known as Hari, is practiced most commonly in Northeast Asia and involves inserting gold needles into the subcutaneous tissues, which are not removed (Fig. 23).[20,21] This is performed repeatedly along predefined meridians and leads to the characteristic radiographic finding of multiple small linear radiodense soft tissue foreign bodies. Although this is an uncommon finding, the appearance is characteristic and should not be confused with other causes of soft tissue foreign bodies, such as metallic staples. Additionally, orthogonal views are important to ensure that the needle tips are indeed in the soft tissues and have not migrated to the viscera.[20,21]

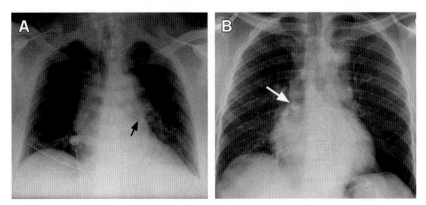

Fig. 21. Tooth aspiration in 2 patients. (A) AP chest radiograph demonstrates radiodensity within the left main-stem bronchus (black arrow) representing an aspirated central incisor, a complication of intubation. (B) PA radiograph in a patient after dental extraction demonstrates a dense object within the right bronchus intermedius (white arrow) representing an aspirated crown of a molar.

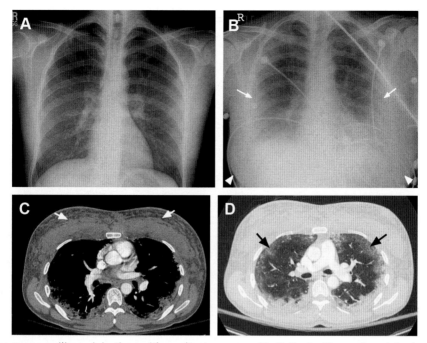

Fig. 22. Subcutaneous silicone injections with resultant pneumonitis. Patient with cough and shortness of breath after undergoing subcutaneous silicone injections for breast augmentation. (*A*) PA radiograph 1 year prior to presentation demonstrating clear lungs and male body habitus. (*B*) AP chest radiograph demonstrates interval change in body habitus with breast shadows (*arrowheads*). The lungs demonstrate increased opacification in a peripheral distribution (*arrows*). (C, D) Axial CT images demonstrate subcutaneous nodules and muscular expansion representing injections of free silicone (*white arrows*). Lung windows demonstrate peripheral patchy opacities (*black arrows*), which are highly consistent with silicone hypersensitivity pneumonitis, similar in appearance to eosinophilic pneumonia/cryptogenic organizing pneumonia.

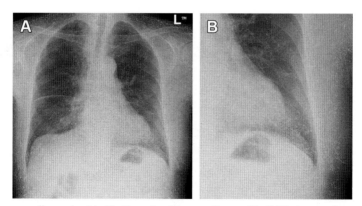

Fig. 23. Acupuncture needles embedded in the subcutaneous tissues. (*A, B*) PA chest radiograph with magnification of the left thorax demonstrates numerous metallic foreign bodies within the subcutaneous tissues. These needle remnants resulted from a specific form of Northeast Asian acupuncture (Hari), where the needles are placed into the subcutaneous tissues, and then broken off at the skin surface. The belief is that the retained needles continue to provide their positive stimuli.

SUMMARY

Radiologists play a critical role in identifying iatrogenic thoracic conditions related to traditional or alternative medical procedures. An understanding of the imaging findings in common iatrogenic thoracic complications can aid in assuring accurate diagnosis to guide appropriate patient management.

REFERENCES

1. Aguilera AL, Volokhina YV, Fisher KL. Radiography of cardiac conduction devices: a comprehensive review. Radiographics 2011;31(6):1669–82.

2. Costelloe CM, Murphy WA Jr, Gladish GW, et al. Radiography of pacemakers and implantable cardioverter defibrillators. AJR Am J Roentgenol 2012; 199(6):1252–8.

3. Hammerstingl C, Lickfett L, Jeong KM, et al. Persistence of iatrogenic atrial septal defect after pulmonary vein isolation–an underestimated risk? Am Heart J 2006;152(2):362.e1–5.

4. Liu E, Shehata M, Liu T, et al. Prevention of esophageal thermal injury during radiofrequency ablation for atrial fibrillation. J Interv Card Electrophysiol 2012;35(1):35–44.

5. Saad EB, Marrouche NF, Saad CP, et al. Pulmonary vein stenosis after catheter ablation of atrial fibrillation: emergence of a new clinical syndrome. Ann Intern Med 2003;138(8):634–8.

6. Dong J, Vasamreddy CR, Jayam V, et al. Incidence and predictors of pulmonary vein stenosis following catheter ablation of atrial fibrillation using the anatomic pulmonary vein ablation approach: results from paired magnetic resonance imaging. J Cardiovasc Electrophysiol 2005;16(8):845–52.

7. Latson LA, Prieto LR. Congenital and acquired pulmonary vein stenosis. Circulation 2007;115(1): 103–8.

8. Poplausky MR, Rozenblit G, Rundback JH, et al. Swan-Ganz catheter-induced pulmonary artery pseudoaneurysm formation: three case reports and a review of the literature. Chest 2001;120(6):2105–11.

9. Kabutey NK, Rastogi N, Kim D. Conservative management of iatrogenic superior vena cava (SVC) perforation after attempted dialysis catheter placement: case report and literature review. Clin Imaging 2013;37(6):1138–41.

10. Tochii M, Takagi Y, Hoshino R, et al. Pseudoaneurysm of ascending aorta 16 years after coronary artery bypass grafting. Ann Thorac Cardiovasc Surg 2011;17(3):323–5.

11. Thurnher S, Cejna M. Imaging of aortic stent-grafts and endoleaks. Radiol Clin North Am 2002;40(4): 799–833.

12. Isasti G, Gomez-Doblas JJ, Olalla E. Aortoesophageal fistula: an uncommon complication after stent-graft repair of an aortic thoracic aneurysm. Interact Cardiovasc Thorac Surg 2009;9(4):683–4.

13. Laredo JD, Hamze B. Complications of percutaneous vertebroplasty and their prevention. Skeletal Radiol 2004;33(9):493–505.

14. Albeldawi M, Makkar R. Images in clinical medicine. Barium aspiration. N Engl J Med 2012;366(11): 1038.

15. Gray C, Sivaloganathan S, Simpkins KC. Aspiration of high-density barium contrast medium causing acute pulmonary inflammation–report of two fatal cases in elderly women with disordered swallowing. Clin Radiol 1989;40(4):397–400.

16. Arai I, Aoki T, Yamazaki H, et al. Pneumomediastinum and subcutaneous emphysema after dental extraction detected incidentally by regular medical checkup: a case report. Oral Surg Oral Med Oral Pathol Oral Radiol Endod 2009; 107(4):e33–8.

17. Hill EE, Rubel B. A practical review of prevention and management of ingested/aspirated dental items. Gen Dent 2008;56(7):691–4.

18. Tiwana KK, Morton T, Tiwana PS. Aspiration and ingestion in dental practice: a 10-year institutional review. J Am Dent Assoc 2004;135(9):1287–91.

19. Zamora AC, Collard HR, Barrera L, et al. Silicone injection causing acute pneumonitis: a case series. Lung 2009;187(4):241–4.

20. Vassiou K, Kelekis NL, Fezoulidis I. Multiple retained acupuncture needle fragments. Eur Radiol 2003; 13(5):1188–9.

21. Park SM, Shim WJ. A hedgehog-like appearance resulting from Hari acupuncture. CMAJ 2011;183(13): E1038.

Imaging of Complications of Thoracic and Cardiovascular Surgery

Jared D. Christensen, MD*, Danielle M. Seaman, MD,
Lacey Washington, MD

KEYWORDS

• Iatrogenic • Complication • Computed tomography • Surgery • Cardiac • Thoracic • Aorta • Valve

KEY POINTS

• Iatrogenic causes of complications following thoracic and cardiovascular surgery are an important source of potentially preventable patient morbidity and mortality.
• Iatrogenic complications common to cardiothoracic surgery, regardless of technique, include hemorrhage, hemothorax, hemopericardium, retained foreign body, lung injury, and nerve damage.
• Most iatrogenic complications manifest in the early postoperative period; however, diagnosis can be challenging because clinical symptoms are often nonspecific.
• Imaging plays a critical role in the diagnosis of thoracic and cardiovascular complications. Early detection often permits timely management to minimize patient morbidity.

INTRODUCTION

Surgery entails risk and, despite advances in technology and patient care, complications are expected in the course of operative treatment. A complication is generally defined as any untoward event that is not part of the expected surgical procedure or postoperative recovery, potentially leading to increased morbidity or mortality. Iatrogenic complications can be considered those directly related to physician error in surgical technique or clinical judgment. Iatrogenic causes constitute a small but important source of complications, in that they are potentially preventable and potentially treatable if identified in the early postoperative course. Given the prevalence of pulmonary and cardiovascular diseases, thoracic and cardiac surgeries represent some of the most commonly performed procedures in the United States and worldwide; therefore, although severe iatrogenic complications are uncommon, a large number of patients are still affected, leading to unnecessary increased morbidity or mortality.

The diagnosis of iatrogenic complications can be challenging. The spectrum of disease and clinical presentation can be diverse. Furthermore, it is often difficult to distinguish iatrogenic complications from those representing normal variations in surgical outcomes. The type of iatrogenic complications may vary by patient population, surgeon, and surgical operative team. It is important for radiologists to consider the iatrogenic etiology of complications in postoperative imaging evaluation. Radiologists should not use accusatory or inflammatory language in reporting, and should work to cultivate close and trusting relationships with their surgical colleagues. Fostering an environment conducive to the free discussion of

Disclosures: None of the authors has a relationship with a commercial company that has a direct financial interest in the subject matter or materials discussed in this article, nor with a company making a competing product.
Department of Radiology, Duke University Medical Center, Box 3808, Durham, NC 27710, USA
* Corresponding author.
E-mail address: jared.christensen@duke.edu

Radiol Clin N Am 52 (2014) 929–959
http://dx.doi.org/10.1016/j.rcl.2014.05.003
0033-8389/14/$ – see front matter © 2014 Elsevier Inc. All rights reserved.

radiologic.theclinics.com

errors, be they diagnostic or surgical, can facilitate improved patient care. This article reviews iatrogenic complications that can be encountered in thoracic and cardiovascular surgery, with an emphasis on their underlying mechanisms and imaging features.

IATROGENIC COMPLICATIONS

Iatrogenic complications constitute a small percentage of the overall complications associated with thoracic and cardiovascular surgery. Although some complications may be unique to specific technical components of an operation, many are ubiquitous and independent of surgical technique. These consequences tend to encompass the complications for which consent is generally obtained before any interventional procedure (bleeding, infection, and injury to surrounding structures), but may have idiosyncratic clinical manifestations in the chest (**Box 1**). Hemorrhage-related complications, retained foreign body, lung injury, and nerve damage are detailed herein, whereas infection is addressed in later sections as it pertains to specific pulmonary and cardiovascular iatrogenic surgical complications.

Hemorrhage

Hemorrhage following thoracic or cardiovascular surgery is typically iatrogenic, but may also be associated with underlying coagulopathy. Whereas venous bleeding is typically self-limited, arterial hemorrhage can be life-threatening. Fortunately, significant bleeding after thoracic surgery is rare, occurring in fewer than 3% of patients after thoracotomy, and in only approximately 1% following video-assisted thoracoscopic surgery (VATS), with an overall mortality rate from hemorrhage of 0.1%.[1,2] The incidence of postoperative bleeding is slightly higher for cardiovascular surgery, with up to 20% of patients requiring blood transfusion for hemorrhage postoperatively.[3] Reoperation rates for bleeding complications after

---

coronary artery bypass grafting (CABG) and open surgical repair of the thoracic aorta are 2% and 8%, respectively.[4,5]

Postoperative hemorrhage following thoracotomy most often results from inadequate hemostasis of a bronchial artery or chest-wall systemic artery. Hemorrhage after cardiac surgery may be attributable to failed vascular anastomoses (coronary, aortic) or inadvertent injury of regional vessels. The manifestations of postsurgical bleeding are variable. For cardiothoracic procedures, common presentations include mediastinal or chest-wall hematoma, hemothorax, and hemopericardium.

Hemothorax

Hemothorax is a common postsurgical complication. A small amount of hemorrhage into the pleural space is anticipated during routine surgery, and some components of blood draining from a chest tube is expected. However, sanguineous chest-tube output of greater than 1500 mL in a 24-hour period, or greater than 200 mL/h for 2 to 4 hours, indicates active bleeding and should prompt surgical exploration.[6] Hemothorax most often presents at imaging as a rapidly enlarging pleural collection in the immediate postoperative period, often appreciable on chest radiography (**Fig. 1**). Noncontrast chest computed tomography (CT) depicts the presence of pleural fluid but confirms hemothorax only in some cases, as the appearance of hemothorax at CT is variable.[7,8] Small amounts of blood may appear as minimal areas of high attenuation within pleural fluid, often with the blood products layering dependently with lower attenuating simple fluid above it, resulting in a fluid-fluid or hematocrit level. If bleeding is extensive, hemothorax may present as a large, complex, loculated collection of mixed attenuation. As hemothorax evolves and becomes defibrinated, the collection can be indistinguishable from simple pleural fluid.

Hemopericardium

Hemopericardium is the presence of blood within the pericardial space. It is most commonly attributable to blunt or penetrating thoracic trauma; however, aortic dissection, ruptured aortic aneurysm, and malignancy are also possible causes. Iatrogenic injury represents an important etiologic mechanism, and is most often encountered after cardiovascular surgery or as a complication of central-line placement (**Fig. 2**). Active hemorrhage into the pericardial space is of particular clinical significance because it can rapidly lead to tamponade and circulatory collapse, even with a relatively low total volume of hemorrhage.

> **Box 1**
> **General iatrogenic complications in thoracic and cardiovascular surgery**
>
> - Hemorrhage
> - Hemothorax
> - Hemopericardium
> - Infection (mediastinitis, empyema)
> - Lung herniation
> - Nerve damage (phrenic, recurrent laryngeal, lateral thoracic, intercostal)

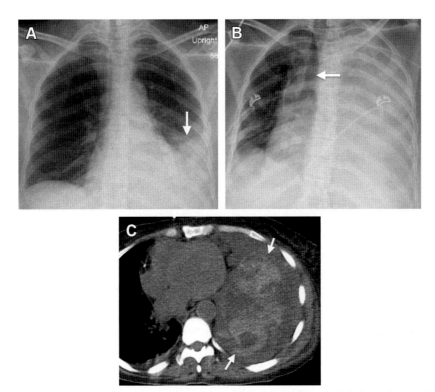

Fig. 1. Hemothorax. A 56-year-old woman after video-assisted thoracoscopic left lung biopsy. (*A*) Anterior-posterior (AP) chest radiograph shows left lower lobe atelectasis and new moderate-sized left pleural collection (*arrow*) following chest-tube removal. A repeat chest radiograph (*B*) obtained 3 hours later following a syncopal episode and hypotension shows complete opacification of the left hemithorax. There are signs of mass effect, with shift of the heart, mediastinum, and trachea (*arrow*) to the right, strongly suggesting increased pleural collection rather than atelectasis. In the interval, the patient's hemoglobin dropped from 9.1 to 7.3 g/dL. (*C*) Single axial image from subsequent noncontrast chest computed tomography (CT) shows mediastinal shift with a large, mixed attenuation left pleural collection, representing a hemothorax (*arrows*).

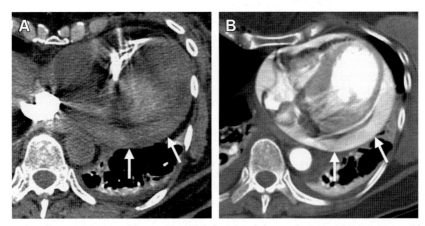

Fig. 2. Hemopericardium. A 74-year-old woman post left upper lobe wedge resection presents with acute hypotension and bradycardia following right central-line placement. Initial axial image on contrast-enhanced CT (*A*) shows high-attenuating fluid in the pericardial space (*arrows*), representing hemopericardium. A delayed axial image from the same scan (*B*) shows extravasated contrast filling the pericardial space (*arrows*). The patient had a cardiac arrest and died during the CT scan. Autopsy revealed pericardial perforation by the central venous catheter resulting in hemopericardium and cardiac tamponade.

Transthoracic echocardiography is the preferred initial imaging modality in the evaluation of suspected hemopericardium, as it is rapid, portable, and permits functional assessment for tamponade. However, CT is often performed in lieu of echocardiography, as symptoms such as hypotension are nonspecific, and hemopericardium may not be suspected. CT can confirm the presence of hemopericardium as pericardial fluid with attenuation typically between 30 and 70 HU. CT also permits evaluation for potential causes of hemopericardium, including aortic dissection.[9] Although CT allows for more thorough characterization of the amount and distribution of blood within the pericardial space than is possible via echocardiography, tamponade cannot be directly diagnosed, but only suggested by secondary signs, which include deformity of the cardiac chambers, flattening or leftward bowing of the interventricular septum, compression of the coronary sinus, narrowing of the intrathoracic inferior vena cava (IVC), and dilation of the superior vena cava and abdominal IVC.[10,11]

Retained Foreign Body

The retention of sponges, instruments, or needles at the time of operation is a relatively rare complication following thoracic and cardiovascular surgery. The incidence in the thorax is difficult to determine, as most series do not discriminate between intrathoracic and intra-abdominal foreign bodies and patients are often asymptomatic; however, estimates are in the range of 1 in 1000 to 1 in 3000 procedures.[12,13] Although relatively rare, retained surgical products can result in serious morbidity. Instrument and materials counts at the end of surgery may first raise the possibility of a retained foreign body, with a count inconsistency prompting intraoperative radiographic or fluoroscopic imaging. However, such counts may not be performed or may fail to identify a discrepancy, and a retained surgical product may be initially unsuspected.

Routine postoperative imaging may be the first indication of a retained surgical foreign body. Most surgical textiles, sponges, and laparotomy pads are radiolucent, but are manufactured with radiodense markers to facilitate detection at imaging. If not identified and removed, retained textiles incite an inflammatory reaction with resultant fibrosis and an inflammatory exudate referred to as a textiloma or gossypiboma; granuloma and abscess formation may develop. Within the thorax, the pleural space is the most common site of retained surgical foreign bodies, but mediastinal and intrapulmonary locations are also described.[14]

The CT imaging appearance is variable but typically consists of focal air, and fluid and/or soft-tissue attenuation; an enhancing rind may be present, and calcifications can develop over time.[12–15] Radiographic and CT findings of gossypiboma often mimic other pathologic conditions including pleural effusion, hemothorax, intrapulmonary abscess, mycetoma, and neoplasm. Most retained foreign bodies are detected in the immediate postoperative period, with a reported mean of 21 days to diagnosis; however, approximately 26% remain undetected for 60 days or more.[16] In a separate series, more than half of retained surgical foreign bodies went undetected for 5 or more years postoperatively.[17] Clinically, patients with retained objects may have pain or signs of infection, or may be completely asymptomatic. The possibility of gossypiboma should be considered in patients with a prior surgical history and infection refractory to appropriate antibiotic therapy. Definitive treatment requires removal of the retained foreign body.

In contrast to textiles, retained needles typically do not incite a pronounced inflammatory response. Surgical needles vary in size and appearance; most are small and may be curved or linear (**Fig. 3**). Despite being radiopaque, needles can be difficult to detect on chest radiographs, particularly if in proximity to surgical clips or in areas that are difficult to evaluate on portable films, such as the posterior costophrenic sulcus. Retained needles within the thorax have been described within the pleural space and mediastinum.[18] If they are within the pleural space, retained needles can migrate and change position at imaging. Although to the authors' knowledge there are no consensus management guidelines, most retained thoracic surgical needles are removed because of the theoretical risk for pneumothorax or vascular injury. Minimally invasive thoracoscopic approaches may be performed depending on needle location.[19]

Lung Herniation

Lung herniation is defined as protrusion of lung parenchyma with pleural membranes through a chest-wall defect. Although rare, it is a recognized complication of thoracic interventional procedures including chest-tube placement, thoracotomy, and minimally invasive thoracic or cardiovascular surgery. In the immediate postoperative period, an intercostal chest-wall defect is typically due to suture failure at the site of thoracotomy or trocar placement for VATS; however, late hernias may develop secondarily from muscle weakness in conjunction with increased intrathoracic

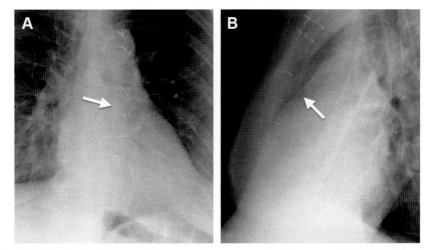

Fig. 3. Retained foreign body. A 48-year-old man post coronary artery bypass grafting (CABG). Posterior-anterior (PA) (*A*) and lateral (*B*) chest radiographs show a retained curved needle (*arrows*) within the anterior mediastinum despite reported correct needle and instrument counts. The patient was taken back to the operating room for removal of the needle.

pressure.[20] Iatrogenic lung herniation most commonly occurs in anterior or posterior locations following intervention at a site of intercostal muscle weakness; the lateral chest wall is a less common site of iatrogenic lung herniation, as it is protected by the serratus and latissimus dorsi in addition to the intercostal muscles.[21]

Physical examination may reveal a palpable mass that changes size with respiration, cough, or Valsalva maneuver. Most patients (up to 75% in one series) present with pain at the hernia site.[22] Lung hernias may strangulate with resultant infarction and hemoptysis. In patients without symptoms, the finding of lung herniation may be incidental. For those with symptoms, imaging evaluation is helpful to confirm the diagnosis, identify associated complications, and assess anatomic considerations for surgical repair. Herniated lung may be demonstrated on chest radiography if large and imaged in profile; however, CT is the imaging examination of choice (**Fig. 4**).[23–25] Lung herniation rarely resolves spontaneously. Large hernias and those that are symptomatic often require surgical repair, consisting of mesh grafts or muscle-flap chest-wall reconstruction.

Phrenic Nerve Injury

Nerve injury complicating thoracic surgery is an uncommon iatrogenic complication following thoracic and cardiovascular surgery, with an overall incidence ranging from 1% to 11%.[26] The phrenic, recurrent laryngeal, vagus, and intercostal nerves are most commonly involved, with clinical presentations corresponding to nerve function. Phrenic nerve injury has been reported to occur after lobectomy, thymectomy, lymph node dissection, lung transplantation, esophagectomy, aortic repair, pericardiotomy, and CABG, among other surgical procedures.[26–29] The highest incidence of phrenic nerve injury is associated with cardiac surgery, with reported complication rates of 10% to 85%.[30]

The risk for nerve injury is primarily related to the type of procedure and the extent of surgery/resection. Iatrogenic injury may result from nerve transection, compression, or excessive traction; in addition, phrenic nerve injury may also result from local hypothermia performed for myocardial protection during cardiac surgery.[31] Phrenic nerve injury is usually unilateral, and produces ipsilateral diaphragmatic paralysis. The left phrenic nerve is more commonly injured than the right, likely because of the more complex anatomic course of the left phrenic nerve and its proximity to the pericardium, left hilum, and thoracic aorta. Phrenic nerve injury is typically first manifest on postoperative chest radiography as a newly elevated hemidiaphragm when directly compared with preoperative imaging (**Fig. 5**). The diagnosis can be confirmed by dynamic fluoroscopy or ultrasonography showing paradoxic movement of the diaphragm during deep inspiration.[32,33] Phrenic nerve conduction studies may also be performed. Treatment is considered when symptoms are present, and involves surgical fixation of the diaphragm at a normal anatomic level to reduce muscular attenuation and to prevent progressive atelectasis and respiratory compromise.[34]

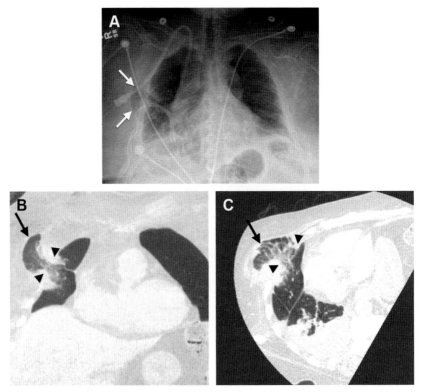

Fig. 4. Lung herniation. A 61-year-old man 5 days after right upper lobe segmentectomy for lung cancer. Frontal chest radiograph (*A*) shows a right chest-wall lucency (*arrows*) concerning for herniated lung at a trocar site. Minimal-intensity projection coronal reconstruction (*B*) and axial image (*C*) in the plane of the defect, from non-contrast CT, confirm herniation of the right middle lobe (*arrows*) through an intercostal chest-wall defect (*arrowheads*) but without evidence of other complication. The patient underwent subsequent repair, owing to the size of the defect and the extent of herniation.

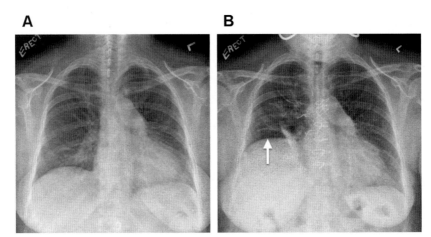

Fig. 5. Phrenic nerve injury. A 53-year-old woman post CABG. Preoperative PA radiograph (*A*) is normal. Postoperative PA radiograph (*B*) shows elevation of the right hemidiaphragm (*arrow*), with confirmed paralysis on dynamic fluoroscopy, representing right phrenic nerve injury.

PULMONARY RESECTION

Indications for pulmonary resection are varied, with the procedure most commonly performed for tumor or infection. Surgical techniques can broadly be categorized as anatomic or nonanatomic. Anatomic resections follow defined anatomic structures and landmarks, and include pneumonectomy, lobectomy, and segmentectomy. Airways, pulmonary arteries, and pulmonary veins supplying the area of resection are carefully identified and ligated, followed by regional parenchymal lymph node dissection. Nonanatomic resections tend to be smaller and independent of anatomy; techniques include wedge resection, bullectomy, and lung volume reduction surgery. In these procedures stapling devices are used to remove portions of the lung, which may be subsegmental or cross-pulmonary segments. Iatrogenic complications associated with lung resection largely depend on the type of surgery (**Box 2**). Thoracostomy with pneumonectomy introduces complications different from those encountered with video-assisted thoracoscopic wedge resection, although there are shared risks such as hemothorax, infection, air leak, and bronchopleural fistula.

Bronchopleural Fistula

Injury to the airways is a commonly encountered complication with pulmonary surgeries. The primary objective for minimizing airway-related complications during pneumonectomy, lobectomy, and sublobar pulmonary resection is to adequately seal the transected airway to prevent an air leak; this is accomplished by stapling across lobar, segmental, or subsegmental bronchioles, or oversewing the mainstem bronchial stump. In the setting of lung transplantation, the objective is to maintain airway patency while preventing stenosis and anastomotic dehiscence. Bronchopleural fistula refers to a direct communication between a bronchus and the pleural space, but is often more generally used to indicate a persistent air leak from either the bronchi or the lung

parenchyma.[35] With the latter classification, a central bronchopleural fistula is defined as an air leak involving a large bronchus and the pleural space, whereas a peripheral bronchopleural fistula indicates a leak from a peripheral bronchus or the lung parenchyma. Although bronchopleural fistulae may have other causes, the most common are iatrogenic,[35,36] with reported incidences of bronchopleural fistula of 4.5% to 20% after pneumonectomy and 0.5% following lobectomy.[37] The condition can result in significant morbidity including chronic pneumothorax, tension pneumothorax, empyema, and aspiration of material from the pleural space. Mortality rates for bronchopleural fistula following thoracic surgery are high, ranging from 18% to 67%.[37,38]

Although most commonly identified in the immediate postoperative period, bronchopleural fistulae can also occur late if infection or necrosis of the bronchial stump leads to dehiscence. Radiographic findings of bronchopleural fistula include a persistent or enlarging pneumothorax or air component of a hydropneumothorax, as well as lack of the anticipated mediastinal shift toward the operated lung to compensate for volume loss.[39] The diagnosis of delayed bronchopleural fistula is based on the spontaneous appearance of air within the pleural space in the absence of interval intervention. CT often demonstrates secondary signs of bronchopleural fistula, including empyema and aspiration.[40] Direct visualization of a communication between the airway and pleural space, once thought to be uncommon, has been reported in both central and peripheral bronchopleural fistulae in up to 50% of cases, the identification of which is aided by thin-section multiplanar CT images (**Fig. 6**).[35,36,41] Precise localization of the air leak, its relative size, and any associated complications are important goals of imaging that may facilitate surgical planning.

Peripheral bronchopleural fistula may occur with segmentectomy or wedge resection, and involve small airways. In the absence of other complications, the resultant air leak can often be managed conservatively with prolonged chest-tube placement. If conservative management is unsuccessful, definitive treatment with minimally invasive techniques, including endoscopic bronchial occlusion with closure devices or glue, may be undertaken.[42–44] Central bronchopleural fistulae occur following lobectomy or pneumonectomy, involve larger airways, and do not respond to conservative therapy. It is reported that central bronchopleural fistula occurs more commonly following right pneumonectomy than left, as the right mainstem bronchus extends into the pleural space.[37] The goals of surgical strategies for the management

---

Box 2
Complications of lung resection

- Bronchopleural fistula
- Infection (mediastinitis, empyema)
- Hemopericardium
- Hemothorax
- Lung injury
- Nerve damage

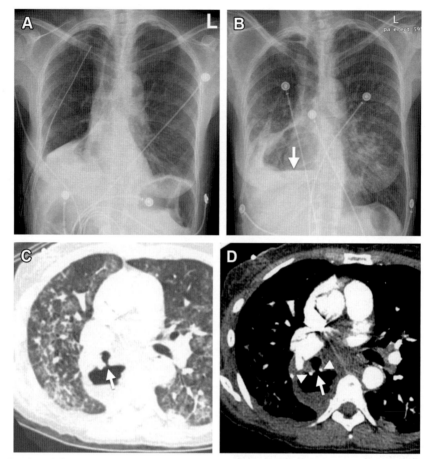

Fig. 6. Bronchopleural fistula. A 53-year-old woman post right lower lobectomy for lung cancer. PA chest radiographs on postoperative days 2 (*A*) and 8 (*B*) show interval development of a large right basilar hydropneumothorax, denoted by an air-fluid level (*arrow*). Noncontrast chest CT images, with lung (*C*) and soft-tissue (*D*) windows, shows dehiscence of the lobectomy staple line (*arrowheads*), with a large bronchopleural fistula (*arrows*) complicated by empyema.

of central bronchopleural fistulae are to occlude the airway and fill the pleural space via thoracotomy or thoracoplasty. The involved airway is repaired with direct closure via stump resection or revision and buttressing with a vascularized tissue flap utilizing muscle, omentum, pericardium, or diaphragm. The pleural space is washed out, debrided, and filled by the flap, reduced by chest-wall resection (thoracoplasty), or left partially open for long-term drainage (Eloesser window thoracostomy or flap) in the case of chronic empyema.

Lung Torsion

Lung torsion occurs by parenchymal rotation around a bronchovascular pedicle. Torsion can occur in association with blunt trauma, pneumothorax, and malignancy, but is a well-described, albeit rare, complication of thoracic surgery.[45–47]

Lobar torsion following lobectomy is most common and has been attributed to increased mobility following division of the pulmonary ligament; however, whole lung torsion can occur, particularly following lung transplantation.[48–50] The risk of torsion is theoretically increased in lung transplantation, owing to division of the pulmonary ligament of the donor lung, potential size discrepancies between the donor lung and recipient thorax, and the complexity of the bronchial and vascular anastomoses that predispose to manipulation and possible rotation of the allograft.

Radiographic findings of torsion are nonspecific, and vary depending on the severity of torsion (ie, whether it is partial or complete). Asymmetric venous congestion of the involved lobe or lung is an early manifestation; however, in cases with more severe airway compromise, consolidation mimicking infection or atelectasis may be present in the immediate postoperative period.[51]

Complete torsion may present as abrupt termination of the bronchial air column on chest radiography, with resultant atelectasis. Venous and/or pulmonary arterial infarction can occur over time if torsion is not identified and surgically corrected by manual detorsion of the affected lobe or lung.

Contrast-enhanced CT is the imaging examination of choice for patients with suspected pulmonary torsion. In addition to the findings described at radiography, CT permits detailed anatomic evaluation of the bronchi and pulmonary vasculature. Reported CT findings of lung torsion include twisting of the airways and vessels (readily evaluated on multiplanar reconstructions), abnormal orientation of the fissures, abrupt airway and/or vascular occlusion, and opacities resulting from hemorrhagic infarction (**Fig. 7**).[46,52,53] Ideally, both arterial-phase and venous-phase imaging should be obtained to evaluate for pulmonary

arterial and venous thrombosis, which can have clinical features similar to torsion, but are distinct on imaging and may not require surgical management.

LUNG TRANSPLANTATION

Lung transplantation was first performed in a human subject in 1963, with the patient only surviving for a few weeks following surgery.[54] Since then, advances in pharmacologic immunosuppression, antibiotic therapies, and surgical techniques have made lung transplantation a viable treatment for many pulmonary conditions, the most common being chronic obstructive pulmonary disease, pulmonary fibrosis, and cystic fibrosis. Lung transplantation may be unilateral or bilateral. Although a discussion regarding the indications for each is beyond the scope of this article, the surgical

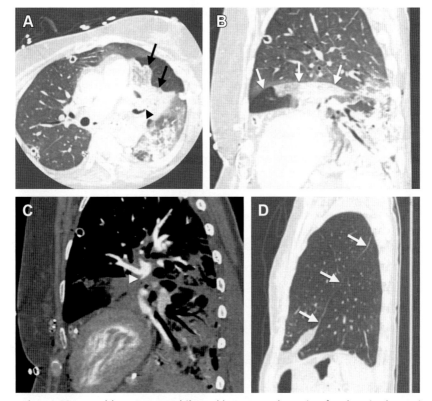

Fig. 7. Lung torsion. A 52-year-old woman post bilateral lung transplantation for chronic obstructive pulmonary disease. A pulmonary embolism protocol CT angiogram was performed on postoperative day 2 for acute hypoxia. Axial image in lung window (*A*) shows tapering and cutoff of the left lower lobe superior segmental bronchus (*arrowhead*), with resultant consolidation and venous congestion of the involved pulmonary segment (*arrows*). Lung (*B*) and soft-tissue (*C*) window sagittal reconstructions show abnormal horizontal orientation of the left major fissure (*arrows*) with anterior displacement of the lower lobe superior segment; the segmental pulmonary artery is also obstructed (*arrowhead*). The patient was taken to the operating room, where the diagnosis of lung torsion was confirmed. Following detorsion, sagittal reconstruction through the left lung (*D*) on repeat CT shows anatomic positioning of the left major fissure (*arrows*) and pulmonary segments with resolution of arterial and venous obstruction.

techniques involved are similar, as are the potential iatrogenic complications.

Bronchial Anastomotic Dehiscence

Bronchial anastomotic complications are common after lung transplantation, occurring in up to 33% of transplant recipients.[55,56] Dehiscence of the bronchial anastomosis represents an important early complication of lung transplantation that, when identified, can be treated and potentially prevent loss of the allograft. The bronchial anastomosis is one of the more technically challenging aspects of lung transplantation, and is the first step in implantation.

Two surgical techniques for establishing an anastomosis between the donor and recipient bronchi have been used: end-to-end and telescoping. The end-to-end technique was used early in the history of lung transplantation, but has fallen out of favor because it was found to be associated with a high failure rate, in part attributed to donor bronchial ischemia.[55] Outcomes were improved by the addition of a muscular or omental wrap, which facilitated healing of the anastomosis; however, these techniques introduced new surgical complications. The telescoping anastomosis was then developed, which negated the need for an omental wrap. With this technique, the donor bronchus is divided between the membranous and cartilaginous layers with the cartilaginous bronchus positioned telescoping into the recipient bronchus, with the anastomosis completed between the full thickness of the donor and recipient bronchi at the level of the membranous dissection.[56]

Regardless of technique, the recipient bronchus maintains the native bronchial arterial supply, whereas the donor bronchus relies on collateral perfusion from the pulmonary arterial circulation. Revascularization of the donor bronchus via the recipient's bronchial arteries can take up to 4 weeks; therefore, the early postoperative period represents a time of airway vulnerability.[57]

Despite improved surgical techniques to minimize anastomotic failure, bronchial dehiscence is reported to occur in 7% to 24% of patients after lung transplantation.[58,59] Bronchial anastomotic dehiscence can be classified as complete or limited. Complete dehiscence is a rare complication with total anastomotic breakdown, and constitutes a surgical emergency requiring open repair for anastomotic revision or retransplantation. Limited dehiscence is more common and may heal with conservative medical management, endobronchial therapy, or more limited surgical repair. Airway defects smaller than 4 mm in size have an overall favorable prognosis with conservative or minimally invasive management.[60]

Bronchoscopy is the preferred technique for definitive bronchial anastomotic evaluation, as it permits direct visualization of the anastomosis and can detect mucosal necrosis; however, the procedure is invasive and carries a risk of disrupting the anastomosis. CT is the preferred noninvasive imaging modality for bronchial anastomotic evaluation. Bronchial dehiscence may be suspected when there is extraluminal air adjacent to the anastomosis with an associated airway defect; direct visualization of communication between the airway and extraluminal air is diagnostic (**Fig. 8**).[61] In the absence of such findings the diagnosis can

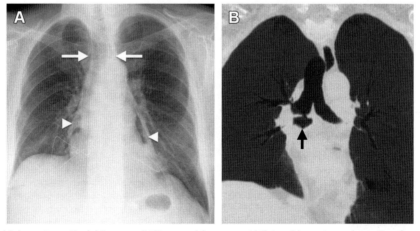

Fig. 8. Bronchial anastomotic dehiscence. A 58-year-old man post bilateral lung transplantation for coal worker's pneumoconiosis. Surveillance chest radiograph (*A*) shows new pneumomediastinum (*arrows*) and pneumopericardium (*arrowheads*). Noncontrast coronal maximum intensity projection reconstructed image (*B*) shows focal bronchial anastomotic dehiscence with communication between the right mainstem bronchus and a mediastinal air collection (*arrow*).

be challenging: airway defects are not always identifiable, and air may not be found adjacent to the airway because it can dissect into the mediastinum and along fascial planes resulting in pneumomediastinum, which is an expected finding up to 2 weeks after lung transplantation.[62] It is important to identify the type of anastomosis (end-to-end or telescoping) as part of the imaging assessment, as air within the lumen adjacent to the telescoping bronchi may appear extraluminal and mimic dehiscence.[63] CT axial images alone are often insufficient for evaluation, and diagnosis is facilitated by multiplanar reconstructions and minimum-intensity projection images.

Bronchial Stenosis

Whereas ischemia resulting in necrosis and anastomotic dehiscence is an early complication, most airway complications occur late following anastomotic healing and tissue remodeling. Bronchial stenosis is the most common late airway complication following lung transplantation, with an incidence ranging between 1.6% and 32%.[59,64] Late stenosis is associated with early complications of necrosis, dehiscence, and airway infection, but can occur in the absence of a history of these predisposing conditions.[60]

Although stenosis most often occurs as an indirect result of iatrogenic complications, it can also occur as a direct result of iatrogenic airway injury. Two primary patterns of bronchial stenosis following lung transplantation have been described: anastomotic and segmental nonanastomotic. The earlier literature reported anastomotic stenosis to be the most common form, with segmental nonanastomotic stenosis believed to represent only approximately 3% of cases.[57] However, more recent data indicate that nonsegmental anastomotic stenosis preferentially involving the bronchus intermedius may actually be more common than anastomotic narrowing, representing 59% of all airway stenoses in one series.[65] Symptomatic severe segmental nonanastomotic stenosis involving the bronchus intermedius has been referred to as vanishing bronchus intermedius syndrome (VBIS), and is associated with high morbidity and mortality.[66] Although the precise etiology is unclear, VBIS has been associated with ischemia, infection, rejection, and mechanical airway injury.[66]

The diagnosis of bronchial stenosis can be suggested clinically when patients present with dyspnea, cough, wheezing, or recurrent postobstructive pneumonia. Symptomatic patients are typically evaluated with bronchoscopy, as it permits direct airway visualization and facilitates

potential treatment at the time of diagnosis. Patients with severe stenosis, such as VBIS, may present with segmental or lobar atelectasis. CT may be used to detect unsuspected cases of airway stenosis as part of routine imaging evaluation after lung transplantation, and can be used to identify other potential causes of clinical symptoms. Dynamic CT can be used to help differentiate stenosis from bronchomalacia, in that the former demonstrates a fixed narrowing on both inspiratory and expiratory phase imaging, whereas malacia consists of luminal narrowing only on expiration.[62] CT is also helpful for characterizing the location, degree, and length of stenosis, as well as patency of distal airways to facilitate treatment planning.

The management of bronchial stenosis depends on the severity and location of disease. Narrowing of the airway diameter of greater than 50% is considered significant and is often treated even in the absence of clinical symptoms.[67] Endoscopic therapies are varied and include balloon bronchoplasty, cryotherapy, laser therapy, and self-expanding stent placement (**Fig. 9**).[57,64] In the event of failed endoscopic treatment, surgical repair may be attempted using techniques including anastomotic revision or bronchial sleeve resection, with or without accompanying lobectomy.

ESOPHAGECTOMY

Esophageal resection is indicated for the management of both benign and malignant conditions, but is most commonly performed for the treatment of esophageal carcinoma. Esophageal cancer is the third most common gastrointestinal malignancy and the sixth leading cause of cancer deaths worldwide.[68] In the United States there are approximately 18,000 new cases annually.[69] Although treatment options include neoadjuvant chemotherapy and radiation therapy, surgical resection remains the standard of care.

Surgical management of esophageal cancer includes esophageal resection, regional lymph node dissection, conduit isolation, and anastomosis of the conduit to the residual esophagus. Each aspect of the surgery presents challenges and potential for complications (**Box 3**). The preferred surgical approach is via thoracotomy. The Ivor Lewis resection consists of a right thoracotomy and laparotomy with lymph node dissection and a thoracic conduit-esophageal anastomosis; it is the most commonly performed surgical technique for the management of esophageal cancer worldwide.[70] The McKeown technique adds a cervical incision, which permits for either a thoracic or cervical esophageal anastomosis, and is the primary

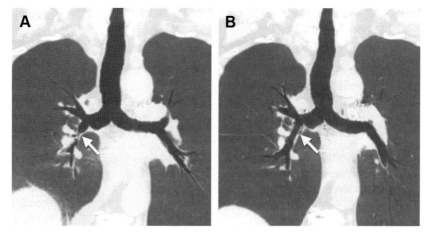

Fig. 9. Bronchial stenosis. A 29-year-old man post bilateral lung transplantation for cystic fibrosis. The patient had abnormal pulmonary function tests, prompting a noncontrast CT to evaluate for infection 4 months following surgery. Coronal minimal-intensity projection reconstruction (A) shows focal narrowing of the bronchus intermedius (arrow). Review of the operative record indicated injury to the bronchus intermedius at the time of organ harvesting. The patient underwent treatment with airway stenting with improved patency (arrow) as illustrated on follow-up CT coronal minimal-intensity projection reconstruction (B).

option for high esophageal tumors. Laparoscopic esophagectomy can also be performed, but is not yet routine. A trans-hiatal approach is preferred for the management of benign disease but is generally not indicated for malignancy, as the approach does not permit thoracic lymph node dissection. The stomach is the ideal conduit and is used whenever possible; it has an excellent blood supply and requires only a single anastomosis. The colon and jejunum may be used as conduits when the stomach cannot be used, such as when tumors involve the gastric fundus and body, or in the event of gastric conduit failure.

Esophagogastric Anastomotic Leak

Leak at the esophagogastric anastomosis is one of the most common complications following esophagectomy, reported to occur in up to 50% of

---

Box 3
Complications of esophagectomy

- Anastomotic leak
- Gastric conduit necrosis
- Bronchogastric fistula
- Gastropleural fistula
- Thoracic duct injury/chylothorax
- Infection (mediastinitis, empyema)
- Hemothorax
- Lung injury
- Nerve damage

---

patients.[71] Anastomotic leak can occur early (2–3 days) as a result of surgical failure of the anastomosis, or late (3–7 days) owing to ischemic changes at or just below the anastomosis secondary to necrosis of the proximal gastric conduit. Early detection is crucial for timely management and to prevent significant morbidity and mortality. Common postsurgical protocols call for an upper gastrointestinal series on the seventh day after surgery, if not sooner, to evaluate for an anastomotic leak.

Findings of an esophageal leak are usually obvious on upper gastrointestinal series, as contrast extends outside of the expected luminal contour (**Fig. 10**). Fluoroscopy has a higher specificity for the diagnosis of anastomotic leak in comparison with CT; however, CT is more sensitive and is a useful companion modality for the identification of the extent of the leak and associated complications including mediastinitis and empyema.[72] Patients with anastomotic leak are also at increased risk of late complications including stricture and fistula formation.

Treatment depends on the size and extent of leak at imaging in addition to the severity of clinical symptoms. Contained leaks are limited to the mediastinum, and may be managed conservatively. Management options include antibiotics, placement of a covered stent across the leak, total parenteral nutrition, and percutaneous drainage if necessary. Large leaks typically have pleural extension and are unlikely to heal with conservative management. Although radiologists may be asked to perform percutaneous drainage of leaks

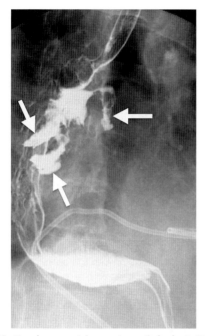

Fig. 10. Esophagogastric anastomotic leak. A 63-year-old man post Ivor Lewis esophagectomy undergoing routine postoperative esophagogram to exclude leak. Single fluoroscopic image following administration of oral contrast shows contrast outside the gastric conduit (*arrows*) but contained within the mediastinum, diagnostic of thoracic esophagogastric anastomotic leak.

communicating with the pleura, this is only a temporary measure until definitive surgical revision can be performed.

Gastric Conduit Necrosis

Although anastomotic leak after esophagectomy can result in significant morbidity, failure of the conduit is devastating and potentially fatal. The reported rate of gastric conduit failure ranges from 0.5% to 3.2%.[73] Ischemia is the most common cause of conduit failure, and several technical factors may contribute to vascular compromise including twisting of the conduit, constriction at the diaphragmatic hiatus, and constriction of the esophagogastric anastomosis.[73,74] Overdistention of the conduit has also been implicated in contributing to ischemia, hence the importance of gastric decompression, particularly in the early postoperative period.[74] The proximal aspect of the stomach is the most common site of necrosis and resultant anastomotic leak.[75] Gastric necrosis should be suspected in the setting of an enlarging leak or failed conservative management of leak. CT findings of gastric necrosis are variable, but the diagnosis can be suggested by wall thickening out of

proportion to lumen distention and lack of conduit enhancement (**Fig. 11**). However, endoscopy is more sensitive and specific than CT for the detection of early gastric necrosis.[76] When necrosis is suspected, early surgical reexploration is recommended to evaluate the conduit; if necrotic, resection of the involved portion of the stomach is performed. If there is sufficient residual length of the gastric conduit, a new cervical esophagogastrostomy is created; if there is insufficient length or if the entire gastric conduit has failed, reconstruction with colonic interposition can be utilized as a salvage technique.[77,78]

Diaphragmatic Hernia

Diaphragmatic hernia is an uncommon but important complication following esophagectomy, with a reported incidence of 0.7% to 15%.[79,80] The esophageal hiatus is stretched or otherwise altered at the time of surgery in the process of transposing the gastric conduit into the thorax, predisposing to the development of diaphragmatic hernias. Herniation of abdominal contents through the diaphragmatic hiatus can result in delayed emptying of the gastric conduit, obstruction, or strangulated bowel. Herniation most commonly occurs in the left hemithorax, with the liver believed to protect against right-sided herniation.[79–81]

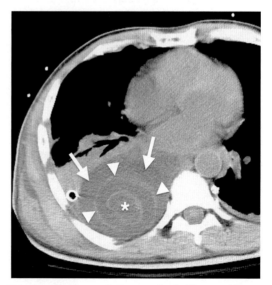

Fig. 11. Gastric conduit necrosis. A 56-year-old man post McKeown esophagectomy with gastric conduit. Noncontrast axial CT image shows diffuse wall thickening of the paravertebral gastric conduit (*arrowheads*), which is concerning for ischemia. The conduit lumen (*asterisk*) has decreased caliber and there is surrounding pleural fluid (*arrows*). Complete gastric conduit necrosis was confirmed at reoperation, with gastric conduit removal and colonic interposition.

Diaphragmatic hernia after esophagectomy can be an early or late complication, with delayed hernias reportedly occurring up to 7 years after esophageal resection.[82] Imaging plays an important role in the evaluation of diaphragmatic hernia, and CT is the preferred imaging modality (**Fig. 12**). The diagnosis is often incidental at the time of routine postoperative surveillance imaging, and may not be reported by radiologists unless large.[83] Although patients may be asymptomatic, the presence of even a small diaphragmatic hernia may prompt closer imaging follow-up, and an increase in size may prompt empiric surgical intervention; therefore, greater attention to the possibility of this complication is probably warranted. Surgical correction involves relocating herniated contents into the abdomen and reducing the hiatal defect with either crural plication or mesh repair.[80]

Bronchogastric Fistula

Fistulae following esophagectomy can involve several anatomic structures including the esophagus, gastric conduit, airway, pleural space, and aorta. Clinical symptoms vary depending on the type of fistula. Bronchogastric fistula is a rare complication that can occur both early and late in the postoperative course, with only a few cases reported in the literature.[84]

Early formation of bronchogastric fistula is most likely attributable to unrecognized thermal or blunt airway injury. The most common mechanism for late formation of bronchogastric fistula is indirectly related to surgical technique. At the time of operation, a staple line is created along the lesser curvature of the stomach with a dual purpose: to elongate the conduit to facilitate creation of the esophagogastric anastomosis, and to reduce conduit volume.[85] Positioning of the conduit in the mediastinum often places the staple line in direct contact with the posterior aspect of the right mainstem bronchus or with the bronchus intermedius. Pressure necrosis with erosion of the gastric staple line into the airway can occur, with resultant bronchogastric fistula. Distention of the conduit and prior infection are believed to be predisposing factors.[84] Patients typically present with clinical symptoms and imaging features of aspiration pneumonitis.

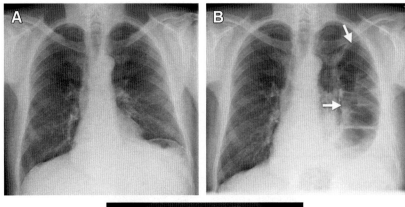

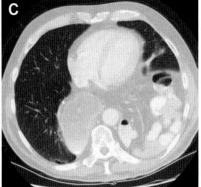

Fig. 12. Diaphragmatic hernia. PA chest radiographs obtained 1 month (*A*) and 6 months (*B*) following esophagectomy show interval herniation of loops of colon (*arrows*) into the left hemithorax with resultant left lung volume loss. Axial image on lung window from contrast-enhanced axial CT (*C*) shows a large hiatal hernia containing fat, colon, and small bowel requiring repair.

A direct fistulous communication may be visualized by CT (**Fig. 13**), bronchoscopy, or via fluoroscopy with oral contrast demonstrated to pass from the conduit into the airway.[86] Initial management may involve placement of a covered stent within the airway and/or gastric conduit.[87] Failed conservative therapy warrants surgical repair, with directed repair of both the conduit and airway. If primary closure of the airway is not possible, reconstruction with the use of mesh, pericardium, omentum, or a muscular flap can be performed.[88,89] Severe cases can result in failure of the gastric conduit, necessitating colonic interposition.

Thoracic Duct Injury

The thoracic duct is a posterior mediastinal structure originating at the cisterna chyli; although the location is highly variable, the second lumbar vertebral body is a common marker for its origin. The duct commonly ascends on the right and crosses to the left at around the fourth thoracic vertebra, eventually emptying into the left subclavian vein. Thoracic duct injury is most often caused by penetrating trauma, with injury during thoracic surgery being the second most common cause.[90] The thoracic duct is routinely ligated or resected during transthoracic esophagectomy, predisposing to potential lymphatic complications; however, the duct can be inadvertently injured during other thoracic procedures. Thoracic duct injury impairs lymphatic drainage and predisposes to development of a lymphatic leak, with a resultant localized lymphocele or chylothorax. The reported incidence of thoracic duct injury following esophagectomy is approximately 4%.[91] Lymphatic injury with chylothorax may be suspected clinically following thoracic surgery with a persistent large-volume chest-tube output (>1000 mL/d) beyond postoperative day 2.[75] Elevated triglycerides (>110 mg/dL) in the pleural fluid is confirmatory for chylothorax.[75,91]

The thoracic duct and lymphatic system are not readily evaluated by routine imaging modalities. Historically, lymphography was performed by cannulation of a lower extremity lymphatic duct and injection of a contrast agent derived from poppy seed oil, followed by radiography. This technique has subsequently been used in conjunction with CT (CT lymphangiography) to define thoracic duct anatomy and identify the specific site of duct injury (**Fig. 14**).[92] Magnetic resonance (MR) lymphangiography has also been described, and may be of future clinical utility in thoracic duct evaluation.[93,94]

Minor thoracic duct injuries with small, contained leaks are typically managed conservatively with percutaneous drainage and dietary restrictions, allowing the leak to heal by reducing lymphatic drainage volumes.[95] Large leaks and small leaks that have failed conservative management generally require definitive treatment with thoracic duct ligation, although minimally invasive techniques such as thoracic duct embolization with glue or coils have been described.[96–98]

CORONARY ARTERY BYPASS GRAFTING

CABG for myocardial revascularization is the preferred management for high-grade and

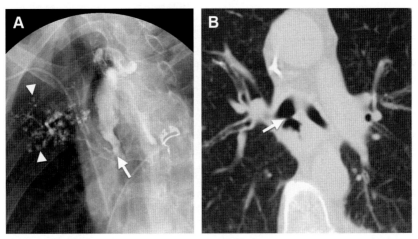

Fig. 13. Bronchogastric fistula. A 53-year-old man post esophagogastrectomy for esophageal cancer presents with recurrent pneumonia and chest pain. Representative image from an upper gastrointestinal examination (*A*) shows a fistula with the right mainstem bronchus (*arrow*) near the upper lobe bronchus origin, as evidenced by contrast filling the alveoli (*arrowheads*). Axial noncontrast CT image (*B*) confirms direct communication between the gastric conduit and the right mainstem bronchus (*arrow*).

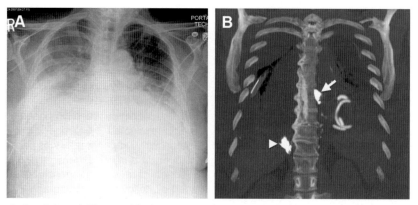

Fig. 14. Thoracic duct injury. A 60-year-old man post esophagectomy presents on postoperative day 5 with persistent bilateral pleural collections on AP chest radiograph (*A*), and a chest-tube output of greater than 1600 mL fluid daily, suggestive of chylothoraces and suspicion for thoracic duct injury. CT lymphangiogram coronal reconstruction (*B*) shows 2 foci of contrast extravasation at approximately T8 on the left (*arrow*) and T12 on the right (*arrowhead*), confirming thoracic duct leaks. The patient underwent subsequent surgical ligation with resolution of the chylothoraces.

obstructive coronary artery atherosclerotic disease. The procedure is performed via median sternotomy to gain access to the heart and coronary arteries in preparation for bypass with either internal mammary or saphenous vein grafts, although radial and gastroepiploic artery grafts may also rarely be used. Clinical outcomes depend directly on long-term patency of the grafts. Although diverse complications are described following CABG, iatrogenic complications are generally associated with the sternotomy site or the bypass graft (**Box 4**). Complication rates for median sternotomy range from 0.5% to 5%, with an overall mortality rate of approximately 7%; higher rates have been reported depending on the patient population.[99] Complications of CABG may present early or late. Most iatrogenic complications manifest early, within days to weeks following surgery.

Graft Occlusion

Early complications involving the graft are most often attributable to endothelial injury at the time of operation, and commonly result in graft occlusion.[100] Vessel injury can occur at the time of saphenous vein graft harvesting, internal mammary artery mobilization, or graft anastomosis. Kinking or twisting of saphenous vein grafts can occur from manipulation during graft positioning and fixation with resultant obstruction; this is particularly an issue with longer grafts.[101] By contrast, grafts that are too short may experience stretching and endothelial damage, predisposing to thrombus and resultant luminal obstruction. Dissection of saphenous vein grafts leading to graft occlusion has also been reported.[102] Early stenosis related to surgical technique can also occur at the graft anastomosis.

The clinical presentation of complications related to bypass grafts is usually nonspecific, with chest pain and dyspnea being the most common symptoms. Conventional cardiac catheterization has historically been the imaging examination of choice in the evaluation of bypass grafts; however, electrocardiography (ECG)-gated multidetector CT (MDCT) with either single-source or dual-source acquisition has become a viable option in the initial evaluation of graft complications, with reported sensitivities and specificities for the detection of graft patency in the range of 95% to 100% for 64-row MDCT.[103–105] Whereas conventional angiography only allows for assessment of the graft lumen, CT angiography permits

---

Box 4
Complications of coronary artery bypass grafting

- Anastomotic leak/dehiscence
- Anastomotic stenosis
- Aneurysm/pseudoaneurysm
- Graft thrombosis with occlusion
- Graft kinking
- Graft dissection
- Aortic dissection
- Infection (mediastinitis, empyema)
- Hemothorax
- Lung injury
- Nerve damage

evaluation of the graft wall and its relationship with adjacent anatomic structures; CT may also be used to identify other potential causes of patient symptomatology, including infection.

Mediastinitis and Sternal Dehiscence

Acute mediastinitis is a relatively rare but potentially life-threatening condition, most commonly caused by spontaneous or iatrogenic esophageal rupture. Although only 1% to 3% of cases occur following CABG, acute mediastinitis represents an important iatrogenic complication, owing to a high associated mortality rate (10%–25%).[106] Numerous factors which increase the risk of mediastinitis following cardiothoracic surgery have been identified. Although most of these are patient comorbid conditions, including diabetes mellitus, obesity, and tobacco use, several contributing iatrogenic causes have been implicated, including improper skin preparation, prolonged time on cardiopulmonary bypass, and contamination of saphenous vein grafts during harvesting, among others.[107] Some studies have also suggested that the use of internal mammary grafts may contribute to sternal ischemia and predispose to mediastinitis.[108] Whatever the cause, the clinical significance of this complication should prompt attention to potential imaging manifestations.

Clinically, affected patients are typically ill, presenting with fever, chills, tachycardia, and chest pain; however, these symptoms may not always be present and the diagnosis may be unsuspected. As with the clinical presentation, the imaging features of mediastinitis are varied. Findings of acute mediastinitis on chest radiography include mediastinal widening and pneumomediastinum. Although these findings may be suggestive in most settings, they are not particularly specific in patients after cardiovascular surgery, as edema, hemorrhage, and air are expected findings in the postoperative period.[109] The diagnosis of mediastinitis may be suggested on the basis of radiography when it is accompanied by sternal dehiscence. A change in alignment of sternotomy wires as a result of expanding fluid and abscess formation has been referred to as the "wandering wire sign," and can lead to wire fracture (Fig. 15).[110] A more subtle finding of mediastinitis is associated with a vertical lucency in the upper aspect of the sternum (midsternal stripe), which may alternatively be a normal finding on a chest radiograph following sternotomy. This stripe should be no more than 2 mm wide and not extend below the first sternal wire; increased lucency or widening of the stripe greater than 3 mm suggests dehiscence.[111]

Clinical signs or symptoms of mediastinitis, with or without chest radiographic abnormalities, should prompt further evaluation with CT. Air, hematomas, and increased attenuation of the anterior mediastinal fat are normal findings up to 2 weeks following sternotomy; the presence of these findings beyond 2 weeks is suggestive of mediastinitis, as are new or enlarging collections of air or fluid.[112] CT is not only helpful for establishing a diagnosis of mediastinitis but also plays an important role in the characterization of the extent of disease, the assessment of fluid collections requiring drainage, and the identification of associated complications including sternal osteomyelitis. Although imaging findings may be suggestive, percutaneous aspiration of fluid collections may be necessary to confirm the diagnosis and assist in directing appropriate antibiotic therapy. Surgical management is indicated for mediastinitis with osteomyelitis, and in the setting of pleural or pericardial involvement.

Saphenous Vein Graft Aneurysm

Saphenous vein graft (SVG) aneurysm is an uncommon complication after CABG, with a reported incidence of 0.07%.[113] However, the true incidence is suspected to be higher, as most aneurysms are asymptomatic, and patients may go undiagnosed for years until aneurysms are incidentally discovered or symptoms develop. True aneurysms are typically late complications, presenting 5 to 7 years after grafting, and are primarily attributable to atherosclerotic disease.[114] False (pseudo)aneurysms are more variable in presentation, but typically occur early in the postoperative period as an iatrogenic complication related to the proximal surgical anastomosis between the graft and the ascending aorta; distal anastomotic pseudoaneurysms have also been described, but are rare.[115]

Pseudoaneurysms may develop secondary to weakness of the saphenous vein wall, injury during harvesting or implantation, dissection, and anastomotic defects such as suture rupture or excessive graft tension.[114] Infection can also be contributory, so the grafts should be carefully evaluated at imaging in the setting of suspected acute mediastinitis. The presence of an SVG pseudoaneurysm can be unsuspected. Although the diagnosis is often incidental, patients may present with chest pain, the onset of clinical symptoms corresponding to thrombosis of the aneurysm sac, with resultant luminal narrowing or occlusion leading to myocardial ischemia and angina.

Chest radiographs in patients with SVG aneurysms or pseudoaneurysms may be normal;

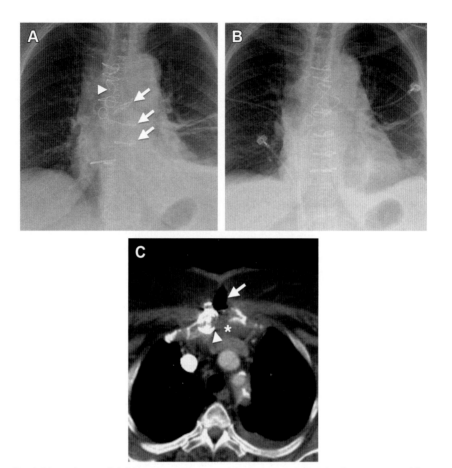

Fig. 15. Mediastinitis and sternal dehiscence. A 63-year-old woman post CABG who presents with new drainage from the sternal incision 3 weeks after surgery. Chest radiograph at the time of presentation (*A*) shows interval fracture and lateral displacement of the fourth through sixth sternotomy wires (*arrows*), with fracture of the third sternotomy wire (*arrowhead*), which is a new finding in comparison with the baseline postoperative chest radiograph (*B*). Axial contrast-enhanced chest CT image (*C*) shows incomplete apposition of the sternum with air (*arrow*) and fluid (*asterisk*) consistent with infection. Note that the sternal wire at this level has migrated into the sternotomy defect (*arrowhead*).

however, if the aneurysm is large a mediastinal mass may be present, prompting further evaluation.[116,117] CT angiography is the optimal imaging examination for the diagnosis and characterization of suspected SVG aneurysm (**Fig. 16**). Conventional angiography may not permit the diagnosis if the aneurysm sac is partially thrombosed with preserved lumen patency, whereas the contour abnormality will be readily evident at CT.[104] The aneurysm may fill completely with contrast, or may be partially or totally thrombosed. Multiplanar CT reconstructions can be beneficial in demonstrating anatomic relationships of the graft and the aneurysm to surrounding structures.

The diagnosis of SVG aneurysm or pseudoaneurysm is important in allowing for early treatment and possibly prevention of potential associated complications, including intraluminal thrombosis with graft occlusion and myocardial infarction, increased graft tension, compression of adjacent structures, rupture with hemothorax or hemopericardium, and fistula formation.[118] Although differentiation between true and false aneurysms can be challenging, a few generalities are noted: true aneurysms tend to be fusiform and can occur at any location along the graft, whereas pseudoaneurysms are more commonly eccentric and saccular, occurring predominantly at the proximal anastomosis. Distinction between true and false aneurysms is important, as pseudoaneurysms can be treated with minimally invasive procedures including coil embolization or covered stent placement, whereas true aneurysms typically require surgical revision.[113,114,119]

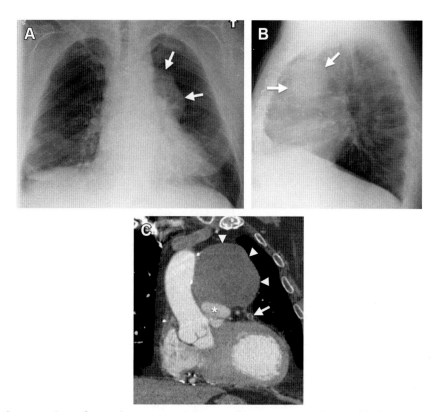

Fig. 16. Saphenous vein graft pseudoaneurysm. A 73-year-old man post CABG × 2, with chest pain and progressive dyspnea. PA (*A*) and lateral (*B*) chest radiographs show a large rounded opacity in the anterior mediastinum (*arrows*). Reformatted coronal image from a subsequent contrast-enhanced CT angiogram (*C*) shows the mass arising from an occluded saphenous vein graft corresponding to a partially thrombosed pseudoaneurysm (*arrowheads*); a small amount of contrast fills the pseudoaneurysm near the graft anastomosis (*asterisk*). The distal unopacified, occluded portion of the graft is also noted (*arrow*).

AORTIC VALVE REPLACEMENT

Open heart surgery with mechanical or porcine bioprosthetic valve replacement is the current standard management for patients with severe aortic valve disease. Replacement of the aortic valve may be performed in isolation or in conjunction with ascending aortic repair. Common surgical indications for aortic valve replacement (AVR) include aortic insufficiency, aortic stenosis, and endocarditis. Newer, minimally invasive techniques are becoming more widely available for high-risk surgical candidates. In particular, transluminal AVR and transapical aortic valve implantation are now possible treatment options, with encouraging outcomes and acceptable risk profiles in otherwise nonsurgical patients with degenerative causes of aortic stenosis.[120,121] However, these new procedures have distinct complications in comparison with open surgical repair, and are not reviewed in this article.

Open surgical repair typically involves median sternotomy, cardiopulmonary bypass, transverse aortotomy with excision of the diseased native valve leaflets, annular debridement, fixation of a mechanical or bioprosthetic valve, and aortotomy closure. AVR involves significant risk and has known, well-described complications, many of which are often attributable to surgical technique or inappropriate valve sizing (**Box 5**). Complications in the early postoperative period requiring emergent management include infective endocarditis, dehiscence, and severe refractory hemolytic anemia. Late complications resulting in valve dysfunction include pannus formation (subprosthetic tissue proliferation), paravalvular leak, and chronic infection.

Paravalvular Leak

Valvular regurgitation is a commonly observed finding following AVR. In the setting of a mechanical valve prosthesis a small amount of regurgitation is necessary to assist in closure of valve leaflets and prevent thrombus formation, whereas little to no regurgitation should be present with

---

Box 5
Complications of aortic valve replacement

- Valvular regurgitation
- Paravalvular leak
- Pseudoaneurysm
- Endocarditis with abscess
- Dehiscence
- Thrombosis with valve obstruction
- Hemolysis
- Aortic dissection
- Infection (mediastinitis, empyema)
- Hemothorax
- Lung injury
- Nerve damage

---

bioprosthetic valves. Mild to moderate regurgitation after AVR can be symptomatic, often worsens, and can lead to heart failure if not corrected. The incidence of clinically significant aortic valve regurgitation after AVR is reported to range from 1% to 17%.[122,123]

Pathologic regurgitation may be classified as valvular or paravalvular depending on the mechanism. Valvular regurgitation is defined as retrograde flow passing between the valve leaflets, and may be central or eccentric. Causes of postoperative valvular regurgitation include structural valve failure and conditions that prevent valve closure, including the development of pannus, vegetations, or thrombus. Paravalvular regurgitation occurs when blood flows through a defect between the prosthetic valve and the native annulus, and may result in both antegrade and retrograde flow during the cardiac cycle. Paravalvular leak, when present in the early postoperative period, is usually due to iatrogenic structural failure of the annulus suture line, whereas late development is most commonly due to infection.[123,124] Inappropriate sizing of the prosthetic valve, which may be either too small or too large, is also believed to be a contributing factor in paravalvular leak when size mismatch results in mechanical and morphologic changes along the annulus.[125]

Current consensus guidelines recommend CT evaluation for patients with suspected valve dysfunction, following an initial echocardiography screening examination.[126] Echocardiography is the preferred initial imaging tool for postoperative valve assessment, as it is rapid, readily available, can be performed at the bedside, and permits both morphologic and functional valve assessment. Unfortunately, the diagnosis can be missed

because of acoustic window limitations. Cardiac CT using retrospective ECG gating has been found to be equivalent to transthoracic echocardiography in the diagnosis of prosthetic valve dysfunction (**Fig. 17**).[127] In addition to functional valve information, gated CT offers simultaneous imaging of the thorax that can be used to identify potential causes of paravalvular leak and associated complications.[128,129] Multiplanar reconstructions demonstrate anatomic relationships of the valve and leaflets in multiple projections throughout the cardiac cycle, and provide important details for diagnosis and surgical planning. Gated cardiac MR imaging offers diagnostic benefits similar to those of CT, but can also be used to precisely quantify the degree of regurgitation with velocity flow mapping (see **Fig. 17C**).[130]

Infection and Valve Dehiscence

Breakdown of the suture line fixing the prosthetic valve to the annulus is a rare but potentially devastating complication, occurring in 0.1% to 1.3 % of patients undergoing AVR. This breakdown is most commonly caused by infection, and may occur early (iatrogenic) or late in the postoperative course. Early infection is typically due to contaminants at the time of operation, and in this setting staphylococci are most common; by contrast, streptococci are the most common pathogens in late infection.[131] Infection typically begins along the suture line and annular cuff before extending to the valves (endocarditis) or into surrounding tissues with abscess formation. The diagnosis of infection can be challenging by echocardiography unless large leaflet vegetations or a perivalvular abscess are present. Dehiscence, when present, may be directly identified or inferred at echocardiography in the presence of paravalvular leak.

CT affords several benefits in the evaluation of suspected infection. Abnormal air and fluid collections around the aortic root are readily identifiable. ECG-gated CT, as previously described, is beneficial in evaluating valve function and can be used to both diagnose and characterize the extent of dehiscence when present. Findings suggestive of prosthetic valve dehiscence include valve displacement, valve dysfunction, paravalvular leak, and pseudoaneurysm formation; ascending aortic aneurysm can occur with untreated small dehiscence (see **Fig. 17; Fig. 18**).[128,130] Recent studies have indicated that ^{18}F-labeled fluorodeoxyglucose positron emission tomography/CT may play an important role in the diagnosis of prosthetic valve infection/endocarditis in the absence of dehiscence. In one large series, the sensitivity of PET/CT for prosthetic valve infection was 97%

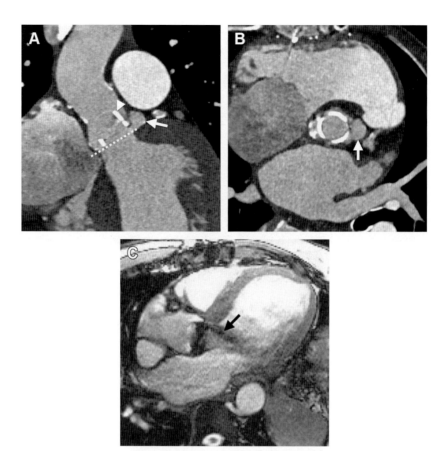

Fig. 17. Paravalvular leak and dehiscence. A 55-year-old man post aortic valve replacement with a bioprosthetic valve presents with increasing dyspnea and chest pain. Echocardiography (ECG) was limited but showed severe aortic regurgitation. An ECG-gated thoracic CT angiogram was obtained for further assessment. Coronal oblique (*A*) and axial (*B*) images in the plane of the valve show upward displacement of the anterior valve strut (*arrowhead*) relative to the annulus (*dotted line*), compatible with partial dehiscence. A small pseudoaneurysm at this level is also present (*arrow*). Steady-state free precession (SSFP) 3-chamber view static magnetic resonance image during diastole (*C*) shows a large, eccentric, dephasing regurgitant jet (*arrow*).

compared with 70% for CT alone, and also resulted in improved diagnostic accuracy.[132] Infective endocarditis after AVR can be treated conservatively with antibiotics; however, if dehiscence is present or conservative management fails, surgical treatment with debridement, washout, and patch repair or valve replacement is indicated.

OPEN REPAIR OF THORACIC AORTA

Numerous conditions of the thoracic aorta, including dissection, aneurysm, and pseudoaneurysm, may require emergent or elective aortic repair. Potential complications of both open and endovascular repair of the thoracoabdominal aortic conditions are discussed here and elsewhere in this issue by Valente and colleagues. Historically, open repair was performed with an inclusion graft: the aorta is incised (aortotomy), a synthetic graft is placed traversing the diseased

segment, and the native aorta is then closed around the graft. This technique produces a potential space within the excluded aorta and is associated with a high complication rate, including leak and rupture.[133] Interposition grafting is an alternative operative repair that involves excision of the diseased aorta with replacement by a synthetic graft. When compared with inclusion grafting, interposition repairs have reduced morbidity and mortality and, even in the era of minimally invasive techniques using endovascular stent grafts, open repair remains the standard of care for disorders involving the aortic root or ascending aorta. There are multiple interposition techniques, with the type of procedure performed depending on which components of the aorta require replacement (**Table 1**). Each aspect of the various interposition procedures lends itself to complications, which may include dissection of the residual native aorta, aneurysm of the

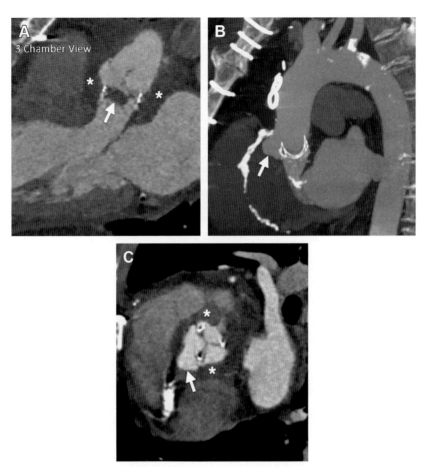

Fig. 18. Endocarditis, prosthetic aortic valve dehiscence, and mycotic pseudoaneurysm. A 66-year-old man post coronary artery bypass grafting × 3 and aortic valve replacement for severe aortic stenosis presents with sudden onset of left-sided weakness, slurred speech, and low-grade fevers. Three-chamber view from cardiac CT angiography (*A*) shows low attenuating material adherent to the aortic valve prosthesis (*arrow*), consistent with aortic valve vegetation. There is surrounding low attenuating fluid (*asterisks*) suggestive of infection. Oblique sagittal maximal-intensity projection CT image through the aorta (*B*) shows a pseudoaneurysm at the level of the aortic valve prosthesis (*arrow*), also visualized on CT image reconstruction in the plane of the aortic valve (*C*), with surrounding fluid (*asterisks*). Dynamic functional imaging (not shown) showed rocking of the prosthetic valve, confirming dehiscence. Blood cultures were positive for coagulase-negative *Staphylococcus aureus*.

native aortic root, pseudoaneurysm formation caused by anastomotic leak, and coronary artery occlusion (**Box 6**).

Anastomotic Dehiscence with Pseudoaneurysm

Perigraft fluid is a normal postoperative finding following open thoracic aorta repair and may show low attenuation on CT, representing seroma or edema, or higher attenuation with hematoma or other mixed blood products, and must be distinguished from leak or pseudoaneurysm. Normal perigraft fluid collections do not enhance on CT imaging following contrast administration, and typically decrease in size over time, although they may not completely resolve.[133] Enlargement

of a perigraft collection should prompt suspicion for infection or dehiscence with contained leak/pseudoaneurysm formation.

Pseudoaneurysm is an uncommon complication following ascending aortic repair, with an incidence of 2% to 3%.[134] Fewer than 10% of all cases are thought to result from technical failure of the anastomosis, with infection being the most common overall cause of pseudoaneurysm (60%).[135] The anastomosis is the most common location of pseudoaneurysm after open repair, followed by aortotomy or cannulation sites.[135] Teflon pledgets are used to reinforce the anastomosis and cannulation sites to minimize the risk of leak and pseudoaneurysm formation.

Pseudoaneurysm formation resulting from anastomotic leak is frequently an incidental finding at

Table 1
Aortic interposition graft repairs

Surgery	Indications	Technique
Supracoronary	Ascending aortic aneurysm or dissection. Normal aortic root, valve, and annulus	The diseased ascending aorta is resected and replaced by a synthetic graft Proximal (supracoronary) and distal (arch) aortic anastomoses are required The root, valve, and coronary arteries remain intact
Wheat	Ascending aortic aneurysm or dissection. The aortic root and annulus are normal, but the valve is diseased (ie, bicuspid valve)	The diseased ascending aorta is resected and replaced by a synthetic supracoronary graft Requires proximal and distal aortic anastomoses The native diseased valve is replaced with a bioprosthetic or mechanical valve
Bentall	Root and ascending aortic aneurysm or dissection with abnormal annulus or valve (ie, insufficiency, bicuspid valve)	Aortic valve, root, and ascending aorta are replaced with a synthetic conduit containing a valve The valve may be bioprosthetic or mechanical The coronary arteries are implanted into the graft Single anastomosis at the arch
Cabrol	Root and ascending aortic aneurysm or dissection with abnormal annulus or valve (ie, insufficiency, bicuspid valve)	Aortic valve, root, and ascending aorta are replaced with a synthetic conduit containing a valve The valve may be bioprosthetic or mechanical The coronary arteries are connected to a synthetic graft, which is then implanted to the aortic graft via side-to-side anastomosis Single anastomosis at the arch
David	Root and ascending aortic aneurysm or dissection with normal annulus and valve	Aortic root and ascending aorta are replaced with a synthetic conduit graft The native aortic valve is resuspended within the conduit The coronary arteries are implanted into the graft Single anastomosis at the arch

Box 6
Complications of open aortic surgery

- Aortic dissection
- Anastomotic leak/dehiscence
- Pseudoaneurysm
- Hemothorax
- Hemopericardium
- Coronary occlusion
- Infection (mediastinitis, empyema)
- Lung injury
- Recurrent laryngeal nerve injury

the time of postsurgical surveillance imaging, and often presents as a mediastinal mass on chest radiography. CT demonstrates a mass adjacent to the surgical anastomosis, which may completely or partially fill with contrast depending on the presence of peripheral thrombus (**Figs. 19** and **20**).[136,137] Open surgical repair with graft replacement is required in most cases because of the risk for rupture or fistula. Endovascular techniques for repair of ascending or arch pseudoaneurysms have been reported; however, its utility is presently limited, and this approach is reserved for patients who are not candidates for conventional open repair.[138,139]

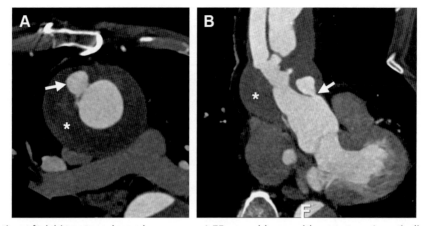

Fig. 19. Aortic graft dehiscence and pseudoaneurysm. A 75-year-old man with acute type A aortic dissection, post supracoronary interposition graft repair. Axial image from an ECG-gated CT angiogram obtained 6 weeks following surgery (A) shows a focal collection of contrast along the right lateral aspect of the ascending thoracic aorta graft (*arrow*), which is consistent with a pseudoaneurysm. Curved-planar reformatted image (B) through the right carotid artery shows the narrow neck of the pseudoaneurysm (*arrow*) at the proximal aortic anasto- mosis, which is suggestive of focal dehiscence. Circumferential perigraft low attenuating collection exhibits a mass effect with narrowing of the graft, which is consistent with thrombus (*asterisk* in A, B).

Aortic Dissection

Iatrogenic aortic dissection is a rare potential complication of cardiovascular surgery including aortic repair, with a reported incidence of 0.06% to 0.23%; however, when present the complication is often fatal, with a mortality rate of 48% in the largest series reported to date.[140,141] Damage to the native aorta at the time of surgery can directly produce an aortic dissection or create a wall injury that subsequently predisposes to dissection in the perioperative period. Manipulation of the aorta, can- nulation, cross-clamping, anastomosis formation, and intra-aortic balloon pump placement are all possible inciting factors. Although iatrogenic dissection may occasionally be detected intraoper- atively, the complication does not typically manifest until the postoperative period following sustained aortic reperfusion.[142] Diagnosis may be delayed, as symptoms of chest pain are common in the post- surgical setting. Serial chest radiographs may demonstrate an enlarging aortic contour; however, CT angiography is the imaging modality of choice, and can be used to document the extent of dissec- tion and involvement of coronary, arch, and visceral arteries (**Fig. 21**).

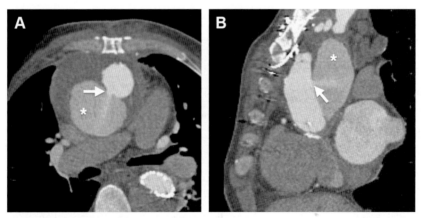

Fig. 20. Aortic graft dehiscence and pseudoaneurysm. A 64-year-old woman post modified David graft repair for type A aortic dissection and aneurysm with endovascular treatment of the descending thoracic aorta presents with chest pain. Axial (A) and oblique sagittal (B) contrast-enhanced CT images show a jet of contrast from the graft (*arrows*) into a large perigraft collection (*asterisks*), consistent with focal anastomotic dehiscence and resultant partially thrombosed pseudoaneurysm.

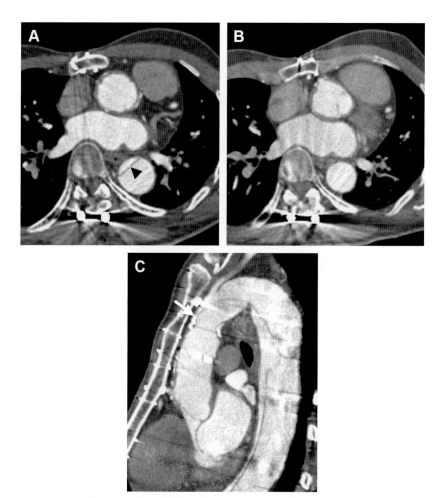

Fig. 21. Aortic dissection. A 60-year-old man 6 weeks after repair of ascending aortic aneurysm presents to the emergency department with acute chest pain. Contrast-enhanced CT angiogram (*A*) shows a new dissection involving the descending thoracic aorta (*arrowhead*) when compared with a postoperative CT angiogram obtained a few weeks earlier (*B*). Curved-planar CT reconstruction (*C*) shows that the dissection begins at the ascending aortic graft anastomosis (*arrow*).

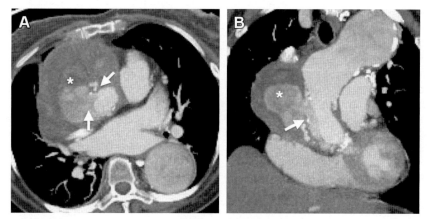

Fig. 22. Coronary implant dehiscence. A 68-year-old man post Bentall procedure for root and ascending aortic aneurysm. Axial (*A*) and coronal oblique (*B*) images from contrast-enhanced CT show dehiscence of the right coronary artery implant (*arrows*), with resultant contained pseudoaneurysm with heterogeneous attenuation representing contrast and thrombus (*asterisk*).

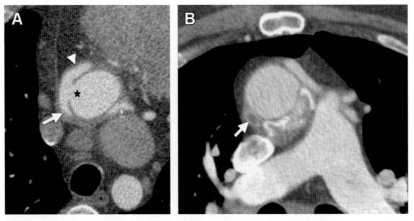

Fig. 23. Coronary graft occlusion. A 72-year-old woman post Cabrol procedure for root and ascending aortic aneurysm. Reconstructed image from contrast-enhanced CT angiogram (*A*) at the level of the coronary-aortic anastomosis (*asterisk*) shows patent left and right coronary graft limbs (*arrowhead* and *arrow*, respectively). Two months later the patient presented with chest pain and ECG abnormalities. Axial image from contrast-enhanced CT (*B*) obtained at that time shows complete thrombosis and occlusion of the right coronary graft (*arrow*).

Coronary Implantation Complications

One of the most challenging technical aspects of aortic root replacement involves reimplantation of the native coronary arteries. In the Bentall procedure, the coronary arteries are directly implanted onto the ascending aortic graft. The original Bentall procedure used an end-to-side anastomosis, which had a high complication rate related to 2 primary causes: coronary artery tension with resultant anastomotic leak (**Fig. 22**) and surgically induced anastomotic stenosis. The procedure was subsequently revised. The modified Bentall, or button Bentall, procedure involves excision of the native coronaries with a wide rim of tissue around the coronary ostia to create sufficient area for suturing to the graft without compromising the coronary artery lumen. The normal postoperative appearance of a button anastomosis at CT is mild dilation of the button with the coronary artery arising centrally. Eccentric origin of the coronary artery may indicate pseudoaneurysm development.[137]

An alternative method for coronary artery implantation is the Cabrol procedure. With this technique the coronary arteries are cut and attached to a synthetic graft via end-to-end anastomoses; the coronary conduit is then sutured to the aortic graft via a side-to-side anastomosis. The Cabrol procedure was originally proposed as an alternative to the Bentall procedure to provide a tension-free coronary anastomosis; however, the coronary conduit is vulnerable to complications including kinking with obstruction, thrombosis, and anastomotic leak (**Fig. 23**).[143] These complications primarily occur in the immediate postoperative period and result in higher failure rates, reoperation rates, morbidity, and mortality than those associated with the button Bentall repair.[144,145] The Cabrol procedure is currently reserved as a salvage technique for failed Bentall procedures, but may be considered as a first-line operation in circumstances where excessive tension on the ostial anastomoses is anticipated, such as with large aneurysms or dissections, or when an adequate coronary button may not be obtained, such as in the setting of severe ostial calcifications and stenosis.[146]

SUMMARY

The operative treatment of thoracic and cardiovascular disease encompasses a diverse range of surgeries including lobectomy, pneumonectomy, esophagectomy, CABG, AVR, and aortic repair, among many others. The complexity of these surgeries in conjunction with a high-risk patient population contributes to a risk of iatrogenic complications, which range in severity from minor, causing discomfort or prolonged hospitalization, to major, resulting in permanent disability or death. Although some iatrogenic complications are common to all surgical techniques, such as hemothorax and infection, some complications are more highly associated with specific surgeries, examples of which are reviewed in this article. The diagnosis of iatrogenic complications has medical and potential legal consequences. Radiologists should be aware of the normal postoperative appearance of thoracic and cardiovascular surgical procedures, the preferred techniques used by their surgical colleagues, and the imaging findings of associated complications, so as to facilitate early diagnosis and timely intervention in an effort to reduce patient morbidity and mortality.

REFERENCES

1. Peterffy A, Henze A. Haemorrhagic complications during pulmonary resection. A retrospective review of 1428 resections with 113 haemorrhagic episodes. Scand J Thorac Cardiovasc Surg 1983; 17(3):283–7.
2. Flores RM, Ihekweazu U, Dycoco J, et al. Video-assisted thoracoscopic surgery (VATS) lobectomy: catastrophic intraoperative complications. J Thorac Cardiovasc Surg 2011;142(6):1412–7.
3. Munoz JJ, Birkmeyer NJ, Dacey LJ, et al. Trends in rates of reexploration for hemorrhage after coronary artery bypass surgery. Northern New England Cardiovascular Disease Study Group. Ann Thorac Surg 1999;68(4):1321–5.
4. Mehta RH, Sheng S, O'Brien SM, et al. Reoperation for bleeding in patients undergoing coronary artery bypass surgery: incidence, risk factors, time trends, and outcomes. Circ Cardiovasc Qual Outcomes 2009;2(6):583–90.
5. Etz CD, Di Luozzo G, Bello R, et al. Pulmonary complications after descending thoracic and thoracoabdominal aortic aneurysm repair: predictors, prevention, and treatment. Ann Thorac Surg 2007;83(2):S870–6 [discussion: S890–2].
6. Mowery NT, Gunter OL, Collier BR, et al. Practice management guidelines for management of hemothorax and occult pneumothorax. J Trauma 2011; 70(2):510–8.
7. Kuhlman JE, Singha NK. Complex disease of the pleural space: radiographic and CT evaluation. Radiographics 1997;17(1):63–79.
8. Kim EA, Lee KS, Shim YM, et al. Radiographic and CT findings in complications following pulmonary resection. Radiographics 2002;22(1):67–86.
9. Bogaert J, Francone M. Pericardial disease: value of CT and MR imaging. Radiology 2013;267(2): 340–56.
10. Krejci CS, Blackmore CC, Nathens A. Hemopericardium: an emergent finding in a case of blunt cardiac injury. AJR Am J Roentgenol 2000;175(1): 250.
11. Restrepo CS, Gutierrez FR, Marmol-Velez JA, et al. Imaging patients with cardiac trauma. Radiographics 2012;32(3):633–49.
12. Suwatanapongched T, Boonkasem S, Sathianpitayakul E, et al. Intrathoracic gossypiboma: radiographic and CT findings. Br J Radiol 2005;78(933):851–3.
13. Madan R, Trotman-Dickenson B, Hunsaker AR. Intrathoracic gossypiboma. AJR Am J Roentgenol 2007;189(2):W90–1.
14. Sheehan RE, Sheppard MN, Hansell DM. Retained intrathoracic surgical swab: CT appearances. J Thorac Imaging 2000;15(1):61–4.
15. Park HJ, Im SA, Chun HJ, et al. Changes in CT appearance of intrathoracic gossypiboma over 10 years. Br J Radiol 2008;81(962):e61–3.
16. Pisal N, Sindos M, Henson G. Risk factors for retained instruments and sponges after surgery. N Engl J Med 2003;348(17):1724–5.
17. Rappaport W, Haynes K. The retained surgical sponge following intra-abdominal surgery. A continuing problem. Arch Surg 1990;125(3):405–7.
18. Whang G, Mogel GT, Tsai J, et al. Left behind: unintentionally retained surgically placed foreign bodies and how to reduce their incidence–self-assessment module. AJR Am J Roentgenol 2009; 193(6 Suppl):S90–3.
19. Liu N, Gilkeson R, Markowitz A, et al. Thoracoscopic removal of a suture needle from the posterior pericardium after coronary artery bypass grafting. Interact Cardiovasc Thorac Surg 2011; 13(3):341–3.
20. Weissberg D, Refaely Y. Hernia of the lung. Ann Thorac Surg 2002;74(6):1963–6.
21. Brock MV, Heitmiller RF. Spontaneous anterior thoracic lung hernias. J Thorac Cardiovasc Surg 2000;119(5):1046–7.
22. Athanassiadi K, Bagaev E, Simon A, et al. Lung herniation: a rare complication in minimally invasive cardiothoracic surgery. Eur J Cardiothorac Surg 2008;33(5):774–6.
23. Bhalla M, Leitman BS, Forcade C, et al. Lung hernia: radiographic features. AJR Am J Roentgenol 1990;154(1):51–3.
24. Sadler MA, Shapiro RS, Wagreich J, et al. CT diagnosis of acquired intercostal lung herniation. Clin Imaging 1997;21(2):104–6.
25. Tamburro F, Grassi R, Romano S, et al. Acquired spontaneous intercostal hernia of the lung diagnosed on helical CT. AJR Am J Roentgenol 2000; 174(3):876–7.
26. Markand ON, Moorthy SS, Mahomed Y, et al. Postoperative phrenic nerve palsy in patients with open-heart surgery. Ann Thorac Surg 1985;39(1):68–73.
27. Ferdinande P, Bruyninckx F, Van Raemdonck D, et al, Leuven Lung Transplant Group. Phrenic nerve dysfunction after heart-lung and lung transplantation. J Heart Lung Transplant 2004;23(1):105–9.
28. Muhyieddeen K, Forouzandeh F. Diaphragmatic paralysis after cardiac surgery. J Am Coll Cardiol 2012;59(18):e35.
29. Maziak DE, Maurer JR, Kesten S. Diaphragmatic paralysis: a complication of lung transplantation. Ann Thorac Surg 1996;61(1):170–3.

30. Dimopoulou I, Daganou M, Dafni U, et al. Phrenic nerve dysfunction after cardiac operations: electrophysiologic evaluation of risk factors. Chest 1998; 113(1):8–14.

31. Beran E, Marzouk JF, Dimitri WR. Bilateral phrenic nerve palsy following aortic valve surgery. J Cardiovasc Surg 2008;23(6):691–2.

32. Sanchez de Toledo J, Munoz R, Landsittel D, et al. Diagnosis of abnormal diaphragm motion after cardiothoracic surgery: ultrasound performed by a cardiac intensivist vs. fluoroscopy. Congenit Heart Dis 2010;5(6):565–72.

33. Ch'en IY, Armstrong JD 2nd. Value of fluoroscopy in patients with suspected bilateral hemidiaphragmatic paralysis. AJR Am J Roentgenol 1993; 160(1):29–31.

34. Ohta M, Ikeda N, Tanaka H, et al. Satisfactory results of diaphragmatic plication for bilateral phrenic nerve paralysis. Ann Thorac Surg 2007;84(3): 1029–31.

35. Gaur P, Dunne R, Colson YL, et al. Bronchopleural fistula and the role of contemporary imaging. J Thorac Cardiovasc Surg 2014;148(1):341–7.

36. Ricci ZJ, Haramati LB, Rosenbaum AT, et al. Role of computed tomography in guiding the management of peripheral bronchopleural fistula. J Thorac Imaging 2002;17(3):214–8.

37. McManigle JE, Fletcher GL, Tenholder MF. Bronchoscopy in the management of bronchopleural fistula. Chest 1990;97(5):1235–8.

38. Hollaus PH, Lax F, el-Nashef BB, et al. Natural history of bronchopleural fistula after pneumonectomy: a review of 96 cases. Ann Thorac Surg 1997;63(5):1391–6 [discussion: 1396–7].

39. Chae EJ, Seo JB, Kim SY, et al. Radiographic and CT findings of thoracic complications after pneumonectomy. Radiographics 2006;26(5): 1449–68.

40. Stern EJ, Sun H, Haramati LB. Peripheral bronchopleural fistulas: CT imaging features. AJR Am J Roentgenol 1996;167(1):117–20.

41. Westcott JL, Volpe JP. Peripheral bronchopleural fistula: CT evaluation in 20 patients with pneumonia, empyema, or postoperative air leak. Radiology 1995;196(1):175–81.

42. Kim KH, Lee KH, Won JY, et al. Bronchopleural fistula treatment with use of a bronchial stent-graft occluder. J Vasc Interv Radiol 2006;17(9):1539–43.

43. Ferguson JS, Sprenger K, Van Natta T. Closure of a bronchopleural fistula using bronchoscopic placement of an endobronchial valve designed for the treatment of emphysema. Chest 2006;129(2): 479–81.

44. Ruttenstock E, Saxena AK, Hollwarth ME. Closure of bronchopleural fistula with porcine dermal collagen and fibrin glue in an infant. Ann Thorac Surg 2012;94(2):659–60.

45. Graham RJ, Heyd RL, Raval VA, et al. Lung torsion after percutaneous needle biopsy of lung. AJR Am J Roentgenol 1992;159(1):35–7.

46. Gilkeson RC, Lange P, Kirby TJ. Lung torsion after lung transplantation: evaluation with helical CT. AJR Am J Roentgenol 2000;174(5):1341–3.

47. Lu MS, Huang YK, Kao CL, et al. Lung torsion associated with complete bronchial transection after blunt chest trauma. J Trauma 2007;63(5):1192.

48. Chan MC, Scott JM, Mercer CD, et al. Intraoperative whole-lung torsion producing pulmonary venous infarction. Ann Thorac Surg 1994;57(5): 1330–1.

49. Nguyen JC, Maloney J, Kanne JP. Bilateral whole-lung torsion after bilateral lung transplantation. J Thorac Imaging 2011;26(1):W17–9.

50. Wong PS, Goldstraw P. Pulmonary torsion: a questionnaire survey and a survey of the literature. Ann Thorac Surg 1992;54(2):286–8.

51. Felson B. Lung torsion: radiographic findings in nine cases. Radiology 1987;162(3):631–8.

52. Farkas EA, Detterbeck FC. Airway complications after pulmonary resection. Thorac Surg Clin 2006; 16(3):243–51.

53. Spizarny DL, Shetty PC, Lewis JW Jr. Lung torsion: preoperative diagnosis with angiography and computed tomography. J Thorac Imaging 1998; 13(1):42–4.

54. Hardy JD, Webb WR, Dalton ML Jr, et al. Lung homotransplantation in man. JAMA 1963;186: 1065–74.

55. Kshettry VR, Kroshus TJ, Hertz MI, et al. Early and late airway complications after lung transplantation: incidence and management. Ann Thorac Surg 1997;63(6):1576–83.

56. FitzSullivan E, Gries CJ, Phelan P, et al. Reduction in airway complications after lung transplantation with novel anastomotic technique. Ann Thorac Surg 2011;92(1):309–15.

57. Santacruz JF, Mehta AC. Airway complications and management after lung transplantation: ischemia, dehiscence, and stenosis. Proc Am Thorac Soc 2009;6(1):79–93.

58. Schmid RA, Boehler A, Speich R, et al. Bronchial anastomotic complications following lung transplantation: still a major cause of morbidity? Eur Respir J 1997;10(12):2872–5.

59. Garfein ES, McGregor CC, Galantowicz ME, et al. Deleterious effects of telescoped bronchial anastomosis in single and bilateral lung transplantation. Ann Transplant 2000;5(1):5–11.

60. Schlueter FJ, Semenkovich JW, Glazer HS, et al. Bronchial dehiscence after lung transplantation: correlation of CT findings with clinical outcome. Radiology 1996;199(3):849–54.

61. Gill RR, Poh AC, Camp PC, et al. MDCT evaluation of central airway and vascular complications of

lung transplantation. AJR Am J Roentgenol 2008; 191(4):1046–56.

62. Krishnam MS, Suh RD, Tomasian A, et al. Postoperative complications of lung transplantation: radiologic findings along a time continuum. Radiographics 2007;27(4):957–74.

63. McAdams HP, Murray JG, Erasmus JJ, et al. Telescoping bronchial anastomoses for unilateral or bilateral sequential lung transplantation: CT appearance. Radiology 1997;203(1):202–6.

64. De Gracia J, Culebras M, Alvarez A, et al. Bronchoscopic balloon dilatation in the management of bronchial stenosis following lung transplantation. Respir Med 2007;101(1):27–33.

65. Lari SM, Gonin F, Colchen A. The management of bronchus intermedius complications after lung transplantation: a retrospective study. J Cardiovasc Surg 2012;7:8.

66. Shah SS, Karnak D, Minai O, et al. Symptomatic narrowing or atresia of bronchus intermedius following lung transplantation vanishing bronchus intermedius syndrome (VBIS). Chest 2006;130 (4_MeetingAbstracts):236S.

67. Thistlethwaite PA, Yung G, Kemp A, et al. Airway stenoses after lung transplantation: incidence, management, and outcome. J Thorac Cardiovasc Surg 2008;136(6):1569–75.

68. Jemal A, Bray F, Center MM, et al. Global cancer statistics. CA Cancer J Clin 2011;61(2):69–90.

69. Siegel R, Naishadham D, Jemal A. Cancer statistics, 2013. CA Cancer J Clin 2013;63(1):11–30.

70. Lee RB, Miller JI. Esophagectomy for cancer. Surg Clin North Am 1997;77(5):1169–96.

71. Bruce J, Krukowski ZH, Al-Khairy G, et al. Systematic review of the definition and measurement of anastomotic leak after gastrointestinal surgery. Br J Surg 2001;88(9):1157–68.

72. Upponi S, Ganeshan A, D'Costa H, et al. Radiological detection of post-oesophagectomy anastomotic leak - a comparison between multidetector CT and fluoroscopy. Br J Radiol 2008;81(967):545–8.

73. Wormuth JK, Heitmiller RF. Esophageal conduit necrosis. Thorac Surg Clin 2006;16(1):11–22.

74. Scheepers JJ, van der Peet DL, Veenhof AA, et al. Systematic approach of postoperative gastric conduit complications after esophageal resection. Dis Esophagus 2010;23(2):117–21.

75. Kim TJ, Lee KH, Kim YH, et al. Postoperative imaging of esophageal cancer: what chest radiologists need to know. Radiographics 2007;27(2):409–29.

76. Oezcelik A, Banki F, Ayazi S, et al. Detection of gastric conduit ischemia or anastomotic breakdown after cervical esophagogastrostomy: the use of computed tomography scan versus early endoscopy. Surg Endosc 2010;24(8):1948–51.

77. Thomas P, Fuentes P, Giudicelli R, et al. Colon interposition for esophageal replacement: current indications and long-term function. Ann Thorac Surg 1997;64(3):757–64.

78. Cerfolio RJ, Allen MS, Deschamps C, et al. Esophageal replacement by colon interposition. Ann Thorac Surg 1995;59(6):1382–4.

79. Price TN, Allen MS, Nichols FC 3rd, et al. Hiatal hernia after esophagectomy: analysis of 2,182 esophagectomies from a single institution. Ann Thorac Surg 2011;92(6):2041–5.

80. Ganeshan DM, Correa AM, Bhosale P, et al. Diaphragmatic hernia after esophagectomy in 440 patients with long-term follow-up. Ann Thorac Surg 2013;96(4):1138–45.

81. Vallbohmer D, Holscher AH, Herbold T, et al. Diaphragmatic hernia after conventional or laparoscopic-assisted transthoracic esophagectomy. Ann Thorac Surg 2007;84(6):1847–52.

82. van Sandick JW, Knegjens JL, van Lanschot JJ, et al. Diaphragmatic herniation following oesophagectomy. Br J Surg 1999;86(1):109–12.

83. Ganeshan DM, Bhosale P, Munden RF, et al. Diaphragmatic hernia after esophagectomy for esophageal malignancy. J Thorac Imaging 2013;28(5): 308–14.

84. Buskens CJ, Hulscher JB, Fockens P, et al. Benign tracheo-neo-esophageal fistulas after subtotal esophagectomy. Ann Thorac Surg 2001;72(1): 221–4.

85. Kim SH, Lee KS, Shim YM, et al. Esophageal resection: indications, techniques, and radiologic assessment. Radiographics 2001;21(5):1119–37 [discussion: 1138–40].

86. Sun JS, Park KJ, Choi JH, et al. Benign bronchogastric fistula as a late complication after transhiatal oesophagogastrostomy: evaluation with multidetector row CT. Br J Radiol 2008;81(970):e255–8.

87. Bennie MJ, Sabharwal T, Dussek J, et al. Bronchogastric fistula successfully treated with the insertion of a covered bronchial stent. Eur Radiol 2003; 13(9):2222–5.

88. Song SW, Lee HS, Kim MS, et al. Repair of gastrotracheal fistula with a pedicled pericardial flap after Ivor Lewis esophagogastrostomy for esophageal cancer. J Thorac Cardiovasc Surg 2006;132(3): 716–7.

89. Reames BN, Lin J. Repair of a complex bronchogastric fistula after esophagectomy with biologic mesh. Ann Thorac Surg 2013;95(3):1096–7.

90. Guzman AE, Rossi L, Witte CL, et al. Traumatic injury of the thoracic duct. Lymphology 2002; 35(1):4–14.

91. Shah RD, Luketich JD, Schuchert MJ, et al. Postesophagectomy chylothorax: incidence, risk factors, and outcomes. Ann Thorac Surg 2012; 93(3):897–903 [discussion: 903–4].

92. Sachs PB, Zelch MG, Rice TW, et al. Diagnosis and localization of laceration of the thoracic

duct: usefulness of lymphangiography and CT. AJR Am J Roentgenol 1991;157(4):703–5.

93. Clement O, Luciani A. Imaging the lymphatic system: possibilities and clinical applications. Eur Radiol 2004;14(8):1498–507.

94. Misselwitz B. MR contrast agents in lymph node imaging. Eur J Radiol 2006;58(3):375–82.

95. Li W, Dan G, Jiang J, et al. A 2-wk conservative treatment regimen preceding thoracic duct ligation is effective and safe for treating post-esophagectomy chylothorax. J Surg Res 2013;185(2):784–9.

96. Tsubokawa N, Hamai Y, Hihara J, et al. Laparoscopic thoracic duct clipping for persistent chylothorax after extrapleural pneumonectomy. Ann Thorac Surg 2012;93(5):e131–2.

97. Koike Y, Hirai C, Nishimura J, et al. Percutaneous transvenous embolization of the thoracic duct in the treatment of chylothorax in two patients. J Vasc Interv Radiol 2013;24(1):135–7.

98. Nadolski GJ, Itkin M. Thoracic duct embolization for nontraumatic chylous effusion: experience in 34 patients. Chest 2013;143(1):158–63.

99. Sarr MG, Gott VL, Townsend TR. Mediastinal infection after cardiac surgery. Ann Thorac Surg 1984; 38(4):415–23.

100. Sabik JF 3rd. Understanding saphenous vein graft patency. Circulation 2011;124(3):273–5.

101. Ricci M, Karamanoukian HL, D'Ancona G, et al. Reoperative "off-pump" circumflex revascularization via left thoracotomy: how to prevent graft kinking. Ann Thorac Surg 2000;70(1):309–10.

102. Roy P, Finci L, Bopp P, et al. Emergency balloon angioplasty and digital subtraction angiography in the management of an acute iatrogenic occlusive dissection of a saphenous vein graft. Cathet Cardiovasc Diagn 1989;16(3):176–9.

103. Nieman K, Pattynama PM, Rensing BJ, et al. Evaluation of patients after coronary artery bypass surgery: CT angiographic assessment of grafts and coronary arteries. Radiology 2003;229(3): 749–56.

104. Weustink AC, Nieman K, Pugliese F, et al. Diagnostic accuracy of computed tomography angiography in patients after bypass grafting: comparison with invasive coronary angiograph. JACC Cardiovasc Imaging 2009;2(7):816–24.

105. von Kiedrowski H, Wiemer M, Franzke K, et al. Noninvasive coronary angiography: the clinical value of multi-slice computed tomography in the assessment of patients with prior coronary bypass surgery. Evaluating grafts and native vessels. Int J Cardiovasc Imaging 2009;25(2):161–70.

106. Sjogren J, Malmsjo M, Gustafsson R, et al. Poststernotomy mediastinitis: a review of conventional surgical treatments, vacuum-assisted closure therapy and presentation of the Lund University

Hospital mediastinitis algorithm. Eur J Cardiothorac Surg 2006;30(6):898–905.

107. Brown PP, Kugelmass AD, Cohen DJ, et al. The frequency and cost of complications associated with coronary artery bypass grafting surgery: results from the United States Medicare program. Ann Thorac Surg 2008;85(6):1980–6.

108. Deo SV, Shah IK, Dunlay SM, et al. Bilateral internal thoracic artery harvest and deep sternal wound infection in diabetic patients. Ann Thorac Surg 2013;95(3):862–9.

109. Boiselle PM, Mansilla AV, White CS, et al. Sternal dehiscence in patients with and without mediastinitis. J Thorac Imaging 2001;16(2):106–10.

110. Boiselle PM, Mansilla AV, Fisher MS, et al. Wandering wires: frequency of sternal wire abnormalities in patients with sternal dehiscence. AJR Am J Roentgenol 1999;173(3):777–80.

111. Boiselle PM, Mansilla AV. A closer look at the midsternal stripe sign. AJR Am J Roentgenol 2002; 178(4):945–8.

112. Li AE, Fishman EK. Evaluation of complications after sternotomy using single- and multidetector CT with three-dimensional volume rendering. AJR Am J Roentgenol 2003;181(4):1065–70.

113. Dieter RS, Patel AK, Yandow D, et al. Conservative vs. invasive treatment of aortocoronary saphenous vein graft aneurysms: treatment algorithm based upon a large series. Cardiovasc Surg 2003;11(6): 507–13.

114. Ramirez FD, Hibbert B, Simard T, et al. Natural history and management of aortocoronary saphenous vein graft aneurysms: a systematic review of published cases. Circulation 2012;126(18):2248–56.

115. Mohara J, Konishi H, Kato M, et al. Saphenous vein graft pseudoaneurysm rupture after coronary artery bypass grafting. Ann Thorac Surg 1998; 65(3):831–2.

116. Gilkeson RC, Markowitz AH. Multislice CT evaluation of coronary artery bypass graft patients. J Thorac Imaging 2007;22(1):56–62.

117. Doyle MT, Spizarny DL, Baker DE. Saphenous vein graft aneurysm after coronary artery bypass surgery. AJR Am J Roentgenol 1997;168(3):747–9.

118. Frazier AA, Qureshi F, Read KM, et al. Coronary artery bypass grafts: assessment with multidetector CT in the early and late postoperative settings. Radiographics 2005;25(4):881–96.

119. Tonelli AR, Desai AK, Anderson RD. Treatment of a ruptured saphenous vein graft pseudoaneurysm using a vascular plug. Catheter Cardiovasc Interv 2008;71(5):587–9.

120. Leon MB, Smith CR, Mack M, et al. Transcatheter aortic-valve implantation for aortic stenosis in patients who cannot undergo surgery. N Engl J Med 2010;363(17):1597–607.

121. Smith CR, Leon MB, Mack MJ, et al. Transcatheter versus surgical aortic-valve replacement in high-risk patients. N Engl J Med 2011;364(23):2187–98.

122. O'Rourke DJ, Palac RT, Malenka DJ, et al. Outcome of mild periprosthetic regurgitation detected by intraoperative transesophageal echocardiography. J Am Coll Cardiol 2001;38(1):163–6.

123. Rallidis LS, Moyssakis IE, Ikonomidis I, et al. Natural history of early aortic paraprosthetic regurgitation: a five-year follow-up. Am Heart J 1999; 138(2 Pt 1):351–7.

124. Sponga S, Perron J, Dagenais F, et al. Impact of residual regurgitation after aortic valve replacement. Eur J Cardiothorac Surg 2012;42(3):486–92.

125. De Cicco G, Lorusso R, Colli A, et al. Aortic valve periprosthetic leakage: anatomic observations and surgical results. Ann Thorac Surg 2005;79(5): 1480–5.

126. Taylor AJ, Cerqueira M, Hodgson JM, et al. ACCF/SCCT/ACR/AHA/ASE/ASNC/NASCI/SCAI/SCMR 2010 appropriate use criteria for cardiac computed tomography. A report of the American College of Cardiology Foundation Appropriate Use Criteria Task Force, the Society of Cardiovascular Computed Tomography, the American College of Radiology, the American Heart Association, the American Society of Echocardiography, the American Society of Nuclear Cardiology, the North American Society for Cardiovascular Imaging, the Society for Cardiovascular Angiography and Interventions, and the Society for Cardiovascular Magnetic Resonance. J Am Coll Cardiol 2010;56(22): 1864–94.

127. Tsai IC, Lin YK, Chang Y, et al. Correctness of multidetector-row computed tomography for diagnosing mechanical prosthetic heart valve disorders using operative findings as a gold standard. Eur Radiol 2009;19(4):857–67.

128. Konen E, Goitein O, Feinberg MS, et al. The role of ECG-gated MDCT in the evaluation of aortic and mitral mechanical valves: initial experience. AJR Am J Roentgenol 2008;191(1):26–31.

129. Habets J, Mali WP, Budde RP. Multidetector CT angiography in evaluation of prosthetic heart valve dysfunction. Radiographics 2012;32(7):1893–905.

130. Pham N, Zaitoun H, Mohammed TL, et al. Complications of aortic valve surgery: manifestations at CT and MR imaging. Radiographics 2012;32(7): 1873–92.

131. Piper C, Korfer R, Horstkotte D. Prosthetic valve endocarditis. Heart 2001;85(5):590–3.

132. Saby L, Laas O, Habib G, et al. Positron emission tomography/computed tomography for diagnosis of prosthetic valve endocarditis: increased valvular ^{18}F-fluorodeoxyglucose uptake as a novel major criterion. J Am Coll Cardiol 2013;61(23):2374–82.

133. Sundaram B, Quint LE, Patel S, et al. CT appearance of thoracic aortic graft complications. AJR Am J Roentgenol 2007;188(5):1273–7.

134. Strauch JT, Spielvogel D, Lansman SL, et al. Long-term integrity of teflon felt-supported suture lines in aortic surgery. Ann Thorac Surg 2005;79(3): 796–800.

135. Sullivan KL, Steiner RM, Smullens SN, et al. Pseudoaneurysm of the ascending aorta following cardiac surgery. Chest 1988;93(1):138–43.

136. Prescott-Focht JA, Martinez-Jimenez S, Hurwitz LM, et al. Ascending thoracic aorta: postoperative imaging evaluation. Radiographics 2013;33:73–85.

137. Hoang JK, Martinez S, Hurwitz LM. MDCT angiography after open thoracic aortic surgery: pearls and pitfalls. AJR Am J Roentgenol 2009;192(1): W20–7.

138. Joyce DL, Singh SK, Mallidi HR, et al. Endovascular management of pseudoaneurysm formation in the ascending aorta following lung transplantation. J Endovasc Ther 2012;19(1):52–7.

139. Mewhort HE, Appoo JJ, Sumner GL, et al. Alternative surgical approach to repair of the ascending aorta. Ann Thorac Surg 2011;92(3):1108–10.

140. Still RJ, Hilgenberg AD, Akins CW, et al. Intraoperative aortic dissection. Ann Thorac Surg 1992; 53(3):374–9 [discussion: 380].

141. Williams ML, Sheng S, Gammie JS, et al. Clark Award. Aortic dissection as a complication of cardiac surgery: report from the Society of Thoracic Surgeons database. Ann Thorac Surg 2010;90(6): 1812–6 [discussion: 1816–7].

142. Leontyev S, Borger MA, Legare JF, et al. Iatrogenic type A aortic dissection during cardiac procedures: early and late outcome in 48 patients. Eur J Cardiothorac Surg 2012;41(3):641–6.

143. Cabrol C, Pavie A, Gandjbakhch I, et al. Complete replacement of the ascending aorta with reimplantation of the coronary arteries: new surgical approach. J Thorac Cardiovasc Surg 1981;81(2): 309–15.

144. Knight J, Baumuller S, Kurtcuoglu V, et al. Long-term follow-up, computed tomography, and computational fluid dynamics of the Cabrol procedure. J Thorac Cardiovasc Surg 2010;139(6): 1602–8.

145. Svensson LG, Crawford ES, Hess KR, et al. Composite valve graft replacement of the proximal aorta: comparison of techniques in 348 patients. Ann Thorac Surg 1992;54(3):427–37 [discussion: 438–9].

146. Kourliouros A, Soni M, Rasoli S, et al. Evolution and current applications of the Cabrol procedure and its modifications. Ann Thorac Surg 2011;91(5): 1636–41.

Multidetector CT Findings of Complications of Surgical and Endovascular Treatment of Aortic Aneurysms

CrossMark

Tullio Valente, MD[a], Giovanni Rossi, MD[a],
Gaetano Rea, MD[a], Antonio Pinto, MD, PhD[b],
Luigia Romano, MD[b], Joseph Davies, MD[c],
Mariano Scaglione, MD[c,d],*

KEYWORDS

- Aorta • Surgical • Adverse effects • Complications • EVAR • TEVAR • Multidetector CT (MDCT)

KEY POINTS

- List the potential complications of aortic open surgery and stent-graft placement.
- Identify normal postprocedural multidetector computed tomography (MDCT) findings related to open thoracic and abdominal aortic surgery and thoracic endovascular aortic repair/endovascular aortic repair (TEVAR/EVAR).
- Describe abnormal postprocedural MDCT findings related to open thoracic and abdominal aortic surgery and TEVAR/EVAR.

INTRODUCTION

Open surgical and endovascular thoracic and abdominal aortic repair techniques (TEVAR/EVAR) can be used to manage aortic disorders, including aneurysms, acute and chronic dissection, intramural hematoma (IMH), penetrating ulcers, traumatic transections, and pseudoaneurysms (PSA) of all types.[1] Hybrid procedures, branched and fenestrated endografts, and percutaneously introduced aortic valves have emerged as potent and viable alternatives to traditional surgeries.[2–4] In the treatment of aortic aneurysms, the extent of aortic resection, surgical vessel reconstruction or endovascular graft placement, as well as the need for ancillary procedures is determined by preoperative testing and intraoperative findings.[5,6]

Following aortic aneurysm repair, a variety of imaging techniques may be used in documenting and assessing after-repair appearances as well as in routine follow-up and investigation of early or late potential complications in which intervention is required.[6] These complications include multidetector computed tomography (MDCT) with 2-dimensional (2D) curved-planar reformation (MPR), full maximum-intensity projection (MIP), 3-dimensional (3D) volume rendering, and electrocardiogram (ECG)-gated time-resolved

Conflicts of Interest: The authors have no conflicts of interest to declare.
[a] Department of Diagnostic Imaging, Section of General Radiology, Azienda Ospedali dei Colli, P.O. Monaldi, Via Leonardo Bianchi, Naples 80131, Italy; [b] Department of Diagnostic Imaging, Section of General and Emergency Radiology, "A. Cardarelli" Hospital, Via Cardarelli 9, Naples 80100, Italy; [c] Department of Radiology, Royal London Hospital, Barts and the London NHS Trust, Whitechapel Road, London E11BB, UK; [d] Department of Diagnostic Imaging, Pineta Grande Medical Center, Via Domiziana Km 30, Castel Volturno, Caserta 81030, Italy
* Corresponding author. Via Mattia Preti 29, Napoli 80127, Italy.
E-mail address: mscaglione@tiscali.it

Radiol Clin N Am 52 (2014) 961–989
http://dx.doi.org/10.1016/j.rcl.2014.05.002
0033-8389/14/$ – see front matter © 2014 Elsevier Inc. All rights reserved.

4-dimensional techniques. This article reviews the normal and abnormal MDCT appearances of the postoperative thoracic and abdominal aorta following open surgical and endovascular repair.

COMPUTED TOMOGRAPHY TECHNIQUE AND NORMAL ANATOMY FOLLOWING OPEN SURGICAL REPAIR

Following aortic aneurysm repair, the computed tomography (CT) protocol should include triphasic CT angiography with unenhanced scans.[7,8] No oral contrast agent should be administered unless gas is identified in the endovascular or perivascular soft tissue or if bronchial/esophageal-vascular fistula is suspected. When feasible and in cases of suspected complications involving the aortic valve or aortic sinus, valve plane, aortic root, or proximal ascending aorta, a contrast-enhanced thoracic acquisition should be obtained with retrospective ECG-gating. These imaging techniques are also of benefit when assessing patency of coronary artery bypass grafts or concomitant disease affecting native coronary arteries or valve pathology (Table 1).[9] The follow-up protocol consists of MDCT performed before hospital discharge (baseline MDCT), at 3 and 12 months, and yearly thereafter.

Knowledge of the specific surgical procedure is often crucial to unambiguously interpret postoperative findings.[6,10] Sites of repair are classified according to the region of the aorta that is repaired, and the following sections are considered separately: the aortic root, ascending aorta, aortic arch, descending aorta, and abdominal aorta (Table 2).

Open Surgery of Thoracic Aortic Aneurysms

When reconstruction of the aortic root and aortic valve is required, the options are either graft repair of the ascending aorta above the level of the coronary arteries with separate valve replacement or a composite graft replacement—that is, an aortic graft directly attached to a mechanical valve.[10] Open repair of the thoracic aorta is performed using an impermeable Dacron tube of variable length, which may be grafted using either the interposition or the inclusion technique.[5,11,12] The interposition technique, which is currently the more commonly performed procedure because of the lower incidence of postoperative complications, involves replacement of the resected diseased aorta with the Dacron graft. In contrast, the inclusion technique involves placement of a graft within the in situ diseased aorta, thus creating a potential space between the graft and the aortic wall that is most commonly of water density. This potential space may, however, be of high density on noncontrast CT due to filling with thrombus or fresh blood. In the case of PSA with active bleeding, both may be apparent with enhancement of fresh blood adjacent to nonenhancing thrombus. Although contrast enhancement in the perigraft potential space raises suspicion for dehiscence and can occur as a result of suture breakdown, this finding

---

Table 1
Multidetector contrast-enhanced (CE) CT acquisition parameters (64-section MDCT)

	CE Spiral CT	CE ECG-gated CT
Section thickness (mm)	0.5–0.625	0.5–0.625
Increment (mm)	0.4	0.4
Tube potential (kV)	100–120	100–120
Collimation	64 × 0.625	64 × 0.625
Pitch	About 1	BPM dependent
Rotation time (s)	0.5	Minimum
Field of view (mm)	210–260	210–260
Matrix	512 × 512	512 × 512
Nonionic CM[a]	50–120 mL (plus saline chaser)	50–120 mL (plus saline chaser)
Polyphasic injection protocol	Yes	Yes
Injection rate (mL/s)	3–6 (18–20 G preferably in right arm)	3–6 (18–20 G preferably in right arm)
Region of interest	Distal AA/Arch (bolus triggering)	Distal AA/Arch (bolus triggering)
Study plan	Lung apices to the groin	Lung apices to diaphragm

Abbreviations: BPM, beats per minute; CM, contrast material; G, gauge.
[a] High-concentration (=/>350 mgI/mL) CM.

Table 2
Surgical repair common technique of the thoracic aorta

Procedure	Ascending Graft	Aortic Root	Aortic Valve	Coronary	Indications	Complications
Wheat	Supracoronary graft	No	Yes	No	Ascending aneurysm, normal sinuses	Dissection or aneurysm of the aorta proximal to the graft
Bentall	Composite graft[a]	Yes	Artificial graft	Reimplanted	Also valvular and sinusal disease	PSA at coronary artery anastomosis
Modified Bentall (button Bentall or Carrel patch)	Composite graft[a]	Yes	Artificial graft	A "button" of the aorta encircling the coronary ostia is removed with the coronary artery, facilitating implantation of the coronary artery into the graft	Also valvular and sinusal disease	PSA at distal aortic anastomosis site; Coronary PSA formation
Ross	Composite graft[a]	Yes	Biologic graft (replaced with his or her own pulmonary valve/proximal artery pulmonary autograft)	Buttons reimplanted into the pulmonary segment	Children and younger adults	(1) Progressive dilatation of the pulmonary autograft; (2) dissection and PSA at proximal or distal anastomosis sites
Cabrol	Composite graft[a]	Yes	Yes	Coronary ostia side-to-side anastomosed to the aortic graft	Severe atherosclerosis precludes good-quality aortic buttons, severe proximal coronary artery disease; failed Ross procedure	Anastomotic leak, coronary graft insufficiency, thrombosis, endocarditis

(continued on next page)

Table 2
(continued)

Procedure	Ascending Graft	Aortic Root	Aortic Valve	Coronary	Indications	Complications
Yacoub (remodeling valve-sparing technique)	Dacron graft (aortic aneurysm fixed at annulus) 2 aortic suture lines	Reconstructed Valsalva sinuses	Native valve intact (avoid anticoagulation)	Reimplanted Carrel "buttons"	(1) Aneurysm of the sinuses of Valsalva or involving STJ, with essentially normal aortic valve leaflets; (2) Marfan syndrome	Dilatation of annulus and valve insufficiency; reoperation for bleeding
David and Feindel (reimplantation valve-sparing technique)	Dacron graft fastened below the native valve at the subannular level (3 aortic suture lines)	Reimplanted valve and commissures within the graft	Native valve intact (avoid anticoagulation)	Reimplanted Carrel "buttons"	Same as Yacoub, but to better stabilize the aortic annulus; especially in acute type A aortic dissection and annuloaortic ectasia	Fewer cases of late aortic insufficiency than remodeling techniques; few coronary or other anastomotic problems
Tirone David Variant technique	Larger graft is used to construct pseudosinuses of Valsalva	—	—	—	Enhance long-term valve durability	Aortic insufficiency
Demers and Miller	Two grafts (an aortic root graft and a smaller distal graft) are sewn together to create pseudosinuses larger than those created in the T. David-V	—	—	—	Enable the native valve to be sutured inside the graft	(1) Late aortic insufficiency; (2) coronary artery anastomoses

Elephant trunk stage I	Graft placed into the ascending and proximal descending aorta (3 anastomoses are created) ± brachiocephalic debranching	—	Decreases the duration of CPB and aortic cross-clamping, minimizes the risk for renal or visceral ischemia, increases the proximal LZ for potential TEVAR	—
Elephant trunk stage II	A second graft is anastomosed with distal graft within the descending or thoracoabdominal aorta by way of a left thoracoab-dominal incision	—	—	(1) Spinal cord ischemia; (2) aortic rupture; (3) death in the interval
"Arch-first"	Arch vessels are reanastomosed to a tubular branched graft (one-stage surgical approach)	—	Early antegrade perfusion of the arch vessels, lower mortality and morbidity rates	—

Abbreviations: CPB, cardiopulmonary bypass; LZ, landing zone; PSA, pseudoaneurysm; STJ, sinotubular junction.
a Composite repair method = graft plus valve.

may be normal in patients treated using older inclusion techniques such as the Cabrol procedure. The Dacron graft is not detectable on chest radiographs but is visualized on nonenhanced MDCT images as a high-density, thin-walled, curvilinear tubular structure with a smooth and uniform appearance. This image is essential to identify as graft material and is key to differentiating what procedure has been performed when the surgical history is obscure. On contrast-enhanced MDCT, the high-density graft is obscured by intraluminal contrast, but the proximal and distal ends of the graft may still be identified if high-density Teflon felt rings are used to reinforce the anastomotic sites (**Fig. 1**). Polytetrafluoroethylene (PTFE) felt material (felt pledgets) also can reinforce sites of arterial cannula placement from cardiopulmonary bypass (CPB), puncture sites used to evacuate air bubbles, and coronary artery reimplantation sites to reduce the tearing of vessels.[13] Pledgets are visualized on MDCT as small, paired, extraluminal densities that are spatially well-defined. Recognition of these appearances is important for differentiating them from areas of calcified atherosclerotic plaque, contrast material (CM)

extravasation, or contrast leak. The high-density felt material in these locations, a normal postoperative imaging finding, can mimic a PSA on MDCT, and unenhanced images must be used to confirm that these areas are surgical materials (**Box 1**).[11,12]

Sometimes a cannula may be placed through a graft side branch and the branch can be oversewn after completion of the CPB procedure used during graft surgery.[13] An oversewn graft side branch may have a felt pledget at the margin and may appear as an outpouching at CT, thereby again mimicking a PSA or leak. In these cases, when the radiologist is uncertain as to whether the imaging findings are within the range of expected or not, the authors recommend reviewing the images in person with the operating surgeon. The interposition graft usually appears smooth and uniform in contour. Occasionally, there can be slight angulation of the aortic graft itself or, where more than one graft is used, at their junction. Graft margins can be seen on sagittal oblique MPR/MIP images as an abrupt change in caliber, contour, or angulations at the junction of the graft and the native aorta, all of which are normal except in the case of significant luminal narrowing.

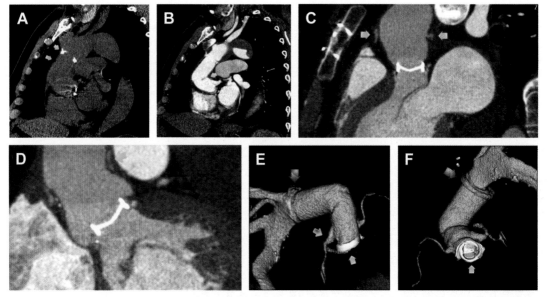

Fig. 1. Bentall procedure. After open surgery. MDCT of the thoracic aorta: normal findings. Unenhanced MDCT (*A*) oblique sagittal thick-slab MIP reformatted image shows a synthetic polyethylene (Dacron) graft (*orange arrow*), which is slightly hyperattenuating compared with the aortic lumen and a high-density felt ring (*green arrow*) used to reinforce the distal anastomosis between the graft and the proximal aortic arch. Enhanced MDCT (*B*) sagittal reformatted image shows that the graft material cannot be appreciated as the intravenous CM is similar high density as the graft. Note angulations at the anastomosis sites (*green arrow*). Wheat procedure. Contrast-enhanced ECG-gated MDCT (*C, D*) oblique sagittal thick-slab MIP reformatted images show felt pledgets material (*orange arrows*) at the proximal anastomosis site; note that there is also a change in contours at the anastomosis of the open graft and native aorta (*green arrow*). Modified button Bentall procedure. Contrast-enhanced ECG-gated MDCT (*E*) oblique sagittal and (*F*) coronal thick-slab volume-rendered projection reformatted images show the graft, coronary buttons (*green arrow*), felt ring at distal anastomosis site (*blue arrow*), and the prosthetic valve (*orange arrows*). Note angulations at the anastomosis sites.

Reformatted images are also helpful in identifying kinks or focal outpouching at the junction of 2 adjacent grafts or at the margin of a single graft. These kinks/outpouchings are regarded as a normal expected postoperative finding but can simulate a dissection flap or a PSA on axial CT images. Similarly, following a stage 1 elephant trunk repair, the free-floating aortic graft in the descending thoracic aorta can mimic a dissection. Another potential pitfall in the interpretation of postoperative CT scans after aortic root reconstruction with a composite graft lies in the variable appearance of the coronary artery anastomosis. With composite graft replacement, the coronary ostia are dissected with a rim of surrounding aorta (button technique) and reanastomosed individually to the composite graft. The buttons along the proximal graft anastomosis can occasionally be rather prominent and may produce a small bulge at the anastomotic site, simulating a PSA.[5,6] The right atrial appendage may appear deformed from a purse-string suture after cannulation, which can mimic clot. Aortic grafts may be covered by a strip of bovine pericardium or, rarely (in the presence of infection), by omentum, to separate them from adjacent structures and prevent fistulas. Bovine pericardium usually has somewhat lower CT attenuation than does soft tissue, whereas the omentum shows fat attenuation. For patients with isolated aortic arch disease, open surgery may range from partial arch (hemiarch) replacement to complete arch replacement with or without debranching and reanastomosis of the arch vessels.[6,10]

Open Surgery of Abdominal Aortic Aneurysms

The most widely practiced technique of open surgical abdominal aortic aneurysm (AAA) repair is the "graft inlay technique." The sac is opened; the aneurysm is repaired with an interposition Dacron graft (tube or bifurcated), and the aneurysm sac is wrapped around the graft to prevent development of adhesions between the graft and the bowel. Ten days postoperatively, normal CT appearances demonstrate a low-density, homogeneous, perigraft fluid collection that does not enhance with intravenous CM. This CM represents seroma, which is commonly seen within the sac up to the first year after repair.[14] The residual sac containing periprosthetic fluid usually has a greater transverse than anteroposterior (AP) diameter (flattened sac). During the initial 6 postoperative months, the sac reduces in transverse and AP diameter with a progressive decrease in the distance between the prosthetic graft and the sac. A small amount of perigraft gas is commonly seen within the aneurysm sac during the first few weeks after open AAA repair, but this usually disappears within 3 months. By 10 years, the prosthetic graft is well "incorporated" with only a thin capsule applied closely around the graft. When the native proximal aorta is friable or severely diseased, a PTFE belt may be used on the outside of the aortic neck to reinforce a potentially friable proximal aortic anastomosis. This belt appears as a high-attenuation ring at CT and should not be confused with an endoleak (EL) or PSA.

Open Surgery Complications

Direct complications of open aortic surgery potentially include[10]

- Nerve injury, most commonly to the phrenic or recurrent laryngeal nerve;
- Postsurgical adhesions, bowel injury, hemopericardium, and tamponade;
- Increased pressure within the left atrium can result from systemic bypass devices leading to pulmonary edema, congestive heart failure, and intracranial hypertension, possibly resulting in stroke;
- Left-ventricular PSA, most often related to myocardial infarction, and cardiac surgery arising from a ventriculotomy site, most commonly at the left ventricular apex, which may be cannulated for arterial perfusion, venting, or deairing[15];
- Ventral abdominal wall incisional hernias after open AAA repair (incidence 5%–35%) and adhesive intestinal obstruction, common to all open intra-abdominal procedures[16];
- Bowel inadvertently damaged by sutures at the time of abdominal wall closure;
- Retrograde ejaculation and impotence may result after AAA repair due to injury to autonomic nerves during aortoiliac dissection.

Graft Infection and Graft Dehiscence

A uniform immediately postsurgical concentric thickening of the lumen near the thoracic graft up to 10 mm is part of the normal postoperative appearance and is mainly seen following the inclusion technique. A periprosthetic hematoma larger than 15 mm at the first postoperative imaging examination indicates an elevated risk for the development of a PSA.[17]

Small to moderate amounts of focal perigraft fluid or blood have been noted on MDCT in up to 50% of cases within the first several weeks following open aortic repair; however, after 3 months, any perigraft hematoma or fluid should have resolved (**Box 2**).

Box 2
Open surgical repair MDCT abnormal findings

Unenhanced

1. Large (>15 mm) periprosthetic fluid/hematomas, usually asymmetric
2. Gas within or adjacent to the graft (pathologic finding if >6–12 wk or increasing on serial scans) by infection, bronchoesophageal or esophageal or enteric/aorta fistula
3. Abscess (infection, mediastinitis, mycotic new aneurysm)
4. Tethering the esophagus or bronchus or bowel adjacent to the aorta by bronchoesophageal or esophageal or enteric/aorta fistula
5. Postsurgical IMH
6. Internal displacement of intimal calcifications (postsurgical dissection)
7. Infected sternal wound, sternal osteomyelitis, infected anterior chest wall fluid collection
8. Large pleural or mediastinal or retro/peritoneal clot/hematoma
9. Malpositioned catheter systems and RSFB

Enhanced

1. Aneurysm sac
   a. Distended and reverts to a circular configuration (growing sac)
   b. Loss of continuity of the aneurysm wall
   c. b + absence of the fat plane between the duodenum and the sac (AEF)
   d. CM outside the prosthetic graft, but within the aneurysm sac (EL or perigraft perfusion)
2. Pronounced stent-graft tortuosity or angulations and stenosis
3. Primary (overtightened suture) or secondary (fibrosis) stenosis, endograft thrombotic filling defect
4. Anastomotic PSA or IV CM leak at graft anastomosis (anastomotic dehiscence), anastomotic thrombosis, confined perforation
5. Paravalvular leaks, ring abscesses, aneurysm, or leak of coronary anastomosis site
6. Native aorta or great arteries iatrogenic dissection flap
7. Periprosthetic area:
   - Large (>10 mm) or increasing size on serial scans of enhancing fluid (seroma)/ soft-tissue attenuation material, or new collection adjacent to the graft (PSA suspected), local hematoma

- Significant increase of the infrarenal aortic neck and new aneurysm

- Extravasation of oral CM (esophageal fistula)

8. Malperfusion syndromes and organ infarction (brain, kidney, bowel)

9. Large pleural and mediastinal effusion, hemothorax, hemoperitoneum

10. Large pericardial effusion or thickening, cardiac tamponade

11. Left lower lobe atelectasis

The low-attenuation material is thought to be secondary to organized fibrous tissue from postoperative hematoma or edema secondary to an allergic immunologic reaction to the aortic graft material. These blood/fluid collections do not enhance with contrast administration and can resolve spontaneously or remain unchanged for years. Although they are most frequently of no clinical significance, a chronic perigraft collection can serve as a site of secondary infection, particularly in patients who are bacteremic, and correlation should be made with clinical indicators of infection. Imaging findings suggestive of an infected perigraft collection include contrast enhancement of the collection, bubble or pockets of air within the collection, increasing size of collection on serial scans, and fistulous connections to other adjacent structures or extension into other compartments (**Fig. 2**).[11,12,17] Ancillary findings may also include stranding of the adjacent fat and soft tissues. The presence of mediastinal air is a common and expected finding during the early postoperative period and can persist for up to 6 to 12 weeks without reported complications. New, persistent (>6–12 weeks), or increasing air near the graft is very suspicious for a developing infection with a gas-producing organism (**Fig. 3**) or a fistula with an adjacent bronchus, the esophagus, or an adherent intestinal loop. Direct signs of a fistula are air or contrast communication between the aorta and adjacent structures. More subtle indirect signs are tethering or distortion of the aorta or adjacent

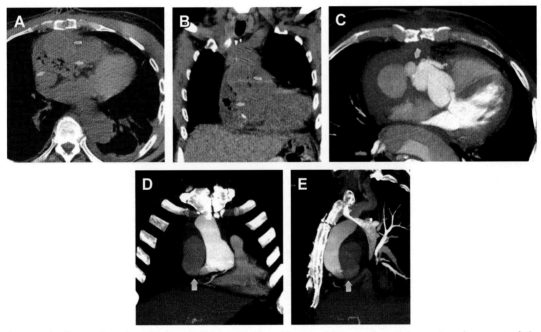

Fig. 2. Infection and graft anastomotic dehiscence in a 70-year-old man who underwent replacement of the ascending aorta for type A dissecting aneurysm 7 months earlier at another institution. A postsurgery 2-month follow-up CT was performed to evaluate the cause of night sweats, mild chills, and fever. Unenhanced MDCT axial (A) and coronal (B) reformatted images show abnormal low-attenuation perigraft material and multiple gas bubbles (*green arrows*) adjacent to the graft anastomosis (*orange arrows*). These findings, suggesting purulent fluid due to graft infection, were initially misinterpreted as normal postoperative findings. After another 2 months, this patient came to observation for fever and worsening dyspnea, and an emergent MDCT scan was performed. Contrast-enhanced axial (C), coronal (D), and sagittal (E) thick-slab MIP reformatted images show active contrast extravasation (*orange arrows*) arising from proximal graft anastomotic dehiscence.

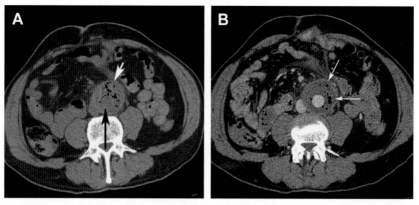

Fig. 3. A 61-year-old man with suspected abdominal graft infection 9 months postoperatively. Unenhanced MDCT axial image (*A*) shows the thin-walled postsurgical aortic graft (*black arrow*) surrounded by gas bubbles (*white arrow*) due to gram-negative prothesis infection. Enhanced MDCT axial image (*B*) confirms gas bubbles spreading into the native aortic sac thrombus (*white arrows*).

mediastinal/enteric structures.[12] Prosthetic valve endocarditis can occur any time postoperatively and is generally classified as early or late by using the cutoff of 2 months. With mechanical prostheses, infection often starts at the sewing cuff or from thrombi near the sewing ring. Common complications include paravalvular leaks, ring abscesses, and extension of the infection into adjacent tissues.[15] MDCT can demonstrate vegetations in the form of small, round, hypoattenuating masses located on the sewing ring or leaflet component, usually on the ventricular surface of the prosthesis. This infected material shows marked contrast enhancement, suggesting a mediastinal and periprosthetic abscess. Rarely, it may invade the wall of the grafted ascending aorta, causing a thrombotic floating pedunculated filling defect in the lumen of the mid-distal aorta with no signs of spreading hemomediastinum or hemopericardium (**Fig. 4**).[18] Anastomotic prosthetic valve or graft dehiscence is often due to advanced perigraft/graft infection and therefore abscess and hematoma may contribute to the CT appearance simultaneously (**Fig. 5**). Valve dehiscence appears as a gap between the aortic annulus and the opposing margin of the artificial valve that allows visualization of a continuous column of CM from the left ventricular cavity into the aortic root.[15,19] MDCT may be used to confirm clinically suspected graft infection in patients presenting with fever or gastrointestinal bleeding following AAA open surgery. This clinically suspected graft infection is confirmed following the visualization of perigraft fluid collection with or without gas content more than 1 year postoperatively, or if the sac progressively enlarges and becomes more circular.[20]

GRAFT DEHISCENCE AND PSA FORMATION

Dehiscence of the suture line can lead to a broad range of complications (anastomotic PSA, perigraft perfusion, confined perforation, suture line failure with hemorrhage). The presence of CM external to an interposition graft is diagnostic of a dehiscence. Partial dehiscence of a suture line can occur at any anastomotic site, but most commonly either proximal or distal to the graft, at cannulation sites. Less frequently dehiscence may occur at the coronary anastomosis site (**Fig. 6**). PSA formation has been reported in 7% to 25% of patients with composite grafts, with mediastinitis and graft infection being the most common risk factor for their formation. Using the Bentall technique, PSA can develop after dehiscence of the suture line at the aortic annulus, coronary ostia, and proximal or distal graft anastomotic site. In this situation, repeat operation is often required unless the PSA becomes thrombosed.[21] Postoperative ascending aortic PSA can occur at an aortotomy site, cannulation site for cardiopulmonary bypass, or needle puncture site (needle inserted for pressure measurement, to purge the aorta of air or to inject cardioplegic solution), or at incompetent suture lines. Crossclamping an atherosclerotic ascending aorta may also cause an iatrogenic aortic dissection, PSA, or shower embolism.[11,12] PSA formation accounts for most late abdominal graft-related complications; however, there is usually a delay of 8 to 10 years before presentation. Timely diagnosis of an aortic PSA is critical, because their natural history includes expansion with a possibility of aortic rupture. At MDCT imaging, a PSA appears as a saccular or fusiform outpouching, usually with a narrow neck that contains CM. Ancillary findings

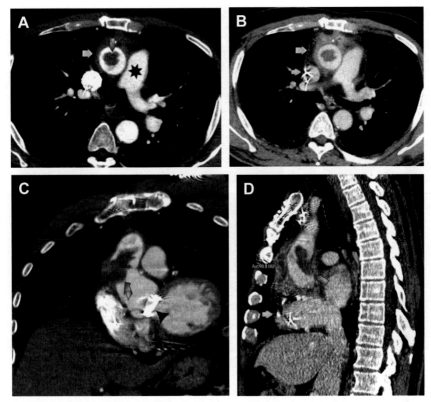

Fig. 4. A 57-year-old immunocompetent man with fever, chest discomfort, leukocytosis, and mildly elevated ESR and CRP, previously surgically treated with the Bentall procedure for a atherosclerotic ascending aorta aneurysm and with a pacemaker (*Candida albicans* graft infection). Contrast-enhanced MDCT axial image (*A*) at level of main pulmonary artery (*asterisk*) shows a perigraft fluid infected collection (*orange arrow*) and a central thrombotic filling defect within the mid-distal ascending aorta lumen (*blue arrow*). Contrast-enhanced MDCT axial image (*B*) shows marked enhancement of the periprosthetic inflammatory tissue (*orange arrow*). Note artifacts from a pacemaker in the superior vena cava (*green arrow*). Contrast-enhanced MDCT coronal MIP reformatted image (*C*) shows thrombosis of the right side aortic wall projecting into the lumen (*blue arrow*) and the mechanical aortic valve (*black triangle*). Contrast-enhanced MDCT oblique sagittal MIP reconstruction image (*D*) shows a perigraft fluid infected collection whose density is of 99 HU, a thrombotic floating filling defect within the lumen of the mid-distal aorta (*blue arrow*), and sternotomy wires and artifacts by pacemaker electrodes (*green arrow*).

include periaortic soft tissue stranding, edema, or periaortic gas. Surgical intervention can be undertaken to repair the PSA depending on several factors, including the absolute size of the PSA and its change over time, the proximity of the PSA to the aortic valve and branch vessels, and the patient's clinical symptoms. Some small sterile PSAs may remain stable for years with conservative management. Less commonly, MDCT findings indicating dehiscence may be simulated by fistula from the graft to adjacent mediastinal structures, such as a bronchus or the esophagus. Significant AAA perigraft dilatation is usually the result of para-anastomotic pseudoaneurysm/true aneurysm formation, which can potentially rupture, thus increasing the risk of death. The reported incidence of para-anastomotic abdominal aneurysms after conventional repair ranges from 1.3% to 27%.

Their cause is multifactorial and includes suture failure, the type of prosthetic material, degeneration of the artery, and infection.[14] Timely diagnosis of para-anastomotic aneurysm is important because of the risk of serious complications, such as rupture, thrombosis, embolism, and pressure onto or erosion into neighboring structures. Most abdominal reoperations following open repair are performed for anastomotic PSAs or true iliac aneurysms and are characterized by high mortality (20%–37.5%) and are therefore now treated by endovascular technique (EVAR). An unconfined extravasation leads to local hematoma formation or to active bleeding into mediastinum or retroperitoneum, which can result in the development of a hemoperitoneum or hemorrhagic pleural or pericardial effusion, potentially causing significant cardiac tamponade (**Fig. 7**).

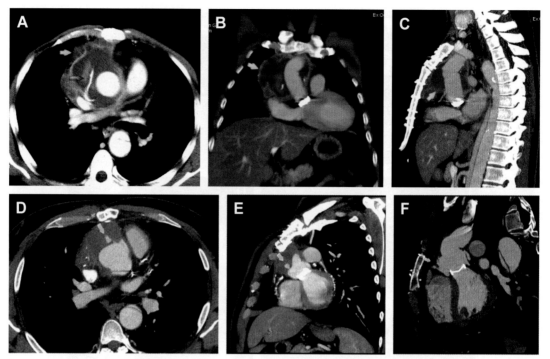

Fig. 5. MDCT findings of graft infection, PSAs, and dehiscence. Two distinct cases. Case 1. A 55-year-old man with Marfan syndrome who presented with PSA secondary to graft infection 5 years after undergoing composite graft repair for type A dissecting aneurysm. Contrast-enhanced MDCT axial (*A*), coronal (*B*), and sagittal (*C*) MIP reformatted images show an infected PSA (*green arrow*) extending into the anterior mediastinum with an open felt ring in the collection (*blue arrow*). Case 2. Perigraft infected fluid and PSA in a 48-year-old man who underwent an emergent Wheat procedure for type A dissecting aneurysm. Contrast-enhanced MDCT axial (*D*) and oblique sagittal (*E, F*) MIP reformatted images show a small focus of CM extravasation into the PSA (*orange arrow*).

AORTO-ENTERIC FISTULA

An aorto-enteric fistula (AEF) may uncommonly occur following open AAA repair, when the graft anastomosis gradually erodes into an adherent intestinal loop, which is usually the third or fourth part of the duodenum, although all parts of small and large bowel are rarely the site of fistula.[14] An AEF should be suspected in patients presenting with gastrointestinal bleeding and a past history of surgical AAA repair. Although endoscopy is important for excluding other causes of gastrointestinal bleeding, it often fails to detect a graft-enteric fistula. MDCT findings that support the diagnosis are a loss of continuity of the aneurysm wall and absence of the fat plane between the duodenum and the aneurysm sac (**Fig. 8**). An active bleeding site is rarely seen on MDCT and is only visible in the presence of continual major bleeding.

NEW ANEURYSMS

Because on average there is progressive enlargement of the infrarenal aortic neck at a rate of 0.16 to 0.57 mm per year, this disease progression can result in the instability of an infrarenal aortic repair by the formation of pseudoaneurysms or recurrent true aneurysms. Approximately 4% to 14% of patients following open repair of AAA subsequently develop a new aneurysm proximal to the original prosthetic graft repair site.[14]

RETAINED SURGICAL FOREIGN BODIES

Surgery requires the placement of foreign material inside the human body. In general, the same 2 types of pathophysiologic responses seen elsewhere in the body apply to RSFB in the chest after aortic surgery (**Fig. 9**). An inflammatory exudative reaction may occur, resulting in an abscess and its possible complications, or may alternatively result in the formation of a predominantly granulomatous response. Textile RSFB have been reported following both thoracotomy and sternotomy procedures.[22]

OTHER LESS COMMON COMPLICATIONS

If the intimal layer of the native vessel at the proximal or distal anastomosis is not stitched properly to the prosthetic graft, dissection flaps can occur and may cause acute limb ischemia or thrombosis immediately following the open repair.

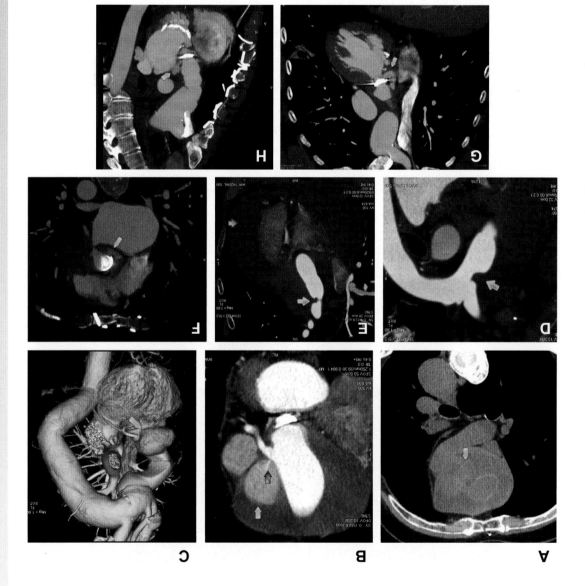

Fig. 6. MDCT findings of perianastomotic sites complications. Three distinct cases. Case 1. A 65-year-old man with ascending aortic interposition graft for aortic aneurysm. Unenhanced MDCT axial image (*A*), contrast-enhanced axial image (*B*), and sagittal volume-rendered projection reformatted image (*C*) show active contrast extravasation (*orange arrow*) arising from left coronary anastomosis site and extending into a large PSA (*orange arrow*) encompassing the ascending aortic graft. Case 2. A 58-year-old man who presented with distal prosthetic anastomosis partial thrombosis 1 month after undergoing aorta interposition graft repair for ascending aorta aneurysm. Contrast-enhanced MDCT oblique sagittal (*D*) and oblique coronal (*E*) MIP reformatted images show partial thrombosis at distal anastomosis sites (*green arrows*) and large pericardial effusion (*blue arrow*). Case 3. Paravalvular leak in a 55-year-old man with a composite aortic graft. ECG-gated contrast-enhanced MDCT axial image (*F*), oblique coronal (*G*), and oblique sagittal (*H*) MIP reformatted images at the level of the left ventricular outflow tract shows a leak (*orange arrows*) below the valve. The defect is continuous with the lumen of the left ventricular outflow tract.

NORMAL ANATOMY FOLLOWING ENDOVASCULAR REPAIR TECHNIQUES

Endovascular repair techniques are focused on 2 main issues:" how to safely deliver the stent-graft

to the target site and place it there" and "how to set a favorable landing zone (LZ)".[23]

Most endovascular stents have an inner metallic skeleton made of nitinol, with a characteristic zigzag appearance causing only mild streak

(PTFE) or polyester graft membrane.[1,24] At MDCT scans, the metallic framework is easily visualized as a metal-density tubular device surrounded by the diseased aorta and adherent to the wall of normal aorta at both ends of the stent. The covering membrane component of the stent-graft is not seen on CT, but it is bordered by circumferential metallic rings at the edges of the metallic stent. Stent-graft position and morphology are best visualized along the long axis in the reformatted sagittal oblique plane. Additional after-processing techniques using a wide window width (>500 WL), MIP, and volume-rendered images improve visualization of the detail of metallic stents.[25] Unlike conventional operative procedures, endovascular repair unfolds within the confines of the aortic inner space and MDCT is widely accepted as an anatomic zone map that highlights the relevant aspects of aortic anatomy from the perspective of endograft therapy.[26]

The most important aspect of stent-graft treatment is to obtain the LZ for the stent on the proximal and distal sides of the aneurysm. When the stent-graft is correctly positioned, the diseased portion (aneurysm sac) of the aorta is covered and excluded from the systemic circulation[25]; at follow-up CT angiography, the endograft should be unchanged in position from that at postoperative angiography and should exclude the entire aortic disease. The stent lumen should be patent without narrowing or sharp angulation. The stent should be closely apposed with no appreciable space between it and the aortic intima along its entire course, particularly near the proximal and distal ends (Box 3, Fig. 10). Flat, straight, long, and cylindrical LZ are ideal for stable stent-graft deployment. Therefore, anatomic complexities at the aortic arch are the most important reasons for early and late stent-graft treatment failure. LZ located near or proximal to the origin of the left subclavian artery (LSA) are associated with a high risk of EL formation, and failure to achieve a proximal seal in the aortic arch resulting in a proximal type I EL remains an Achilles' heel of the TEVAR procedure. Aortic debranching extends the anatomic LZ and expands the number of potential patients who are candidates for TEVAR. In such cases where the LSA is intentionally covered, but not bypassed, it is crucial to document a

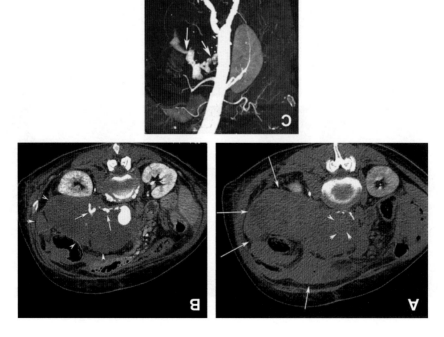

Fig. 7. A 61-year-old man who presented with acute abdominal pain and active hemorrhage after a postsurgical aortic graft dehiscence. Unenhanced MDCT axial image (A) shows a thin-walled postsurgical aortic graft (arrowheads) with an adjacent wide retroperitoneal hematoma (arrows). Contrast-enhanced MDCT axial image (B) demonstrates aortic graft dehiscence with active bleeding (arrows) from the graft lumen into the periaortic hematoma (arrowheads). Contrast-enhanced MDCT sagittal MIP reformatted image (C) gives a further perspective to the active periaortic hemorrhage (arrows).

patent circle of Willis to maintain limb perfusion and avoid neurologic complications. The chimney technique consists of endovascular stent or stent-graft placement parallel to the main aortic stent-graft to preserve or rescue flow to aortic branch vessels and to allow proximal extension of endog-raft fixation zones (Fig. 11).[27] Initial success of en-dovascular stent grafting for aneurysms depends on complete thrombosis in and exclusion of the aneurysm; concerning mid- and long-term results, the most important review criteria for the evalua-tion of results is change in the aneurysm diameter. No changes or a decrease in the aneurysm diam-eter indicates favorable results. An increase in aneurysm diameter should prompt a thorough search for a potential cause should additional treatment be necessary.[28]

In EVAR, the proximal neck of the aneurysm should not be excessively conical or flared and should be free of excessive atherothrombosis

because during stent fixation angiographic bal-loons are used to deploy the main graft, which uses barbs or hooks to achieve satisfactory fixa-tion. These barbs or hooks may disrupt local athe-rothrombotic disease causing distal embolic phenomena. The ipsilateral and contralateral iliac limbs are deployed in a similar fashion, albeit through their respective common femoral arteries. Aortoiliac aneurysms, where the common iliac aneurysm component extends to the iliac artery bifurcation, require the use of a bifurcated endo-vascular stent-graft with extenders into the external iliac artery on the involved side. Fenestra-tion allows the stent-graft to overlay the renal artery ostia while providing for transgraft flow to the renal artery, which improves sealing every-where except the area immediately around the fenestration. Multiple measurements are required in EVAR follow-up MDCT to assess the condition of the graft.

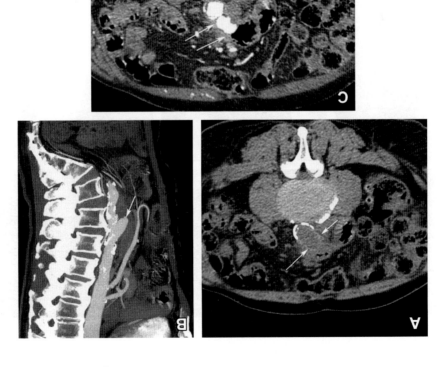

Fig. 8. Graft PSA and AEF in a 67-year-old man presenting with melena and with a history of surgical AAA repair. Unenhanced MDCT axial scan (A) shows a thin-walled postsurgical aortic graft (arrows). Contrast-enhanced MDCT sagittal maximum intensity projection reformatted image (B) shows a PSA arising from the graft wall (arrow). Contrast-enhanced MDCT axial scan (C) demonstrates an AEF resulting from the tight connection between graft PSA and the small bowel wall (arrows).

The external AP and transverse dimensions of the aneurysm sac in addition to the endoluminal measurements of the aortic stent-graft and its 2 limbs are required. It is also important to measure the distance between the proximal margin of the stent-graft and the inferior margin of the most inferior renal artery, and the lower margin of the stent-graft and the iliac artery bifurcation of each side. Diameter measurements are most accurate if performed orthogonal to a centerline through the aorta, but volume assessment has been proven to be more accurate than diameter measurements in the early detection of aneurysm growth, although it is time-consuming, requires advanced processing (although semi-automated vessel tracking programs are available on many workstation), dedicated equipment, and skilled operators.

ENDOVASCULAR REPAIR TECHNIQUES (TEVAR/EVAR) COMPLICATIONS

Although early results compare favorably with those of conventional open surgery, several procedure-related complications or adverse events have been described[29,30] that can be divided into 2 categories: implantation and post-implantation (Box 4). Lifelong clinical and morphologic surveillance is mandatory after TEVAR/EVAR because late treatment failure may develop even years after the initial treatment (Box 5).[25]

ELs

An EL is defined as a persistent blood flow within the sac outside the stent-graft and is classified into types I to V according to its cause. Early or primary ELs occur in the first 30 days following an endovascular procedure, whereas ELs that fail to seal within 30 days are called persistent or secondary ELs and represent the main failure of the endovascular treatment.[31] Accurate diameter measurements of the access vessels and the sealing zones are important to determine the feasibility of the procedure and appropriate graft sizes. An undersized endograft can result in an EL or migration, while excessive oversizing may cause

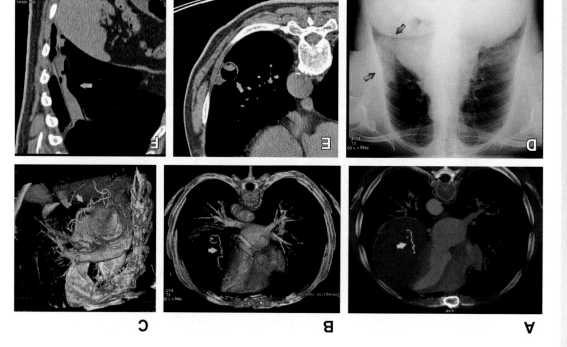

Fig. 9. RSFB. Two distinct cases. Case 1. A 67-year-old man with unremitting mediastinitis 4 months after an ascending aorta replacement for aortic aneurysm performed at another institution. Contrast-enhanced MDCT axial (A), axial volume-rendered projection (B), and oblique sagittal volume-rendered projection (C) reformatted images show an abnormal paracardiac low-attenuation collection caused by a textile-based type foreign body (a lap sponge, gauzoma) with an inner "whorled" texture of radio-opaque marker (green arrows). Case 2. A 70-year-old man presenting with left atypical chest pain 15 months after an ascending aortic graft replacement for aortic aneurysm. Chest radiograph (D) shows peripheral opacification of left lower hemithorax (blue arrows). Unenhanced MDCT axial image (E) and oblique sagittal MIP reformatted image (F) show a syringe plunger within the left pleural space (orange arrows).

Box 3
EVAR/TEVAR MDCT normal findings

Unenhanced

1. Stent-graft: uniform metallic zigzag appearance of framework bordered by circumferential metallic rings at the edges of the metallic stent; straight, aorto-uni-iliac grafts and bifurcated

   - Position
   - No angulations
   - Detail and continuity of metallic stents (infrarenal/suprarenal fixation and fenestrated devices)
   - Joint between the stent-grafts

2. Native aorta

   - IMH
   - Calcium in the aortic wall or in thrombus (vs EL)

3. Periprosthetic area

   - Moderate soft-tissue attenuation material adjacent to the graft (its maximum diameter)

Enhanced

1. Stent-graft

   - Homogeneously opacified patent lumen
   - Aneurysm dimensions (diameters, 3D volume)
   - Uniform wall adherence (good apposition)
   - Position versus anatomic arch zone map
   - Distal and proximal LZ
   - Stent-grafts margins (no appreciable space between stent-graft and the aortic intima)
   - Distance of the proximal end of the stent from the nearest major branch

2. Intact native aorta

3. Homogeneously opacified side branch lumen

4. Periprosthetic area

   - Enhancing soft-tissue attenuation material adjacent to the graft (its maximum diameter)

---

infolding, poor sealing, and excessive radial force with accelerated degeneration of the neck. ELs have been divided into 5 types on the basis of the source of blood flow: type I, leak at the attachment site; type II, leak from a branch artery; type III, graft defect; type IV, graft porosity; and type V, endotension (**Fig. 12**). Unlike in the infrarenal aorta, type II EL is uncommon in the thoracic aorta and type I is prevalent. There are several CT findings that may help distinguish between different types of ELs. *Type I*, due to inadequate seal between the stent-graft and the host aorta, is seen communicating with the proximal (IA) or distal (IB) attachment site of the stent-graft with reperfusion of the aneurysm sac; an EVAR *type I* EL may also be due to inadequate seal of an iliac occluder (IC). Anatomic problems (eg, a short, irregular, ulcerated, or angulated LZ or proximal neck without an optimal conformation of the stent-graft to the curved aortic contour) may cause separation of the device from the arterial wall. Bird-beak aortic arch wall configuration is defined as the incomplete apposition of the proximal endograft with a wedge-shaped gap between the device and the aortic arch wall. Thoracoabdominal junction curvature increases the risk of type IB EL.[32,33] *Type II* or "a side branch" EL, accompanied by retrograde flow from side branches of an aortic aneurysm, is located in the periphery of the aneurysm sac without contact with the stent. In the abdominal aorta, type II EL is commonly located in a posterior or lateral position and is associated with opacification of the lumbar arteries. If an EL is located in the anterior position, retrograde flow into the sac by the inferior mesenteric artery must be suspected. CT can also help visualize vessels in communication with the stent-graft cavity; however, contrast enhancement in these vessels may represent inflow (as in type II EL) or outflow (from EL other than type II). Most frequently, type II ELs connect an inflow source with an outflow vessel, thus limiting the increase of sac pressure. When an outflow path does not exist, the net effect is a higher mean pressure in the sac with a potential risk for complication. *Type III*, also called a connection leak or fabric leak, occurs where the leakage is accompanied by an inadequate joint between the modular or multimodular devices or damage to the stent-graft itself and usually manifests around the graft while sparing the sac periphery. These ELs are more likely when multiple prostheses with short overlapping areas are used. When type III leaks are suspected, MDCT can be used to evaluate for stent-graft integrity as well. *Type IV* ELs secondary to graft porosity are uncommon with today's stent-grafts and are identified as a "blush" on the immediate after-deployment angiogram when the patient is fully anticoagulated. The diagnosis of type IV EL is one of exclusion, because other types of EL can be present on the postimplantation angiogram and should be excluded. Identification of the correct type of EL has important treatment implications. In general,

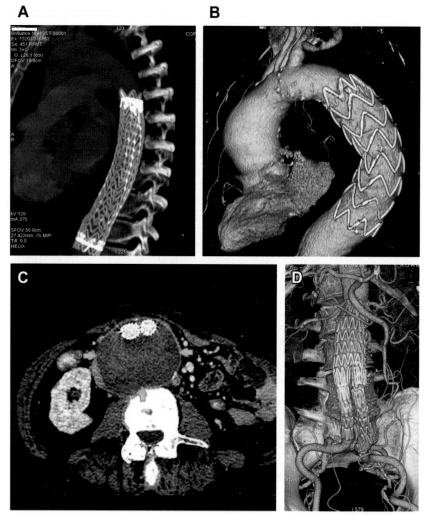

Fig. 10. Normal MDCT findings in TEVAR and EVAR. Contrast-enhanced MDCT sagittal (*A*) MIP and sagittal (*B*) volume-rendered projection reformatted images show normal appearance of the endograft, which is tightly apposed to the thoracic aorta without narrowing or sharp angulation. Contrast-enhanced MDCT axial image (*C*) shows normal opacified lumen of the endograft limbs surrounded by a homogeneous hypodense thrombus of the native AAA (*green arrows*) without EL signs. Contrast-enhanced MDCT coronal volume-rendered projection reformatted image (*D*) shows aortic endograft appropriately sited into the lumen of an aortic aneurysm. The superior attachment is localized below the origin of the renal arteries and the extensions are positioned in the lumen of the common iliac arteries.

high-pressure leaks (type I and type III) require urgent management because of the relatively high short-term risk of sac rupture. The former are managed by securing the attachment sites with angioplasty balloons, stents, or stent-graft extensions, and the latter are managed by covering the defect with a stent-graft extension.[7,34] The management of type II EL, generally a low-pressure lesion, is controversial and, although some authors recommend conservative management for stable aneurysms, others prefer to repair it by coil embolization, plug occlusion, or surgical ligation. Type IV ELs are self-limiting, require no

treatment, and resolve with normalization of the patient's coagulation status. Aneurysm expansion without demonstrable reperfusion defects is known as endotension or *type V* EL. Although the exact cause of endotension is unknown, possible causes include an EL that cannot be visualized with traditional imaging techniques, ultrafiltration of blood across the graft, and thrombus providing an ineffective barrier to pressure transmission. Most ELs can be avoided by careful selection, particularly with regard to important morphologic details such as the length of the LZ, use of multiple stents, length of overlapping segments, as well as

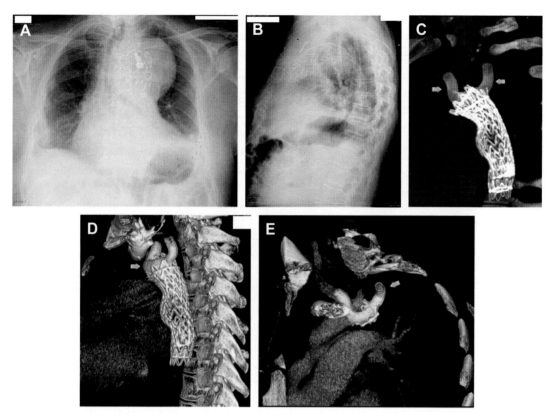

Fig. 11. Aortic debranching and chimney graft complication. Two distinct cases. Case 1. A 75-year-old man presenting with chest pain. Chest radiographs, postero-anterior (*A*), and lateral (*B*) views show an arch aortic atherosclerotic aneurysm treated with hybrid arch debranching approach. Case 2. A 28-year-old woman presenting 4 months after TEVAR for traumatic aortic injury treated with Chimney technique to preserve the flow into the LSA. Follow-up contrast-enhanced MDCT oblique coronal (*C*) MIP and oblique sagittal (*D, E*) volume-rendered projection reformatted images show U-shaped LSA stent-graft migration into the left carotid artery with vessel stenosis (*orange arrows*).

severe angulation and massive aortic calcification (porcelain aorta).[35] Recently, type IV and type V ELs have been considered historical phenomena, no longer observed with more recent technology.[36] Because ELs have variable flow rates, they can be detected at variable times after CM injection. For this reason, a delayed phase has been recommended to increase the sensitivity of detection of ELs not visualized during the arterial phase, the so-called less conspicuous low-flow ELs, but this increases radiation dose exposure, especially on serial CT imaging. Because there is no general agreement on the use of follow-up MDCT, the authors recommend contrast-enhanced ultrasound in the case of sac stability/shrinkage and when there is no more evidence of ELs at the last MDCT follow-up examinations.

STENT-GRAFT INFOLDING, COLLAPSE, MIGRATION

Risk factors for stent-graft infolding or (proximal/distal) collapse are a small aortic lumen and a small radius of the aortic arch curvature (young patients), as well as stent oversizing. MDCT findings of stent infolding and collapse include focal narrowing of the endoluminal stent diameter and loss of contact by the side of the stent with the aortic wall (**Fig. 13**). Stent-graft collapse requires urgent intervention only when there is clinically significant narrowing of the aortic lumen.[37,38] Stent-graft migration (more than 5 mm is generally considered significant) occurs as a result of poor attachment of the stent to the aortic wall, which can cause sac reperfusion and subsequent aneurysm rupture (**Fig. 14**)[39]; in EVAR, proximal neck length, diameter, and angulation (>45°) are predisposing factors.[40]

STENT-GRAFT RUPTURE OR A CONNECTING-BAR FRACTURE

Stent-graft rupture has been described as a possible consequence of graft fatigue, fabric defects, or an abnormal joint between stent-grafts (EL type III) (**Fig. 15**).[41,42]

Box 4
List of endovascular repair techniques (TEVAR/EVAR) main complications/adverse events

Implantation

- Procedure-related
  - Neurologic (stroke, spinal-cord-related problems)
  - Vascular-access (spasm, vessel trauma, rupture, dissection, thrombosis, interruption, bleeding, PSA, lymphoceles)
  - Ischemic (lower extremity ischemia, retrograde dissection, colon necrosis)
  - Contrast-induced renal failure
  - Death
- Device-related (deployment-related)
  - Endograft migration, type I/III/IV ELs, graft limb stenosis/kinking
  - Aneurysm rupture, aorta dissection, perforation
  - Brain injury (by excessive device manipulation or overstenting of the great vessel)
  - Bleeding (requiring transfusion)

Postimplantation

- Endoleak, sac enlargement
- Branch vessel occlusion
- Retrograde type A dissection/IMH
- Anterograde dissection
- Collapse
- Stent-graft (limb) thrombosis/occlusion
- Endograft migration
- Paraplegia
- Coverage of vital vessels (spinal cord ischemia)
- Medical complications (pneumonia, pulmonary embolism, myocardial infarction)
- Aneurysm late rupture
- Stent-graft twisting/kinking
- Loss of stent-graft integrity
- ABF
- AEF
- Endograft infection and mediastinitis
- In-stent-graft dissection
- PSA formation
- Surgical conversion
- Renal complications
- Postimplantation syndrome
- Abdominal compartment syndrome

Box 5
TEVAR/EVAR MDCT complications/adverse events findings

Unenhanced

1. Stent-graft
   - Position (misplacement, migration)
   - Margins (collapse)
   - Marked angulations (fracture or distortions)
   - Collapse/twisting/breakage of the metal portion of the device
2. Distance of the stent ends from the nearest major branch
3. Native aorta IMH
4. Periprosthetic area
   - Large soft-tissue attenuation material adjacent to the graft (its maximum diameter), perigraft hematomas
   - Gas within or adjacent to the graft (pathologic finding if >6 weeks; infection, suspected broncho-esophageal or esophageal/aorta fistula)

Enhanced

1. Stent graft and/or graft limb
   - Inhomogeneously opacified lumen with narrowing (unfolding/collapse/twisting/kinking/thrombosis/in stent-graft dissection) or sharp angulations, occlusion
   - Lack of apposition (ELs)
   - Anatomic zone map position (side branch coverage, migration)
2. EL(s) and aneurysm reperfusion with sac enlargement: high-/low-pressure or high/low-volume flow in the excluded aortic lumen
   - IA: proximal LZ IV CM leak; bird-beak configuration
   - IB: distal LZ IV CM leak
   - II: from a side-branch artery (subclavian, bronchial, intercostals, a persistent patent ductus arteriosus, lumbar, inferior mesenteric artery, accessory renal arteries)
   - III: by inadequate joint between the stent-grafts or damage to stent-graft
2. Native aorta dissection flap/IMH/rupture/new true aneurysm
3. Collateral (epi-aortic, visceral abdominal vessels) stenosis/obstruction/dysfunction and malperfusion syndromes
4. Periprosthetic area
   - Enhancing soft-tissue attenuation material adjacent to the graft (infection, mediastinitis)

- Gas within or adjacent to the stent-graft and mediastinal (infection, broncho-esophageal or esophageal/aorta fistula)
- Oral CM leak (aortoesophageal fistula)
- Large pleural, pericardial, and mediastinal effusion

5. Shower pulmonary embolism
6. Major visceral infarction
7. Injury to adjacent structures (ureter, iliac veins, parasympathetic nerves)

STENT-GRAFT THROMBOSIS/OCCLUSION

Acute retrograde dissection, extending to the thoracic aorta, is the result of abnormal maneuvers during EVAR. Any distortion of the limbs of the stent-graft used in EVAR may result in graft limb thrombosis. On contrast-enhanced CT scans, graft thrombosis is recognized as an intraluminal parietal circular or semicircular area within the stent-graft. Thrombi within the stent-graft are reported to occur at rates of 3% to 19%. Stenosis of the iliac graft limb is reported in a series of bifurcated grafts not fully supported by stents, but graft occlusion is a relatively rare event after stent-graft implantation (**Fig. 16**). Percutaneous local thrombolysis or open surgical conversion depends on the severity of the vascular occlusion.[1,2,43] Patent symptomatic distorted or kinked stent-grafts can usually be treated by an additional stenting, whereas an occluded limb typically requires surgery with construction of a femoro-femoral cross-over bypass.

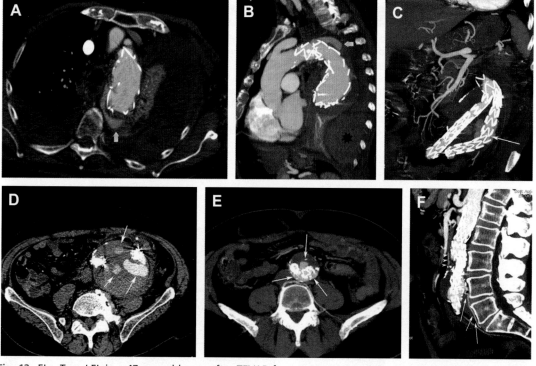

Fig. 12. ELs. *Type I* EL in a 47-year-old man after TEVAR for emergent traumatic aortic PSA. Contrast-enhanced MDCT axial image (*A*) and oblique sagittal (*B*) MIP reformatted image of the thoracic aorta show a jet of contrast medium extravasation from the stented aorta into the excluded aortic lumen (*orange arrows*) directly communicating with the native aorta, consistent with a type IA EL. Large pleural effusions are noted (*asterisk*). *Type III* EL in a 76-year-old man at 1-year follow-up after EVAR. Contrast-enhanced MDCT oblique coronal MIP reformatted image (*C*) shows wire diastasis of the left limb extension with angulation (*arrow*). MIP image (*D*) demonstrates a large type III EL (*arrows*) within the native aortic sac thrombus, adjacent to the endograft. *Type II* EL in an 85-year-old man with an aorto-bi-iliac endovascular stent-graft. Contrast-enhanced MDCT axial scan (*E*) shows CM extravasation into the thrombus in the native aneurysm (*arrows*). Contrast-enhanced MDCT sagittal multiplanar reformatted image (*F*) demonstrates type II EL supplied by a superior mesenteric arterial branch (*arrowheads*) and by a lumbar artery (*arrows*).

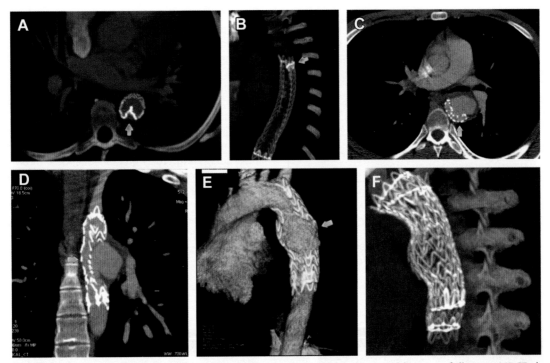

Fig. 13. Stent-graft infolding and collapse. Two distinct cases. Case 1. A 65-year-old woman follow-up MDCT obtained 3 weeks after TEVAR for descending aorta aneurysm. Contrast-enhanced MDCT axial image (*A*) and oblique sagittal MIP reformatted image (*B*) show stent-graft focal infolding (*green arrows*). Case 2. A 31-year-old woman on follow-up MDCT obtained 3 weeks after TEVAR for traumatic aortic PSA. Contrast-enhanced MDCT axial (*C*), oblique coronal (*D*) MIP, and sagittal (*E*) volume-rendered projection reformatted images show that, at level of the PSA, the stent is not expanded (*orange arrows*). This feature is consistent with extensive stent collapse. Thus, a new stent-graft was sited. Contrast-enhanced MDCT oblique sagittal MIP reformatted image (*F*) shows subsequent endograft expansion with normal configuration.

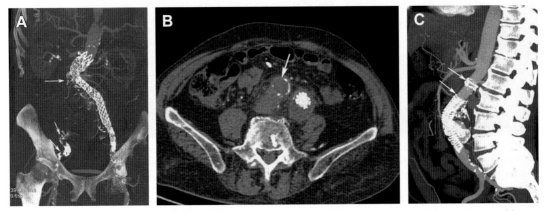

Fig. 14. Rupture and migration of the graft associated with an iliac vein thrombosis in a 68-year-old man, 6 months after EVAR. Contrast-enhanced MDCT coronal MIP reformatted image (*A*) shows detachment and migration of the right extension of the aortic endograft toward the external iliac artery lumen (*arrows*). Contrast-enhanced MDCT axial image (*B*) demonstrates a thrombosis of the right common iliac artery lumen in which the graft extension was previously positioned (*arrow*). Contrast-enhanced MDCT MIP sagittal reformatted image (*C*) shows rupture and migration of the aortic endoprosthesis (*arrows*).

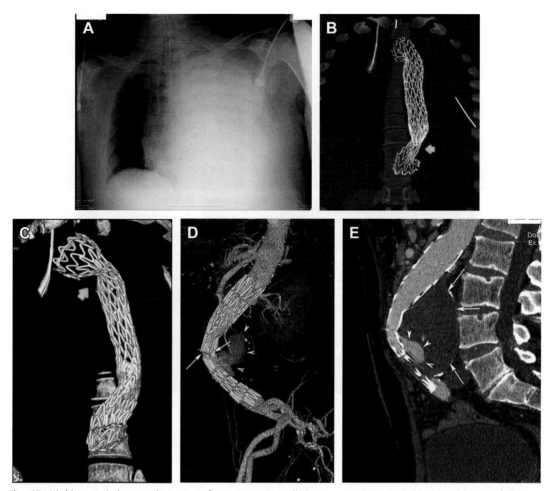

Fig. 15. Kinking, twisting, and stent-graft rupture. Two distinct cases. Case 1. A 63-year-old man, follow-up 2 weeks after TEVAR for a large atherosclerotic aneurysm. Chest radiograph (*A*), contrast-enhanced MDCT coronal (*B*) MIP, and oblique coronal (*C*) volume-rendered projection reformatted images show a large left hemothorax and mediastinal hematoma due to the endograft rupture, which was related to an inadequate joint between the stent-grafts, kinking, mild twisting (*green arrows*). These findings were confirmed at surgery. Case 2. Contrast-enhanced MDCT oblique coronal volume-rendered projection image (*D*) shows an aortic endograft rupture (*arrows*) associated with CM extravasation (*arrowheads*). Contrast-enhanced MDCT MIP sagittal reformatted image (*E*) confirms active hemorrhage (*arrowheads*) within the sac of the native aortic aneurysm, resulting in a *type III* EL (*arrows*).

NATIVE AORTA (PROXIMAL TYPE A/DISTAL TYPE B) DISSECTION/IMH/PAU POSTENDOVASCULAR REPAIR

Published data include TEVAR in the list of procedures resulting in iatrogenic dissection. The remaining question is whether dissection/IMH/penetrating atherosclerotic ulcer is a true complication of the procedure or the natural progression of the disease itself. Patients may have an appropriately placed stent; however, given the fragility of the aortic wall, they can develop a retrograde or anterograde dissection/IMH at either end of the endostent.[1,2,24,44] Steep arch angulation (>90°) is associated with increased risk of retrograde type A dissection and type IA EL.

IN-STENT-GRAFT DISSECTION

Monitoring neointima formation within the stent-graft incorporated onto the aortic wall is not yet possible with current CT/magnetic resonance (MR) imaging. In young patients with TEVAR devices in situ, increased physical activity may result in in-stent-graft dissection and a subsequent reduction in flow downstream (**Fig. 17**).[24,45]

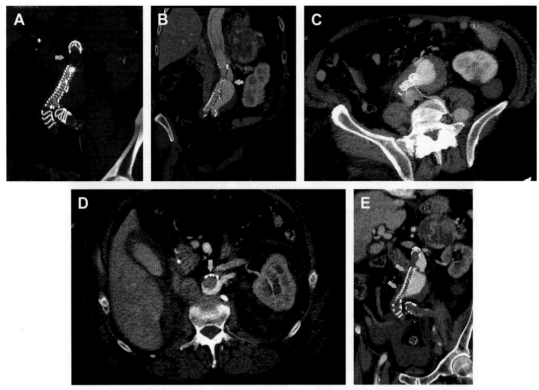

Fig. 16. Thoracoabdominal retrograde dissection and stent-graft thrombosis/occlusion after EVAR in an atherosclerotic abdominal aorta aneurysm. Images obtained in a 72-year-old man with recurrent renal cancer and widespread metastases who underwent EVAR for unstable atherosclerotic AAA. Unenhanced MDCT oblique coronal MIP reformatted image (*A*) shows that the proximal part of the main body endograft consists of 2 nitinol rings at a variable distance from each other according to the vascular diameter; the distal one is unsupported by other stents or longitudinal bars and is more radiolucent (*orange arrow*). At day 1, post-EVAR emergency contrast-enhanced MDCT oblique coronal MIP reformatted image (*B*) shows retrograde thoracoabdominal iatrogenic dissection (actually dissecting type aneurysm), with entry tear located at the proximal part of the stent-graft's main body (*green arrow*). A type III high-pressure EL supplies the aneurysm's false lumen. In a more caudal enhanced MDCT MIP axial reformatted image (*C*), a lumbar artery is feeding a hypervascular metastasis to the left psoas muscle, which potentially may be confused with a type II EL (*blue arrow*). However, its density is lower than that of the false lumen. At day 4, paraparesis and acute renal failure occurred. Contrast-enhanced MDCT axial image (*D*) and oblique coronal MIP reformatted image (*E*) show complete thrombosis of the prosthesis due to poor outflow, which is appreciable either at the aortic component or at the iliac limbs (*orange arrows*).

ENDOPERIGRAFT INFECTIONS/SEPSIS, AORTO-BRONCHOPULMONARY, AORTO-ESOPHAGEAL FISTULA

Time from a TEVAR procedure to diagnosis of infection is 243.6 ± 74.5 days.[46] Patients with graft infection can present with nonspecific clinical findings, including leukocytosis, fever, and chest pain. Infection of the abdominal endograft is rare but devastating, with mortality approaching 75%.[47] CT findings suggestive of endograft infection after TEVAR/EVAR are aortic-wall thickening, perigraft soft tissue or fluid collection, PSA, perigraft air or an increasing amount of air on serial imaging examinations, adjacent soft-tissue stranding, or abscess formation, and graft thrombosis or expansion.[48] In the thoracic aorta, greater than 5 mm of perigraft soft tissue between an adjacent organ or vessel and the graft is abnormal and may suggest infection. Further investigation with MR imaging, fluorine-18 fluorodeoxyglucose positron emission tomography, or tagged white blood cell scanning may be helpful in differentiating endograft infection from other pathologic conditions. TEVAR-associated aorto-esophageal fistula (AEF) occurs in less than 1% of endovascular repair procedures, usually relatively early after the procedure, is uniformly fatal, and is thus probably not widely known within the medical community.[49] When it occurs, it is an early to midterm complication, encountered within 1 to 16 months after TEVAR, presenting as either hematemesis or

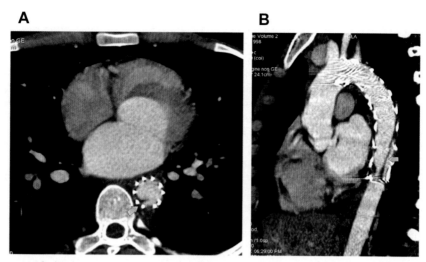

Fig. 17. In-stent-graft dissection. A 26-year-old man 1 year after TEVAR for posttraumatic aortic PSA with a recent history of a fall from 50 cm in height and an acute sudden onset of ischemia in both legs with weak femoral pulses, numbness, and renal function deterioration. Contrast-enhanced MDCT axial image (*A*) and sagittal MIP reformatted image (*B*) shows an intimal flap in the distal part of the stent-graft and narrowing of the aortic lumen (*orange arrows*). In-stent-graft dissection was successfully treated by an additional endograft placement.

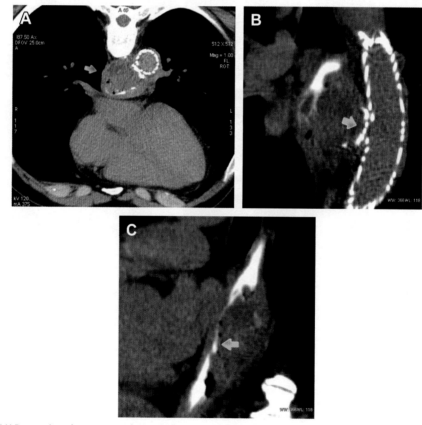

Fig. 18. TEVAR-associated aorto-esophageal fistula. MDCT in a 52-year-old man urgently transferred from another hospital for massive hematemesis, 6 weeks after TEVAR for elective repair of a descending aortic aneurysm. Unenhanced MDCT prone axial image (*A*) and oblique (*B*) and sagittal (*C*) MIP reformatted images after oral contrast medium ingestion show a partially calcified PSA wall (*green arrows*) with a very large thrombus extensively communicating with the esophageal lumen through a fistula with the subcarinal esophagus.

new-onset fever accompanied by elevated inflammation markers, and may herald the onset of imminent rupture of the aorta into the esophagus, followed by sepsis.[50] This presentation is frequently complicated by hypovolemic shock or infectious complications. CT is particularly helpful as an initial imaging modality because evidence of a relatively characteristic new heterogeneous mass between the descending thoracic aorta and esophagus with or without air entrapment in the arterial wall gives an early clue to the diagnosis. Use of oral contrast medium may help show the site and extent of esophageal tear, often to assist the therapeutic planning (**Fig. 18**). When periprosthetic air is appreciable, water-soluble oral contrast media should always be given.

Aorto-bronchial fistulae (ABFs) are connections between the aorta (more often descending aorta) and a bronchus (more often left bronchus), which are rare and fatal if untreated.[51] Open surgery for TAA is the most common cause, responsible for at least 50% to 60% of ABFs reported in the literature. Incidence of ABFs after TEVAR is rare but not negligible (0.8%). Hemoptysis is the first (and often the only) symptom and may be massive or intermittent, depending on the size of the opening.[52] CT may help to identify abnormalities in the descending thoracic aorta (endovascular repairs of aortic coarctation, aneurysms, dissections) or secondary changes of the adjacent lung, often represented by consolidation. Rarely, extravasation of intravenously administered CM from the aorta into

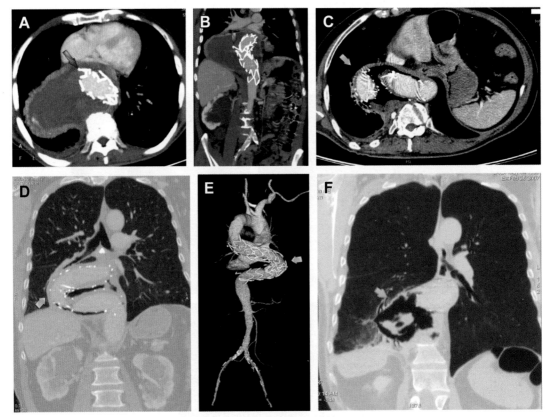

Fig. 19. Two-stage aorto-broncho-pulmonary fistula. A 76-year-old man with a history of hypertension, diabetes mellitus, and peripheral vascular disease, 8 months after TEVAR for descending thoracic aorta inflammatory aneurysm. Recurrent episodes of hemoptysis and chest pain. Before discharge, a contrast-enhanced MDCT was performed. Axial image (*A*) and a coronal MIP reformatted image (*B*) show 2 endovascular stent-grafts obliterating a large, thick-walled aneurysm at a tortuous descending thoracic aorta. Note a nitinol ring protruding into the point of maximum convexity of the vessel (*blue arrow*). Six-month contrast-enhanced MDCT follow-up was performed. Axial image (*C*), coronal MIP image (*D*), and volume-rendered projection (*E*) reformatted image show shrinkage of the aneurysm sac and markedly increased stent-graft right-angle convexity. The proximal end of the stent-graft lies in close proximity to the right lower lobe bronchus, and a large amount of air surrounds the aneurysm and stent-graft (*orange arrows*). MDCT coronal oblique minimum intensity projection reformatted image (*F*) demonstrates multiple large fistulous communications between basilar bronchi and the perigraft thrombus (*green arrow*). The aorto-broncho-pulmonary fistula was confirmed at surgery.

the lung tissue or airways can be seen. Occasionally, intragraft or perigraft air surrounding the aneurysm and stent-graft is the presenting feature of an ABF, whereas a fistula between bronchus and graft almost never is seen (**Fig. 19**).

SUMMARY

Current evidence has demonstrated that endovascular treatment is a feasible alternative to open aortic surgery. As endovascular repair use grows, clinicians as well as general radiologists should be aware of the more frequent as well as of uncommon and rare potential adverse events or complications to avoid delayed diagnosis in patients following open surgery and EVAR/TEVAR. Imaging has an important role in monitoring and detecting complications and the postoperative thoracoabdominal imaging appearance will vary depending on the surgical technique used.

The informed radiologist with a knowledge of the structural features of the prosthesis used, in addition to information provided by the surgeon relating to specific operative techniques, should reliably differentiate the range of normal and abnormal postoperative MDCT findings. They thus can respond to specific and sophisticated diagnostic requests concerning the follow-up of thoracic and abdominal aortic repair to identify significant postoperative complications. The radiologist may then assist in the selection of the most appropriate therapy for the pathologic condition requiring intervention, taking into account the specific risk characteristics of the patient and the locally available open and interventional vascular surgery devices. Finally, MDCT imaging has in particular made a key contribution to the planning, initial success, and long-term durability of these vascular interventions in this complex area of vascular surgery.

REFERENCES

1. Hiratzka LF, Bakris GL, Beckman JA, et al. 2010 ACCF/AHA/AATS/ACR/ASA/SCA/SCAI/SIR/STS/SVM Guidelines for the diagnosis and management of patients with thoracic aortic disease. A report of the American College of Cardiology Foundation/American Heart Association Task Force on Practice Guidelines, American Association for Thoracic Surgery, American College of Radiology, American Stroke Association, Society of Cardiovascular Anesthesiologists, Society for Cardiovascular Angiography and Interventions, Society of Interventional Radiology, Society of Thoracic Surgeons, and Society for Vascular Medicine. J Am Coll Cardiol 2010;121(13):e266–369.

2. Fattori R, Napoli G, Lovato L, et al. Descending thoracic aortic diseases: stent-graft repair. Radiology 2003;229(1):176–83.

3. Therasse E, Soulez G, Giroux MF, et al. Stent-graft placement for the treatment of thoracic aortic diseases. Radiographics 2005;25(1):157–73.

4. Ueda T, Fleischmann D, Rubin GD, et al. Imaging of the thoracic aorta before and after stent-graft repair of aneurysms and dissections. Semin Thorac Cardiovasc Surg 2008;20(4):348–57.

5. Sundaram B, Quint LE, Patel S, et al. CT appearance of thoracic aortic graft complications. AJR Am J Roentgenol 2007;188(5):1273–7.

6. Prescott-Focht JA, Martinez-Jimenez S, Hurwitz LM, et al. Ascending thoracic aorta: postoperative imaging evaluation. Radiographics 2013;33(1):73–85.

7. Stavropoulos SW, Charagundla SR. Imaging techniques for detection and management of endoleaks after endovascular aortic aneurysm repair. Radiology 2007;243(3):641–55.

8. Lehmkuhl L, Andres C, Lücke C, et al. Dynamic CT angiography after abdominal aortic endovascular aneurysm repair: influence of enhancement patterns and optimal bolus timing on endoleak detection. Radiology 2013;268(3):890–9.

9. Johnson PT, Horton KM, Fishman EK. Aortic valve and ascending thoracic aorta: Evaluation with isotropic MDCT. AJR Am J Roentgenol 2010;195(5):1072–81.

10. Gardner TJ, Spray TL, Rob C. Operative cardiac surgery. London; New York: Arnold (distributed in the USA by Oxford University Press); 2004.

11. Quint LE, Francis IR, Williams DM, et al. Synthetic interposition grafts of the thoracic aorta: postoperative appearance on serial CT studies. Radiology 1999;211(2):317–24.

12. Hoang JK, Martinez S, Hurwitz LM. MDCT angiography after open thoracic aortic surgery: pearls and pitfalls. AJR Am J Roentgenol 2009;192(1):W20–7.

13. El-Sherief AH, Wu CC, Schoenhagen P, et al. Basics of cardiopulmonary bypass: normal and abnormal postoperative CT appearances. Radiographics 2013;33(1):63–72.

14. Nayeemuddin M, Pherwani AD, Asquith JR. Imaging and management of complications of open surgical repair of abdominal aortic aneurysms. Clin Radiol 2012;67(8):802–14.

15. Bennett CJ, Maleszewski JJ, Araoz PA. CT and MR imaging of the aortic valve: radiologic-pathologic correlation. Radiographics 2012;32(5):1399–420.

16. Papadimitriou D, Pitoulias G, Papaziogas B, et al. Incidence of abdominal wall hernias in patients undergoing aortic surgery for aneurysm or occlusive disease. Vasa 2002;31(2):111–4.

17. Hoang JK, Martinez S, Hurwitz LM. Imaging of the postoperative thoracic aorta: the spectrum of normal and abnormal findings. Semin Roentgenol 2009;44(1):52–62.

18. Piffaretti G, Tozzi M, Mariscalco G, et al. Mobile thrombus of the thoracic aorta: management and treatment review. Vasc Endovascular Surg 2008; 42(5):405–11.

19. Pham N, Zaitoun H, Mohammed TL, et al. Complications of aortic valve surgery: manifestations at CT and MR imaging. Radiographics 2012;32(7): 1873–92.

20. Mantoni M, Neergaard K, Christoffersen JK, et al. Long-term computed tomography follow-up after open surgical repair of abdominal aortic aneurysms. Acta Radiol 2006;47(6):549–53.

21. Milano AD, Pratali S, Mecozzi G, et al. Fate of coronary ostial anastomoses after the modified Bentall procedure. Ann Thorac Surg 2003;75(6):1797–801.

22. Whang G, Mogel GT, Tsai J, et al. Left behind: unintentionally retained surgically placed foreign bodies and how to reduce their incidence – pictorial review. AJR Am J Roentgenol 2009;193(Suppl 6):S79–89.

23. JCS Joint Working Group. Guidelines for diagnosis and treatment of aortic aneurysm and aortic dissection (JCS 2011): digest version. Circ J 2013;77(3):789–828.

24. Morgan TA, Steenburg SD, Siegel EL, et al. Acute traumatic aortic injuries: posttherapy multidetector CT findings. Radiographics 2010;30(4):851–67.

25. Valente T, Rossi G, Lassandro F, et al. Unusual complications of endovascular repair of the thoracic aorta: MDCT findings. Radiol Med 2012; 117(5):831–54.

26. Criado FJ. Mapping the aorta: a new look at vascular anatomy in the era of endograft repair. J Endovasc Ther 2010;17(1):68–72.

27. Criado FJ, McKendrick C, Criado FR. Technical solutions for common problems in TEVAR: managing access and aortic branches. J Endovasc Ther 2009;16(Suppl 1):I63–79.

28. Booher AM, Eagle KA. Diagnosis and management issues in thoracic aortic aneurysm. Am Heart J 2011;162(1):38–46.

29. Dumfarth J, Michel M, Schmidli J, et al. Mechanisms of failure and outcome of secondary surgical interventions after thoracic endovascular aortic repair (TEVAR). Ann Thorac Surg 2011;91(4): 1141–6.

30. Gopaldas RR, Huh J, Dao TK, et al. Superior nationwide outcomes of endovascular versus open repair for isolated descending thoracic aortic aneurysm in 11,669 patients. J Thorac Cardiovasc Surg 2010;140(5):1001–10.

31. White GH, Yu W, May J, et al. Endoleak as a complication of endoluminal grafting of abdominal aortic aneurysms: Classification, incidence, diagnosis, and management. J Endovasc Surg 1997; 4(2):152–68.

32. Ueda T, Fleischmann D, Dake MD, et al. Incomplete endograft apposition to the aortic arch: bird-beak configuration increases risk of endoleak formation after thoracic endovascular aortic repair. Radiology 2010;255(2):645–52.

33. Kawajiri H, Oka K, Kanda K, et al. Aneurysm formation at both ends of an endograft associated with maladaptive aortic changes after endovascular aortic repair in a healthy patient. Interact CardioVasc Thorac Surg 2013. http://dx.doi.org/10.1093/icvts/ivt336.

34. Stavropoulos SW, Carpenter JP. Postoperative imaging surveillance and endoleak management after endovascular repair of thoracic aortic aneurysms. J Vasc Surg 2006;43(Suppl A): 89A–93A.

35. Fillinger MF, Greenberg RK, McKinsey JF, et al, Society for Vascular Surgery Ad Hoc Committee on TEVAR Reporting Standards. Reporting standards for thoracic endovascular aortic repair (TEVAR). J Vasc Surg 2010;52(4):1022–33.

36. Grabenwoger M, Alfonso F, Bachet J, et al. Thoracic Endovascular Aortic Repair (TEVAR) for the treatment of aortic diseases: a position statement from the European Association for Cardio-Thoracic Surgery (EACTS) and the European Society of Cardiology (ESC), in collaboration with the European Association of Percutaneous Cardiovascular Interventions (EAPCI). Eur Heart J 2012;33(13):1558–63.

37. Canaud L, Alric P, Desgranges P, et al. Factors favoring stent-graft collapse after thoracic endovascular aortic repair. J Thorac Cardiovasc Surg 2010;139(5):1153–7.

38. Bandorski D, Bruck M, Gunther HU, et al. Endograft collapse after endovascular treatment for thoracic aortic disease. Cardiovasc Intervent Radiol 2010;33(3):492–7.

39. Iezzi R, Santoro M, Dattesi R, et al. Multi-detector CT angiographic imaging in the follow-up of patients after endovascular abdominal aortic aneurysm repair (EVAR). Insights Imaging 2012;3(4): 313–21.

40. Moll FL, Powell JT, Fraedrich G, et al. Management of abdominal aortic aneurysms clinical practice guidelines of the European Society for Vascular Surgery. Eur J Vasc Endovasc Surg 2011; 41(Suppl 1):S1–58.

41. Dialetto G, Bortone AS, Covino FE, et al. Fracture of the connecting bar of a stent graft in the thoracic aorta: a diagnosis by echocardiography. J Am Soc Echocardiogr 2004;17(2):189–91.

42. Major A, Guidoin R, Soulez G, et al. Implant degradation and poor healing after endovascular repair

of abdominal aortic aneurysms: an analysis of ex-planted stent-grafts. J Endovasc Ther 2006;13(4): 457–67.

43. Aziz ZA, Naidu PR, Prasad J, et al. Role of multide-tector computed tomography in evaluating compli-cations following endovascular repair of aortic aneurysm. J Cardiovasc Dis Res 2010;1(3):125–9.

44. Yu T, Zhu X, Tang L, et al. Review of CT angiog-raphy of aorta. Radiol Clin North Am 2007;45(3): 461–83.

45. Vulev I, Klepanec A, Balázs T, et al. Endovascular treatment of late in-stent-graft dissection after thoracic endovascular aneurysm repair. Cardio-vasc Intervent Radiol 2011;34(4):864–7.

46. Fiorani P, Speziale F, Calisti A, et al. Endovascu-lar graft infection: preliminary results of an inter-national enquiry. J Endovasc Ther 2003;10(5): 919–27.

47. Calligaro KD, Veith FJ. Diagnosis and management of infected prosthetic aortic grafts. Surgery 1991; 110(5):805–13.

48. Orton DF, LeVeen RF, Saigh JA, et al. Aortic pros-thetic graft infections: radiologic manifestations and implications for management. Radiographics 2000;20(4):977–93.

49. Chiesa R, Melissano G, Marone EM, et al. Aorto-oe-sophageal and aortobronchial fistulae following thoracic endovascular aortic repair: a national sur-vey. Eur J Vasc Endovasc Surg 2010;39(3):273–9.

50. Eggebrecht H, Mehta RH, Dechene A, et al. Aortoesophageal fistula after thoracic aortic stent-graft placement: a rare but catastrophic complication of a novel emerging technique. JACC Cardiovasc Interv 2009;2(6):570–6.

51. Picichè M, De Paulis R, Fabbri A, et al. Postoperative aortic fistulas into the airways: etiology, pathogen-esis, presentation, diagnosis, and management. Ann Thorac Surg 2003;75(5):1998–2006.

52. VonFricken K, Karamanoukian HL, Ricci M, et al. Aortobronchial fistula after endovascular stent graft repair of the thoracic aorta. Ann Thorac Surg 2000; 70(4):1407–9.

Imaging of Abdominal and Pelvic Surgical and Postprocedural Foreign Bodies

CrossMark

Gabriela Gayer, MD[a,b,*], Meghan G. Lubner, MD[c], Sanjeev Bhalla, MD[d], Perry J. Pickhardt, MD[c]

KEYWORDS

- Surgical foreign bodies • Iatrogenic complication • Iatrogenic injury • Implanted devices
- Postprocedural complications • Computed tomography

KEY POINTS

- An intraoperative radiograph obtained to diagnose or exclude a retained foreign object should be carefully scrutinized with particular attention to objects partially visualized at the periphery of the film.
- Radiologists must familiarize themselves with the imaging findings of surgical materials to recognize them as such and raise suspicion of unintentionally retained objects in the appropriate setting.
- Imaging plays a critical role in assessing the proper positioning and function of a wide array of implanted medical devices.
- Postprocedural imaging is useful in the setting of suspected complications stemming from implanted devices.
- Appropriate knowledge of the underlying device in question, including route of placement and expected appearance, is vital when assessing for potential complications.

INTRODUCTION

Every form of medical and surgical treatment, even the most trivial one, carries with it some chance of complications. This risk is usually small, and the benefit of the treatment should clearly outweigh the risk. Treatment-related complications may occur, however, presenting either soon after the intervention or remote from it. In the latter case, the challenge of diagnosing a complication is significant because presenting symptoms are often nonspecific and clinical suspicion of a treatment-related complication is low. It is then the task of the radiologist to recognize such complications, and this can only be achieved if he/she is familiar with the spectrum of normal and abnormal imaging findings pertaining to the treatment the patient had undergone. In this review, the focus is on imaging findings of surgical materials used in abdominal surgery, and of a wide array of implanted abdominal devices. The pertinent complications of these devices and of retained surgical objects are highlighted and illustrated.

SURGICAL FOREIGN BODIES AND MATERIALS

Abdominopelvic surgery makes use of materials such as sponges, needles, and instruments. Many of these remain in the abdominal cavity only temporarily and are removed before its closure. However, some materials or devices are placed in the abdominal cavity for therapeutic

a Department of Radiology, Sheba Medical Center, Sackler School of Medicine, Tel Aviv University, 2 Derech Sheba, Ramat-Gan 52621, Israel; b Department of Radiology, Stanford University Medical Center, 300 Pasteur Drive, Stanford, CA 94304, USA; c Department of Radiology, University of Wisconsin School of Medicine & Public Health, 600 Highland Avenue, Madison, WI 53792-3252, USA; d Mallinckrodt Institute of Radiology, Washington University School of Medicine, 510 South Kingshighway, St Louis, MO 63110, USA
* Corresponding author. Department of Radiology, Sheba Medical Center, Ramat-Gan, Israel 52621.
E-mail address: gayer@post.tau.ac.il

Radiol Clin N Am 52 (2014) 991–1027
http://dx.doi.org/10.1016/j.rcl.2014.05.006
0033-8389/14/$ – see front matter © 2014 Elsevier Inc. All rights reserved.

purposes during surgery and remain there. Radiologists may encounter such items on imaging examinations performed postoperatively and must familiarize themselves with the characteristic findings of these paraphernalia. The first part of this review focuses on imaging findings of surgical objects retained unintentionally in the abdominal cavity. The second part highlights the surgical objects placed there on purpose, with therapeutic intention.

Unintended Retained Surgical Foreign Objects

The unintended retention of a foreign object in a patient after surgery is one of the most devastating errors that affect both patients and health professionals. It is associated with significant morbidity and mortality for the former and with malpractice risk for the latter.[1,2] The exact incidence of such an event has not been determined, but estimates suggest that it occurs in 1 of every 1000 to 1500 intra-abdominal operations.[1] Reports of the most frequently retained items reveal that sponges, followed by instruments, top the list.[1,3]

The current approach to the prevention of a retained foreign object (RFO) relies on a standardized counting protocol of surgical items. However, counting procedures have limitations. One study found that a final count was erroneously thought to be correct in 88% of cases wherein RFOs were detected.[1] Various technological innovations (bar-code scanning, radiofrequency identification detection) may serve to improve or replace the standard sponge-counting protocol and reduce the risk of RFOs. However, these techniques are still undergoing development and evaluation and are not yet widely implemented.

The radiologist may become involved in the detection of a RFO in 2 completely different situations: at the time of surgery and remote from surgery, as discussed below in detail.

The intraoperative, acute phase

When retention of a foreign object is suspected at the end of surgery, a radiograph of the operative site is obtained, and the radiologist is requested to rule out an RFO. This request is most frequently triggered by a mismatch between the preoperative and postoperative sponge/instrument count; that is, when not all materials are accounted for (**Fig. 1**).

Some institutions (eg, Mayo Clinic College of Medicine, Rochester, MN, USA) have implemented the routine screening of all patients who undergo operations involving a body cavity with a postoperative radiograph. The screening takes place in a dedicated radiography suite, before the patients enter the recovery room.[3] However, this procedure has not become common practice worldwide, and most surgical facilities do not routinely obtain postoperative radiographs to look for the radiopaque marker in sponges, and for instruments.

Factors adversely affecting the results of the intraoperative radiograph Intraoperative radiographs currently form the main tool for ruling out a suspected RFO. However, they have several shortcomings that limit their value.[3]

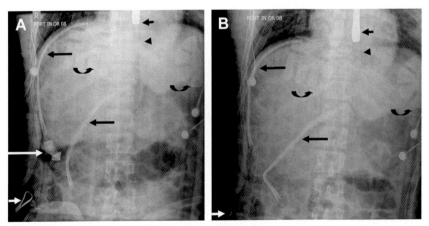

Fig. 1. Retained sponge identified on intraoperative radiograph. (*A*) Radiograph obtained at the end of laparotomy because of a mismatch in sponge count shows multiple radiopaque densities: an esophageal Doppler probe (*short black arrow*), a nasogastric tube (*black arrowhead*), 2 drains (*long black arrows*), several overlying external defibrillator/pacer pads (*curved black arrows*), clamp (*short white arrow*), and a radiopaque marker within a sponge (*long white arrow*) in the right mid abdomen. (*B*) Subsequent radiograph after removal of the sponge shows all previously noted radiopaque densities except for the radiopaque marker within a sponge.

Quality of the radiograph Intraoperative as well as portable early postoperative radiographs may be of suboptimal quality, and therefore, require digital magnification and manipulation of soft copy images to facilitate detection.

The presence of multiple radiopaque foreign objects in the field should be minimized before acquiring the radiograph, because these may obscure the presence of a radiopaque marker (**Fig. 2**).

The adequacy of the field of view should also be evaluated, giving particular attention to partially imaged sponges at the periphery of the film (**Fig. 3**). The radiologist should report to the surgical team if any part of the abdomen is obscured and request a repeat radiograph if possible.

Familiarity with the appearance of the missing object It is imperative that the surgical team requesting the radiograph inform the radiologist not only of a discrepancy in numbers of sponges/instruments but also of the exact nature of the missing object. Most sponges are detectable because they incorporate a radiopaque marker. The body of the sponge itself may be faintly radiodense on ex vivo radiographs, but is unlikely to be visible in vivo. Sponges come in different sizes and with various radiopaque markers embedded or attached to them, and therefore, have different appearances on radiography (**Fig. 4**). Consequently, it is important that the radiologist be notified regarding the type of

the missing sponge and that he/she be familiar with the expected appearance of the specific type of sponge on the radiograph. To this end, radiologists in one center have adopted a strategy to radiograph a duplicate of the missing item at the same time as the patient is radiographed in the operating room. Both images are uploaded together into the picture archiving and communication system side-by-side, thus facilitating perception of the missing object.[4]

Accurate and prompt communication Effective and timely communication between the surgical team and the radiologist is of utmost importance and cannot be overstressed. This communication needs to be bidirectional and requires commitment from both the surgical team and the radiologist. The surgical team needs to communicate the purpose of the radiograph to the interpreting radiologist and provide precise information regarding the missing object. The radiologist needs to prioritize the interpretation and report back promptly to the surgeon before wound closure. Communication should be particularly rapid in case a reason arises to repeat the radiograph, for example, when the image does not display the entire surgical field or when the film reveals artifacts.

Remote from surgery
Suspicion of a RFO in the postoperative period usually arises when a patient undergoes

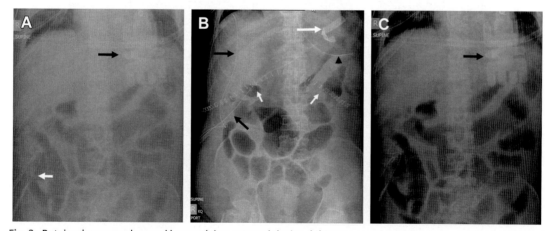

Fig. 2. Retained sponge obscured by overlying external device. (*A*) Intraoperative radiograph obtained at the end of liver transplant surgery because of a mismatch in sponge count shows drains overlying the right mid abdomen (*white arrow*). An external defibrillator/pacer pad (*black arrow*) overlies and partially obscures the left upper abdomen. No additional radiopaque marker within a sponge is visualized. (*B*) Radiograph of the abdomen obtained several hours after closure of the incision shows surgical staples (*short white arrows*). The previously noted external defibrillator/pacer pad has been removed from the left upper quadrant, revealing a radiopaque marker of a retained sponge (*long white arrow*). A nasogastric tube (*black arrowhead*) and drains (*black arrows*) are now present. (*C*) Digital manipulation of the original radiograph did not enable retrospective detection of the radiopaque marker obscured by the external defibrillator/pacer pad (*black arrow*), underscoring the importance of removing external overlying objects before obtaining an intraoperative radiograph.

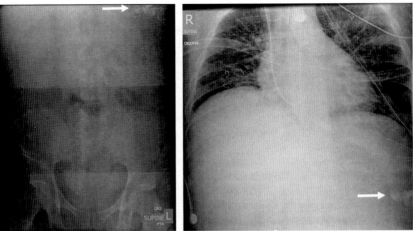

Fig. 3. Overlooked sponge marker at the periphery of an abdominal radiograph. (*A*) Intraoperative radiograph obtained at the end of laparotomy and resection of a very large paraganglioma shows a folded sponge marker (*arrow*) at the left upper edge. This density was overlooked, resulting in closure of abdominal cavity without removal of the sponge. Note the background "bubbly" appearance, typical of a warming blanket. (*B*) Chest radiograph obtained after closure of the abdominal cavity shows the retained sponge marker (*arrow*) in the left upper quadrant of the abdomen.

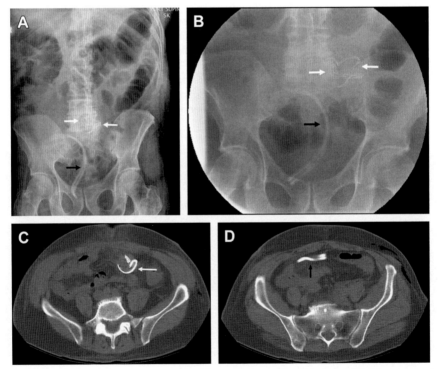

Fig. 4. Retained sponge and a drain in a 71-year-old man 5 days after robotic-assisted laparoscopic prostatectomy. (*A*) Radiograph of the abdomen shows 2 curvilinear opacities: a fine twirled density overlying the lower lumbar spine (*white arrows*) and a wider and denser opacity (*black arrow*) overlying the pelvis. The twirled density is more visible on a subsequent radiograph obtained during fluoroscopy (*B*). This appearance is typical of a radiopaque marker in a sponge that contains 2 barium sulfate blue monofilaments. The wider linear opacity is that of a drain. (*C*) Axial CT shows the dense marker (*arrow*) within a soft-tissue mass containing small air bubbles, a typical appearance of a retained sponge. (*D*) Axial CT at a slightly lower level shows the linear density (*arrow*) representing the drain. Unlike the retained sponge, this linear opacity has no adjacent soft-tissue spongiform mass. This example highlights the importance of familiarity with the radiologic appearance of radiopaque markers of various sponges and differentiating them from intentionally placed surgical objects (eg, a drain).

cross-sectional imaging, mainly computed tomography (CT),[5] and less frequently, magnetic resonance (MR) imaging, ultrasonography, and positron emission tomography–computed tomography (PET/CT). To consider the diagnosis of an RFO remote from surgery, the radiologist must suspect this possibility and also have the expertise to recognize the imaging features of RFOs on these modalities.

Imaging features of retained objects remote from surgery

Sponges

The most common RFO is a surgical sponge, also referred to as a gossypiboma or a textiloma. Retained sponges tend to occur most frequently after emergency surgery, after an unexpected change in the surgical procedure, or in patients with a higher body mass index (BMI).[1,6]

Variable reactions can occur in response to the foreign body. The first kind of body reaction is exudative in nature and often leads to abscess formation, fistula, bowel obstruction, or erosion into adjacent structures.[7,8] Septic complications, mainly abscess formation, are more likely to occur in the early postoperative period.[5] The second kind of body reaction is an aseptic foreign body granuloma with fibroblastic reaction and complete encapsulation. This form usually has no clinically significant symptoms; however, patients can present years later with abdominal pain resulting from mass effect on other abdominal organs.[5,6]

Radiographs The radiological diagnosis of sponges can be difficult because the radiopaque markers on the sponges may become twisted or folded and present an unusual image. If surgery had been in the distant past, a sponge or towel without a marker could have been left behind.[5] As in the case of the intraoperative radiograph, here too artifacts or suboptimal image quality may prevent recognition of the marker (**Fig. 5**).

Computed tomography A retained sponge may have various appearances on CT. It usually appears as a well-circumscribed mass with soft tissue attenuation, a whorled texture, and low-attenuation foci related to gas trapped in the fiber meshwork.[5,8,9] The spongiform pattern with small gas bubbles is a typical CT sign of a textiloma (see **Fig. 4**C; **Fig. 6**).[7-9] The presence of gas bubbles inside the textiloma should therefore not necessarily be interpreted as a sign of a severe complication, particularly an abscess or perforation of the intestine.[7] Associated abscess may be seen appearing as a loculated fluid collection with thick rim enhancement (**Fig. 7**). The radiopaque marker

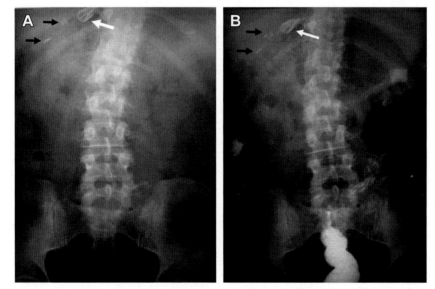

Fig. 5. Overlooked sponge marker at the periphery of a radiograph several weeks after surgery. (*A*) Radiograph of the abdomen in a patient with persistent abdominal pain 6 weeks after cholecystectomy shows a partially imaged laparotomy sponge marker (*white arrow*) medial to cholecystectomy clips (*black arrows*). The main contributing factors as to why this marker was overlooked were the location of the sponge marker at the edge of the film and the low index of suspicion for a retained sponge several weeks after surgery. (*B*) The patient subsequently underwent a barium enema to evaluate his symptoms. Radiograph of the abdomen again shows the radiopaque marker (*white arrow*) medial to cholecystectomy clips (*black arrows*), but various additional dense opacities (contrast material in colon, artifact in left mid abdomen) render the marker less noticeable. The marker was noticed on subsequent reevaluation of the patient's imaging examinations.

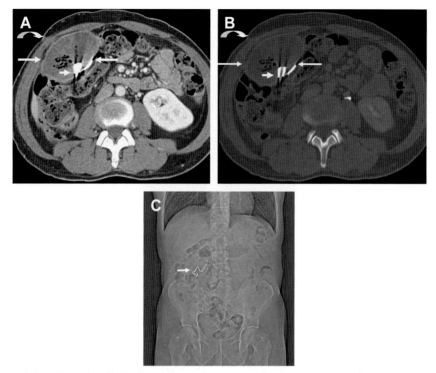

Fig. 6. Sponge left unintentionally in the abdomen. Patient underwent resection of a retroperitoneal liposarcoma 2 months earlier and was asymptomatic. (*A*) Axial contrast-enhanced CT images demonstrates an encapsulated soft-tissue mass (*long arrows*), a retained sponge, with multiple small central air bubbles and a peripheral radiopaque marker (*short arrow*) with associated beam-hardening artifact. Note the adjacent surgical scar at the right abdominal wall (*curved arrow*). (*B*) Bone window shows more clearly the folded radiopaque marker (*short arrow*) within the sponge (*long arrows*). Curved arrow points to surgical scar. (*C*) Scout film of the scan clearly shows the classic appearance of a radiopaque marker (*arrow*).

inside the sponge may not be as obvious on CT as it is on radiographs. Careful inspection of the CT scout is often very helpful in confirming suspicion of a sponge, because the radiopaque marker, which can be obscured by beam-hardening artifacts, is more apparent on the scout (see **Figs. 6**C and **7**E).[7] Clinical correlation is critical in differentiating a retained sterile sponge from a sponge with an associated abscess.

Magnetic resonance A retained sponge typically appears on MR as a well-circumscribed round soft-tissue intensity mass, with T1-weighted intermediate signal intensity, similar to that of skeletal muscle. On T2-weighted images, the mass may have internal high-signal-intensity fluid. Internal wavy low-signal-intensity nonenhancing structures that have a "whorled" appearance, due to the sponge material, are considered indicative of a retained sponge. Postcontrast T1-weighted images show smooth, thick rim enhancement without internal enhancement (**Fig. 8**).[5,8,10]

Ultrasonography The ultrasonographic findings of a retained sponge have been described in a

few case reports as hyperechoic wavy structures with posterior acoustic shadowing.[11,12]

PET/CT A few descriptions of a retained sponge on PET/CT note uneven fluorodeoxyglucose (FDG) uptake at the periphery of a mass. The rim-shaped FDG uptake corresponds to a thick wall with an aseptic fibroblastic reaction and complete encapsulation, while the center of the mass without FDG uptake represents the cavity packed with hematoma and the sponge.[13,14]

Possible pitfalls on cross-sectional imaging Cross-sectional imaging remote from surgery often results in misinterpretations of retained surgical sponges.[7,11,12,15] Several factors contribute to such errors. Most commonly, a retained sponge is completely unexpected and therefore not identified. Other factors concern the embedded radiopaque marker, which is usually the hallmark of a sponge. The marker, that is usually evident on radiographs and CT, is not visible on MR imaging. Another possible pitfall occurs when the radiopaque marker remains unrecognized on CT or is erroneously considered a calcification or

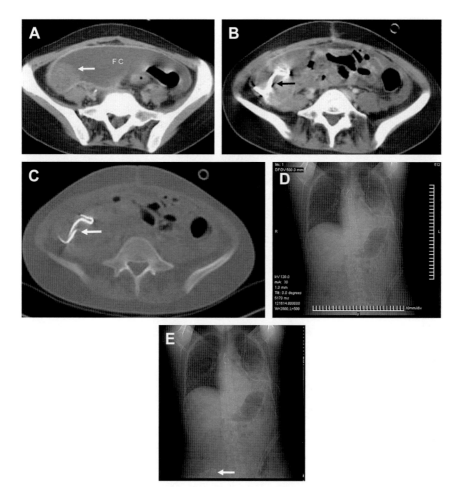

Fig. 7. Retained sponge within a large abscess in a 20-year-old woman presenting with fever and abdominal pain after resection of a large retroperitoneal mass. (*A*) Axial CT shows a large fluid collection (FC) surrounded by enhancing peritoneum. A round soft-tissue mass is present (*arrow*), containing a retained sponge at the periphery of the collection. This mass may potentially be mistaken for a large blood clot. (*B*) Axial CT at a slightly more cranial level shows a linear radiopaque density (*arrow*), which could be mistaken for a drain within a large fluid collection. (*C*) Bone window clearly shows the folded radiopaque marker (*arrow*) within the sponge. (*D*) Scout film of the scan does not clearly show the radiopaque marker. However, after removal of the graphic overlay (*E*), the radiopaque marker is clearly seen (*arrow*).

intestinal contrast material.[7] In addition, old sponges may not have had an embedded radiopaque marker.

The 2 most common misinterpretations of a retained sponge on cross-sectional imaging are the following:

- Tumor: The round, well-defined "masslike" appearance of a retained sponge has been mistaken in the past for various tumors. When found in the peritoneal cavity, the most frequent erroneous diagnosis based on CT has been a gastrointestinal (GI) stromal tumor.[16–18] When encountered in the retroperitoneum in patients who had undergone various procedures related to the kidney

(partial nephrectomy, surgery for urolithiasis), it has been mistaken for renal cell carcinoma, leading in some instances to nephrectomy.[11,12,15]

- Abscess: The appearance of a soft-tissue mass containing gas bubbles, while often considered typical of a retained sponge, may be mistaken for an abscess. Clinical information is important in determining the nature of the mass.

Mimickers of retained sponge on cross-sectional imaging

- Heterotopic ossification in surgical scar: Heterotopic ossification in surgical incisions of the abdomen is thought to represent a

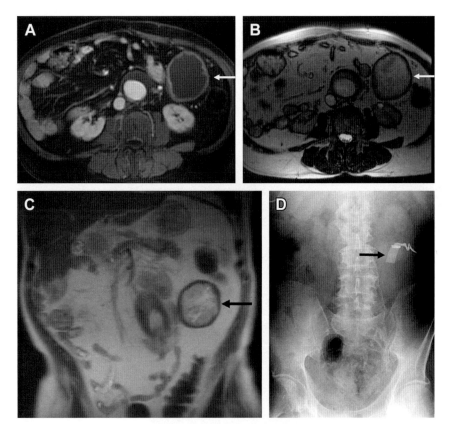

Fig. 8. Retained sponge in a 75-year-old asymptomatic man many years after abdominal aortic aneurysm repair. (*A*) Axial gadolinium-enhanced fat-suppressed T1-weighted gradient echo MR image obtained through the mid abdomen demonstrates a round lesion with smooth thick rim enhancement without internal enhancement (*arrow*). (*B*) Axial T2-weighted single-shot fast spin-echo MR image at the same level shows high-signal intensity fluid with wavy low-signal-intensity structures internally (*arrow*), indicating a retained sponge. (*C*) Coronal T2-weighted single-shot fast spin-echo MR image shows high-signal intensity fluid with wavy low-signal-intensity structures internally (*arrow*), indicating a retained sponge. (*D*) Abdominal radiograph obtained subsequently clearly shows the typical appearance of a radiopaque marker (*arrow*) that is not visible at MR, thus establishing the diagnosis of a retained sponge.

subtype of traumatic myositis ossificans. It usually occurs in midline scars in the upper abdomen and has a heterogeneous appearance with peripheral high density, reflecting heterotopic ossification. The radiologic characteristics as well as the fact the ossification was not present preoperatively may give rise to the erroneous conclusion that it represents an RFO (**Fig. 9**).[19]

• Failed renal transplant: A renal transplant which has failed is not removed, but is usually left in place. Such a failed graft commonly loses its original size and reniform shape, undergoes global shrinkage, and often calcifies heterogeneously. At CT, a failed allograft often appears as an oval soft-tissue mass with coarse calcifications (**Fig. 10**).

This appearance can be confused with a retained sponge. The main clues for the correct diagnosis of the failed transplant are the location of the mass in the iliac fossa and the shrunken native kidneys.[20]

Drains

Retained intraperitoneal drain secondary to fracture is a rare but probably underestimated surgical complication.[21] The diagnosis cannot be accurately established from abdominal radiographs, but is straightforward on CT if the entire course of each drain is carefully evaluated (**Fig. 11**).

Instruments

Instruments are far less frequently retained than sponges, due to their large size. Surgical instruments (eg, clamps) are usually radiopaque and

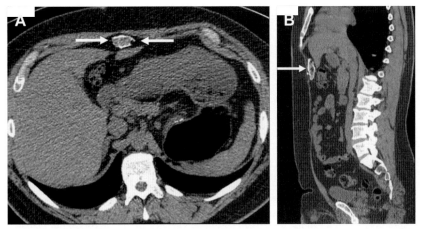

Fig. 9. Mimicker of a retained sponge: heterotopic ossification in a surgical scar. Axial (*A*) and sagittal (*B*) CT images obtained 2 months after surgery show an oval masslike lesion (*arrows*) with a dense calcified rim, located in the midline, caudal to the sternal xiphoid process and anterior to the liver. This lesion may easily be mistaken for a retained foreign body. The midline location of the lesion and its bone density are helpful in correctly identifying heterotopic ossification in the scar.

therefore easily established radiographically (**Figs. 12** and **13**).[22] Most of the known cases have been published in the lay press.[23]

Needles Reports of retained needles are sparse. Surgical needles less than 10 mm are not detectable or are detected with low frequency on intraoperative radiographs.[3]

Intentionally Placed Surgical Materials

Abdominal sponges for packing
Abdominal packing is a life-saving technique for temporary control of severe injury, mainly for liver

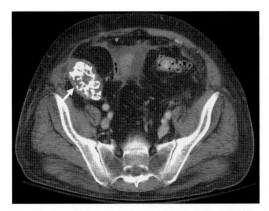

Fig. 10. Mimicker of a retained sponge: a failed renal allograft. Axial unenhanced CT shows an oval soft-tissue mass with coarse calcifications in the right iliac fossa (*arrow*), a shrunken failed renal allograft. The calcifications have a different appearance than the linear density of a sponge marker.

and spleen lacerations. Packing with several large abdominal packs must exert enough pressure to tamponade and slow the bleeding without stopping blood flow through the organ. These packing sponges are typically removed within 48 to 72 hours in the operating room.[24,25] The sponges usually contain radiopaque markers and appear on abdominal radiograph or CT similar to inadvertently retained sponges (**Fig. 14**). The patient might undergo an abdominal radiograph or CT in the interim between placement and removal of the abdominal sponges. Recognition and awareness of the purpose of the sponges are important so as not to mistake them for retained sponges.

Hemostatic agents
It is increasingly common for surgeons to place absorbable hemostatic sponges in the operative cavity. Therefore, the radiologist's familiarity with a sponge's appearance is essential, to recognize it and avoid its misinterpretation as an abscess, a residual tumor, or the recurrence of a tumor.

Absorbable hemostatic sponges may be made of gelatin (Gelfoam; Surgifoam) or oxidized cellulose (Surgicel). These materials appear on CT in the early postoperative period as mixed or low-attenuation masses, often containing collections of gas, either centrally or peripherally (**Figs. 15** and **16**).[26,27] These packing agents are usually absorbed within 7 to 14 days (see **Fig. 16**), but they can mimic the appearance of an abscess at imaging performed before absorption. Abscess formation can also complicate a surgically packed operative site,[26] and therefore, the radiologist's knowledge that absorbable hemostatic sponges

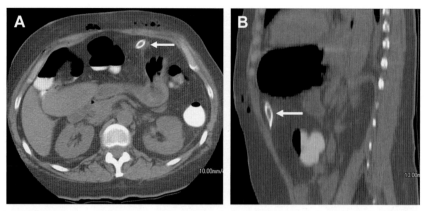

Fig. 11. Fractured drain 2 days after laparoscopic repair of a large hiatal hernia. Axial (*A*) and sagittal (*B*) CT images show a peripherally opaque tubular structure (*arrow*), typical of a drain. On subsequent levels, this drain was seen to dwell entirely within the abdominal cavity. Subcutaneous air bubbles were present due to recent laparoscopic surgery. The retained fractured drain was removed on subsequent laparoscopy. This case underscores the importance of following each drain and tube along their entire course.

have been used should not deter further investigation in the appropriate clinical setting (**Fig. 17**). The usual presence of a radiopaque marker in surgical sponges enables their differentiation from unmarked absorbable hemostatic sponges. Although most hemostatic sponges get absorbed within days or weeks, some of these remain for prolonged periods and may still be encountered many months after surgery (**Fig. 18**).

Prosthetic mesh

Implantation of a prosthetic mesh is frequently used for ventral hernia repair.[28] The mesh is composed of nonabsorbable, inert, sterile, and porous material, with a thickness of up to a millimeter. Its structure ensures early fixation to host tissue with minimal foreign body reaction. The mesh is not visible on radiographs. At CT, some meshes (polypropylene mesh) are seen as a line with attenuation similar to that of the adjacent muscles (**Fig. 19A**), while others (polytetrafluoroethylene mesh) appear as a line of increased attenuation (see **Fig. 19B**).[28]

Bogotá bag

A Bogotá bag is a sterile plastic bag used for temporary closure of the abdominal wall when additional surgical procedures are required, such as

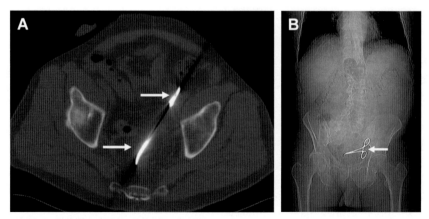

Fig. 12. Retained surgical clamp in a patient presenting with vague abdominal pain 9 months after laparotomy and ileostomy. (*A*) Noncontrast CT soft-tissue window shows 2 adjacent linear opacities of very high attenuation (*arrows*) and associated beam hardening artifact. (*B*) The exact nature of this metallic density, a clamp (*arrow*), is obvious on the scout radiograph. (*Reprinted from* Gayer G, Petrovitch I, Jeffrey RB. Foreign objects encountered in the abdominal cavity at CT. Radiographics 2011;31:421; with permission.)

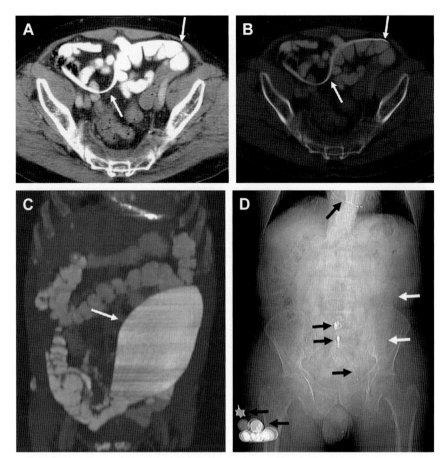

Fig. 13. Unintentionally retained viscera retainer. (*A*) Contrast-enhanced CT scan reveals a curvilinear structure (*arrows*) within the pelvis. Its anterior portion is almost indistinguishable from the contrast material within adjacent bowel loops and is more readily visible on bone window settings (*B*). (*C*) Coronal contrast-enhanced maximum intensity projection image helps to identify the object (*arrow*) as a retained SurgiFish Viscera Retainer (Greer Medical). (*D*) The scout radiograph shows that although the viscera retainer contains barium, it is only mildly radiopaque (*white arrows*) and its presence is not obvious. Black arrows point to multiple incidentally seen radiopaque items (pacer electrode, zipper, surgical clips, coins, and charm). (*Reprinted from* Gayer G, Petrovitch I, Jeffrey RB. Foreign objects encountered in the abdominal cavity at CT. Radiographics 2011;31:422; with permission.)

in case of peritonitis or necrotizing pancreatitis.[29] It is generally a sterilized genitourinary irrigation bag that is sewn to the skin or fascia of the anterior abdominal wall. Use of this technique mandates a subsequent procedure to remove the Bogotá bag and perform a more definitive closure. At CT, the Bogotá bag appears as a linear high-attenuation area in the abdominal wall (**Fig. 20**).

IMPLANTED DEVICES AND POSTPROCEDURAL COMPLICATIONS

A wide array of implanted devices is commonly placed throughout the body to treat or temporize a variety of medical conditions and diseases. Regardless of whether these medical devices are placed under imaging guidance or via percutaneous, endoscopic, or surgical approaches, imaging often plays a critical role in assessing proper positioning and function. Although knowledge of the normal appearance is also important, this section focuses primarily on the imaging diagnosis of device malposition and related postprocedural complications. Conventional radiography, contrast fluoroscopy, ultrasound, and CT may all play an important role in individual cases. A variety of GI, hepatobiliary/pancreatic, genitourinary, vascular, and neurologic devices are considered below.

Gastrointestinal Devices

Several enteric catheters, stents, and bands are in common use. Inappropriate positioning,

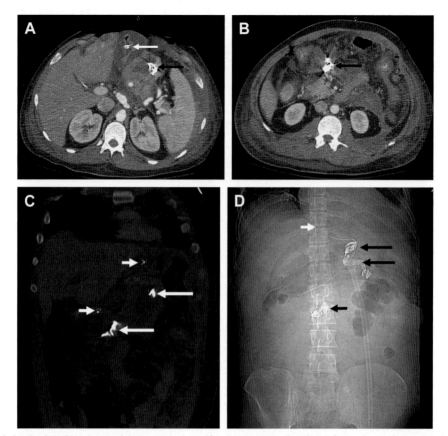

Fig. 14. Abdominal packing in a multitrauma patient after laparotomy. (*A, B*) Axial contrast-enhanced CT images at 2 different levels of the mid abdomen show 2 separate dense sponge markers (*black arrow*). A tubular density (*white arrow, A*) corresponds to a nasogastric tube within the stomach. Note perisplenic hemorrhage and the open abdominal wall (*A*) and left retroperitoneal hemorrhage (*B*). (*C*) Coronal CT reformat, bone window, clearly shows the dense opacity of the 2 sponge markers (*long white arrows*) and the tubular density of the nasogastric tube (*short white arrows*). (*D*) Scout radiograph shows several sponge markers in the left upper quadrant (*long black arrows*) and an additional sponge overlying L3 vertebral body (*short black arrow*). White arrow points to the nasogastric tube.

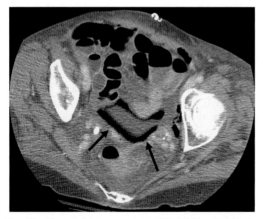

Fig. 15. Absorbable sponges used to achieve hemostasis. Axial contrast-enhanced CT scan 6 days after hysterectomy. A well-defined mouth-shaped hypodensity is present, outlined by peripheral tiny air bubbles in the post-hysterectomy bed, an absorbable sponge (*arrows*).

migration, erosion, occlusion, and perforation all constitute potential complications associated with these devices. This section focuses on the imaging appearances of such complications related to bariatric gastric bands, specific enteric tubes (eg, gastrostomy and nasoenteric), and endoluminal GI stents.

Bariatric gastric bands

Laparoscopic gastric banding is a frequently performed bariatric operation for morbid obesity (BMI>40 kg/m^2) or obesity complicated by other conditions and/or failure of nonsurgical therapy. Although less invasive than a Roux-en-Y gastrojejunal bypass, gastric bands are associated with a relatively high rate of both early and delayed complications that require revision. Band slippage resulting in excessive outlet obstruction and band migration resulting in erosion of the device are

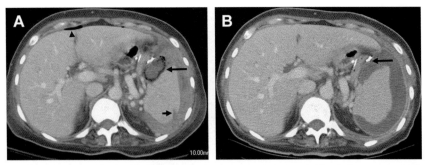

Fig. 16. Absorbable sponge used to achieve hemostasis. Contrast-enhanced CT scan in a patient after Roux-en-Y gastric bypass revision. (A) Axial contrast-enhanced CT image on the sixth postoperative day shows a well-defined oval-shaped hypodensity outlined by peripheral tiny air bubbles, an absorbable sponge (*long arrow*), adjacent to surgical clips. Without the appropriate surgical correlation, such a sponge may be mistaken for a postoperative abscess. Note small peripheral splenic laceration and subcapsular splenic hematoma (*short arrow*), indicating hemorrhage during surgery. A small volume of residual free air is seen anterior to the liver (*arrowhead*). (B) Follow-up CT 8 days later shows complete interval absorption of the sponge (*arrow*). The subcapsular splenic hematoma has liquefied and the residual free air has been absorbed.

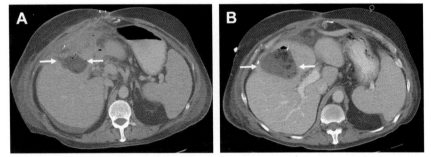

Fig. 17. Absorbable hemostatic sponge (Surgicel) applied during laparoscopic cholecystectomy for gangrenous cholecystitis. (A) Axial contrast-enhanced CT images on the fourth postoperative day shows a well-defined oval-shaped hypodensity outlined by peripheral tiny air bubbles (*arrows*), corresponding to the applied absorbable sponge. (B) Follow-up CT 5 days later shows interval increase in size of the fluid collection in gallbladder bed, compatible with development of an abscess (*arrows*).

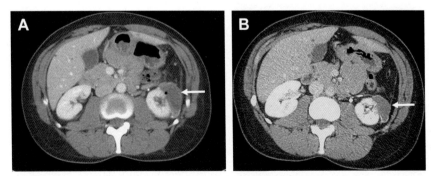

Fig. 18. Unusually long persistence of multiple absorbable hemostatic agents (Surgicel, Floseal, and Tisseel) applied during laparoscopic nephron-sparing surgery for renal cell carcinoma. (A) Axial contrast-enhanced CT 3 months after surgery reveals a round hypodense masslike lesion containing small air bubbles (*arrow*) along the resection line at the periphery of the left kidney. This line corresponds to the applied hemostatic agents. (B) Follow-up CT 1.5 years later shows persistent large hypodense area, only minimally smaller (*arrow*) than on the prior CT examination. Air bubbles are no longer seen and a linear peripheral high density (possibly calcification) is more conspicuous.

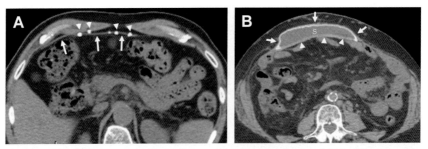

Fig. 19. Different types of mesh used for repair of ventral hernia (hernioplasty) in 2 different patients. (*A*) Axial contrast-enhanced CT shows the mesh as a fine linear density along the anterior abdominal wall (*arrows*). It is attached to the tissues around the hernia site with high-density tacks (*arrowheads*). (*B*) Mesh complicated by development of an adjacent seroma. Axial contrast-enhanced CT shows the mesh as a high-density linear structure (*arrows*) and a low-density seroma (*S*) deep to it. The posterior wall of the seroma consists of enhancing granulation tissue (*arrowheads*) that is of lower density than the mesh.

serious complications that generally necessitate surgical repair.[30]

Normal positioning of the laparoscopic band results in a small gastric pouch. The band itself is typically seen in profile with a slight tilt on abdominal radiographs. Diagnosis of asymptomatic or mildly symptomatic inferior displacement (slippage) of the gastric band may be suggested at radiography but often requires more advanced fluoroscopic and/or CT evaluation (**Fig. 21**). With more advanced symptomatic slippage, an abnormal en face orientation of the band may become evident on the frontal radiograph, termed the "O sign" (**Fig. 22**).[31] An abnormally dilated gastric pouch may also be more apparent on conventional radiographs in advanced cases, but can be readily confirmed at fluoroscopy or CT (see **Fig. 22**). Contrast fluoroscopy allows for functional assessment that can be used to grade the degree

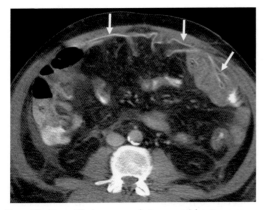

Fig. 20. Bogotá bag, used to provide temporary abdominal closure, when additional laparotomy is indicated. Axial contrast-enhanced CT scan shows a Bogotá bag (*arrows*) as a curvilinear high-attenuation band along the anterior abdominal wall.

of outlet obstruction in cases of band slippage (see **Fig. 22**).

Erosion of the band into the gastric wall is a serious complication. CT evaluation may provide the first clue of subserosal erosion, as nonspecific reactive thickening typically develops adjacent to the band (**Fig. 23**). More advanced endoluminal erosion of the band may result in a greater degree of soft-tissue thickening and air adjacent to the band (see **Fig. 23**), and often extraluminal air or contrast. Frank luminal erosion of the device through the gastric mucosa can be confirmed by endoscopy (see **Fig. 23**) and often requires urgent surgical management.

Enteric tubes

Nasogastric, nasoenteric, gastrostomy, and a variety of other enteric tubes can provide a route for supplemental nutrition or for luminal decompression. The primary complications of these devices relate to malposition, usually related to initial placement. Radiologic evaluation plays a central role in confirming appropriate positioning and detecting complications related to placement. Complications related to mucosal and deeper intramural injury may include ulceration, hemorrhage, and perforation.

Radiologic confirmation of appropriate positioning of enteric feeding tubes is generally required before use. Malpositioning of nasally or orally inserted feeding tubes into the tracheobronchial tree represents a relatively common complication and is easy to recognize with conventional radiography (**Fig. 24**).[32,33] Such airway placement can be completely avoided with the use of real-time fluoroscopy to guide initial placement. A malpositioned enteric tube related to GI perforation will have a less predictable course and may require more advanced imaging for definitive diagnosis (**Fig. 25**). Misplaced percutaneous gastrostomy

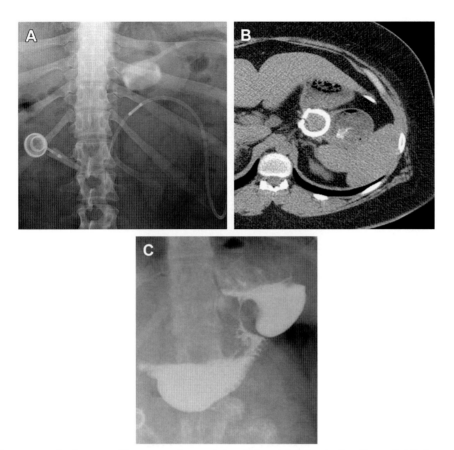

Fig. 21. Asymptomatic slippage of laparoscopic gastric band. Frontal abdominal radiograph (*A*) shows an intact band device with essentially normal orientation. CT (*B*) and contrast fluoroscopic (*C*) examinations show a dilated gastric pouch above the band. Debris is seen within the dilated pouch at CT. Fluoroscopy allows for assessment of dynamic emptying.

tubes often involve the transverse colon because of its proximity to the stomach. Gastrocolic fistula formation is more common with endoscopic placement (percutaneous endoscopic gastrostomy [PEG] tubes) given the lack of radiologic visualization at placement (**Fig. 26**).[34] Malpositioning of a gastrostomy within the transverse colon can be easily confirmed with contrast administration (**Fig. 27**). Some other less common complications may require CT evaluation for proper assessment (**Fig. 28**). Regardless, radiologic confirmation of appropriate positioning should always precede tube feeds (see **Figs. 24** and **28**).

Endoluminal GI stents

Endoscopic placement of metallic stents within the esophagus, gastroduodenum, and colorectum is usually a palliative measure for inoperable malignant strictures, perforations, or fistulae (**Fig. 29**).[35–37] Stent complications are fairly common and include migration, occlusion, bleeding, and perforation. Radiographs can be used to suggest stent migration (**Fig. 30**) or detect discontinuity, but contrast fluoroscopy, CT, or endoscopy is often required to adequately assess for complications.

Hepatobiliary and Pancreatic Devices

A variety of hepatobiliary and pancreatic stents is commonly used in the setting of portal hypertension, biliary obstruction, or biliary/pancreatic leak. As with GI devices, misplacement, occlusion, migration, erosion/fistulization, or perforation represents potential complications of these devices. This section focuses on the use of transjugular intrahepatic portosystemic shunts (TIPS), biliary endoprostheses, and pancreatic stents.

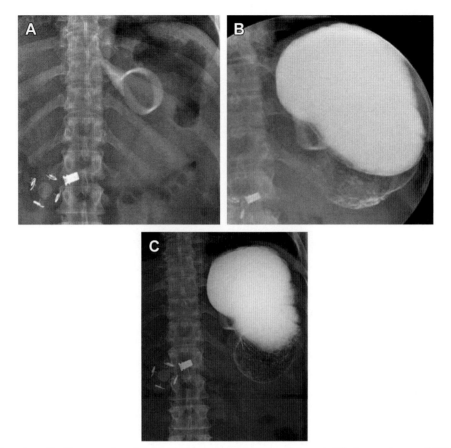

Fig. 22. Symptomatic slippage of gastric band. Frontal abdominal radiograph (*A*) shows abnormal tilting of the gastric band with en face orientation (the "O" sign), suggesting significant slippage, which is confirmed at contrast fluoroscopy (*B*) demonstrating a markedly dilated gastric pouch. A 2-hour delayed radiograph (*C*) shows lack of emptying through the band, consistent with high-grade obstruction.

TIPS

TIPS placement is an effective means for treating complications of portal hypertension, particularly refractory variceal bleeding or ascites. However, shunt dysfunction is relatively common. Causes of early shunt dysfunction (<30 days) include stent shortening, migration (**Fig. 31**), and stenosis/ thrombosis, which can be related to transection of a bile duct, and TIPS-biliary fistula when bare stents are used (**Fig. 32**).[38,39] Later causes of shunt dysfunction include nonthrombogenic parenchymal stenosis or pseudointimal hyperplasia, which occurs most commonly in the cephalic or hepatic venous end of the stent (**Fig. 33**). The fibroblasts of the hepatic parenchyma differentiate into myofibroblasts, which migrate from the adjacent parenchyma into the stent, leading to tissue overgrowth of the lumen.[40] In addition, leaving the proximal portion of the hepatic vein uncovered by the stent can predispose to development of hepatic venous stenosis, because of vascular intimal hyperplasia from shear stress related to turbulent, high-velocity blood flow.[41] These intimal and pseudointimal stenoses can form months to years after stent placement. A less common cause of late stent stenosis or occlusion is tumor thrombus related to hepatocellular carcinoma.[42] Hypercoagulable states (as seen with Budd-Chiari) and extrahepatic hemodynamic flow-stealing states such as varices or spontaneous mesocaval shunts can also lead to shunt dysfunction.

Imaging with conventional venography and measurement of portosystemic pressures represent the reference standard for determination of TIPS dysfunction, with demonstration of a portocaval pressure gradient greater than 12 mm Hg and focal

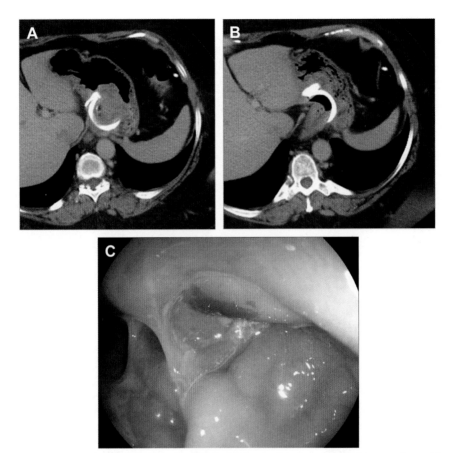

Fig. 23. Erosion of gastric band into lumen of stomach. Abdominal CT images (*A, B*) in a patient with worsening abdominal pain and dysphagia show asymmetric gastric wall thickening along a portion of the band (*A*) and luminal gas immediately adjacent to another portion (*B*). Same-day upper endoscopy (*C*) confirmed erosion of the band into the gastric lumen, which required surgical exploration.

luminal narrowing seen in the setting of stenosis.[43] Sonography is the most frequently used screening tool for detecting early shunt dysfunction. Ultrasound is often performed 1 week to 1 month following TIPS placement to document baseline velocity values. Abnormal velocities include portal vein flow of less than 30 cm/s, flow within the TIPS less than 90 cm/s or greater than 190 cm/s, or a change in velocity of greater than 50 cm/s compared with a prior examination. Reversal of flow direction in the portal vein (away from the TIPS), recanalization of varices, and recurrent ascites can also suggest TIPS dysfunction.[44,45]

Biliary endoprostheses
Biliary stents are placed for biliary decompression in the setting of biliary obstruction related to both benign and malignant causes, as well as for treatment of bile leak.[46,47] The most common reason

for biliary stent placement is choledocholithiasis.[47] These stents may vary in diameter and length and may be plastic or metallic, depending on the indication for use. Complications of these stents include misplacement or displacement, bleeding (**Fig. 34**), occlusion, cholangitis, stent fracture or collapse, and bowel perforation or obstruction (**Figs. 35** and **36**).[48–51] Malignant stenoses are more prone to complications than benign types. Endoscopic retrograde cholangiopancreatography (ERCP) images are often used to guide stent placement, and complications related to stent location may be recognized immediately on these images. However, many complications may be discovered on or confirmed with multi-detector CT. Stent dislocation or migration is estimated to occur 6% of the time.[51] Bowel perforation (most commonly duodenal), which is estimated to occur 1% of the time, is a surgical emergency and may

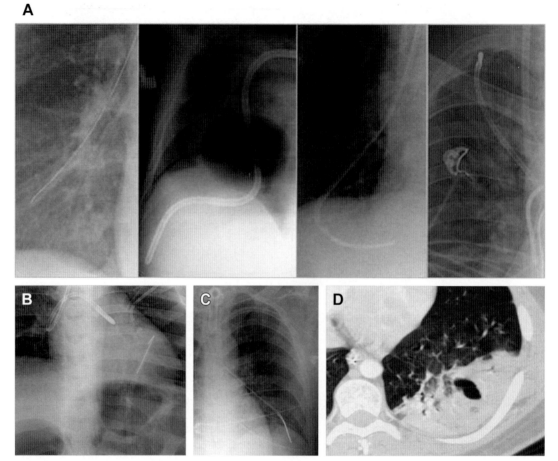

Fig. 24. Tracheobronchial placement of feeding tubes. Collage of radiographic images (*A*) showing tube placement in the right lower lobe (*first 3 images*) and right upper lobe (*last image*). Coiling of the tube at the carina is shown in *B*. Left lower lobe placement in *C* was not corrected before initiating tube feeds, resulting in air-space filling (*D*).

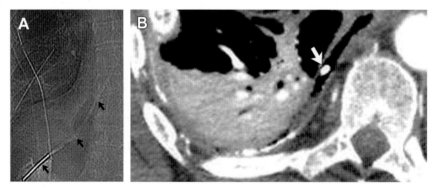

Fig. 25. Feeding tube extending through an esophageal perforation related to endoscopic treatment of Barrett esophagus. Frontal radiograph (*A*) shows an abnormal course of the feeding tube (*arrows*), which does not correspond to the tracheobronchial tree. CT (*B*) confirms pleural location of tube (*arrow*).

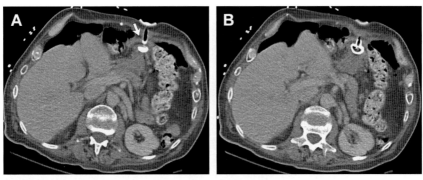

Fig. 26. Gastrocolic fistula related to endoscopic placement of a gastrostomy tube. CT images (*A, B*) show the PEG tube piercing the transverse colon (*arrow, A*) en route to the stomach.

demonstrate leak of contrast on ERCP, and retro-peritoneal air and an extraluminal stent on CT (see **Fig. 36**).

Pancreatic stents

Pancreatic stents are used in the setting of pancreatic duct leak or fistula, most commonly related to acute or chronic pancreatitis, trauma, surgery, or malignancy.[52] Pancreatic stents are most effective when the leak is able to be bridged by the stent.[53] Complications include migration, persistent ductal leak (**Fig. 37**), and stent occlusion. The stents are often placed during ERCP, but can be visualized on radiographs or CT.

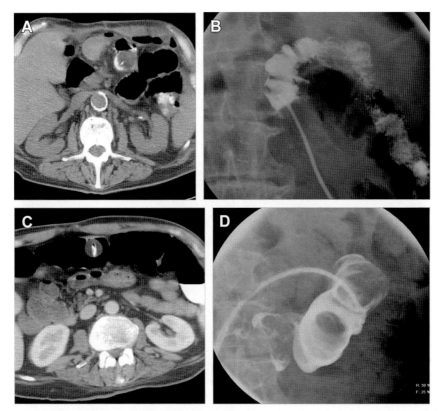

Fig. 27. Malpositioning of PEG tube within the transverse colon. CT image (*A*) shows the balloon of the gastrostomy tube adjacent to the gas-filled stomach. Fluoroscopic image after contrast injection (*B*) confirms location within the transverse colon. CT (*C*) and fluoroscopic contrast (*D*) images in 2 additional different patients show transverse colon malposition of gastrostomy tubes.

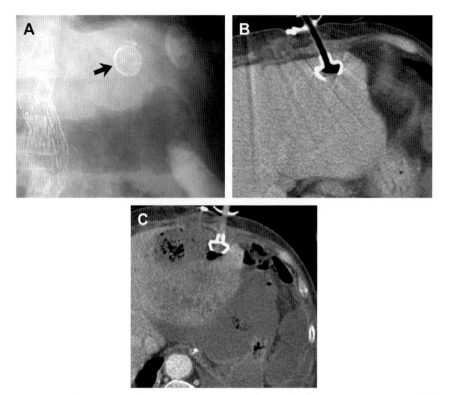

Fig. 28. Displacement of PEG tube within the liver. Frontal radiograph of the upper abdomen (*A*) shows a PEG tube (*arrow*) that appears to overlie the liver. CT image (*B*) confirms that the tip projects into the left hepatic lobe. Unfortunately, malpositioning was ignored and tube feeds were started, resulting in intrahepatic and peri-hepatic abscess formation (*C*).

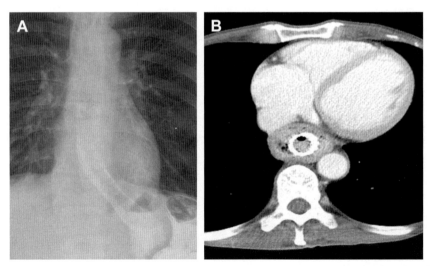

Fig. 29. Palliative esophageal stent placement for inoperable cancer. Frontal radiograph (*A*) and CT (*B*) shows an esophageal stent in good position, although intraluminal debris and/or tumor ingrowth later caused stent occlusion.

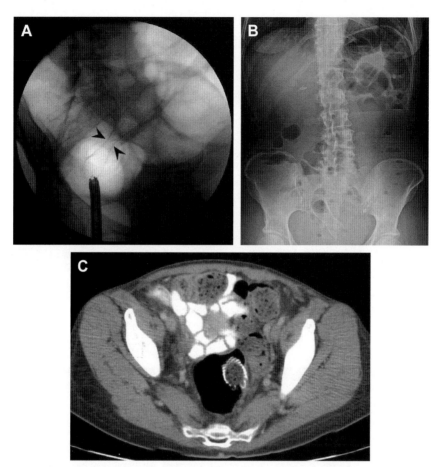

Fig. 30. Migration of a colonic stent in patient with occlusive cancer. Fluoroscopic image obtained during endoscopic stent placement (*A*) shows waistlike narrowing (*arrowheads*) related to the annular-constricting cancer. Subsequent radiograph (*B*) shows interval change in the orientation of the stent, as well as inferior displacement, with associated findings of developing obstruction. CT (*C*) shows inferior displacement of the stent, as well as debris within its lumen.

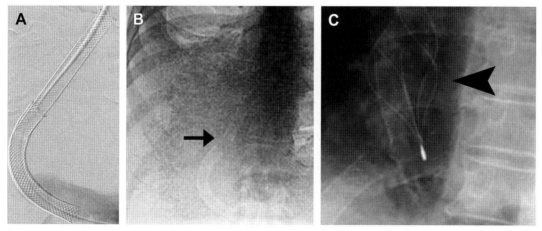

Fig. 31. Stent migration. Digital subtraction angiography (DSA) image at the conclusion of TIPS placement (*A*) demonstrates 2 overlapping stents. Follow-up bone subtraction radiograph (*B*) demonstrates separation of the stents with migration of the cephalad stent into the region of the right atrium (*arrow*). Intraoperative fluoroscopic image (*C*) during stent retrieval demonstrates a basket capturing the migrated stent (*arrowhead*), which was successfully removed.

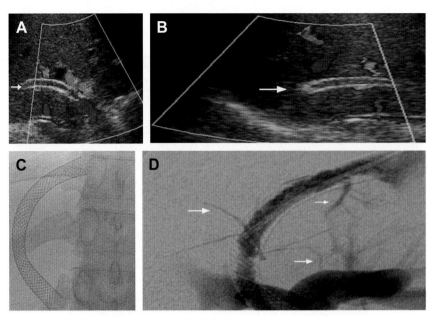

Fig. 32. Stent occlusion due to biliary-TIPS fistula. Color Doppler ultrasound (US) images (*A, B*) demonstrate absent flow throughout the shunt 1 week following placement (*arrows*), representing thrombosis. Scout (*C*) and DS image from portohepatic venography (*D*) demonstrate narrowing of the TIPS lumen due to circumferential thrombus, with opacification of multiple small biliary radicles (*arrows*), indicating a biliary-TIPS fistula.

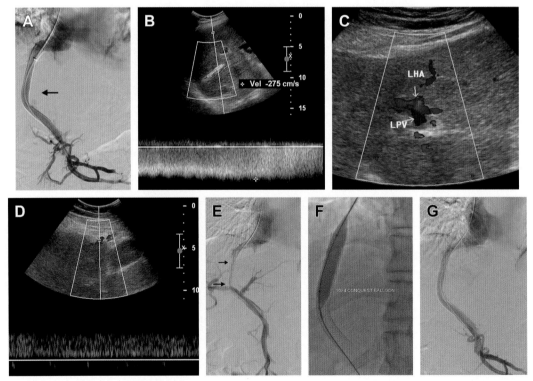

Fig. 33. TIPS stenosis from pseudointimal hyperplasia. Digital subtraction portal venogram image (*A*) demonstrates initial placement of TIPS (*arrow*). Follow-up US demonstrates focal flow abnormality in the mid shunt with velocities up to 275 cm/s on pulsed Doppler (*B*), as well as reversal of flow in the left portal vein (away from the TIPS) on color Doppler (*C*), and flow out of a recanalized umbilical vein (*D*), suggestive of shunt dysfunction. Repeat portal venogram image (*E*) demonstrates diffuse luminal narrowing involving the mid and distal portions of the stent (*arrows*) with elevated portosystemic gradient of 22 mm Hg, consistent with pseudointimal stenosis. Balloon dilation was performed (*F*) with improved luminal patency (*G*) and decreased gradient to 14 mm Hg.

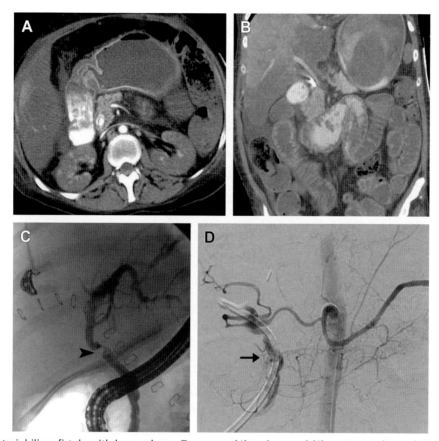

Fig. 34. Arteriobiliary fistula with hemorrhage. Transverse (*A*) and coronal (*B*) contrast-enhanced CT images in a patient following liver transplantation demonstrate a large amount of high attenuation material in the stomach and proximal small bowel, caused by active extravasation of intravenous contrast into the biliary tract (ie, severe, active hemobilia). ERCP image (*C*) obtained earlier demonstrates a chronic anastomotic stricture (*arrowhead*) treated with long-term indwelling biliary stent. DSA image from celiac injection, obtained immediately after CT (*D*), demonstrates active extravasation of contrast along the course of the biliary stent (*arrow*) caused by erosion of the stent into the adjacent hepatic arterial structures.

Persistent pancreatic leak may manifest as a focal fluid collection, pancreatic ascites, or a pleural effusion.

Genitourinary Devices

A variety of devices can be used in the genitourinary system with a spectrum of complications related to stent location/migration, obstruction/infection, and perforation. This section focuses on intrauterine devices (IUDs) and urinary stents.

IUDs

IUDs are commonly used for contraception. IUDs consist of a T-shaped polyethylene frame with a copper wire or levonorgestrel-containing collar along the stem with a monofilament string at the base of the stem. Complications related to IUD migration from the expected location in the endometrial cavity at the uterine fundus are commonly encountered and range in severity.[54,55] Commonly encountered complications include expulsion, displacement, and uterine perforation. Late complications include infection, specifically with *actinomycosis* species in patients with long-term IUDs (**Fig. 38**).[56]

Various imaging modalities can be used for evaluation of IUDs. Ultrasound can be used to easily determine IUD position and can demonstrate displacement or myometrial perforation. 3D ultrasound images can be a helpful adjunct in determining IUD position and are becoming part of the routine evaluation of IUDs (**Fig. 39**). At ultrasound, the stem of a properly placed IUD is straight and

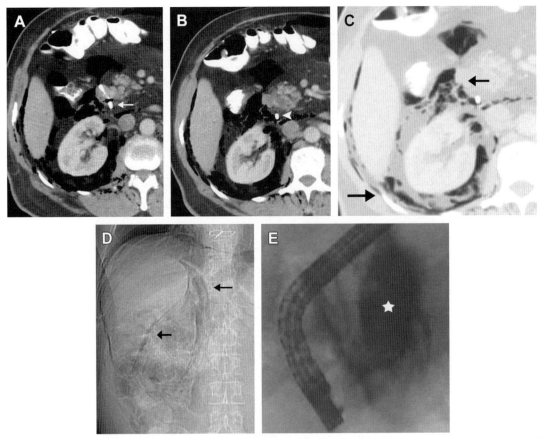

Fig. 35. Biliary stent perforation. Transverse CT images (*A, B*) demonstrate a biliary stent in the duodenum (*arrow*) with the tip extending outside the duodenal lumen (*arrowhead, B*), with retroperitoneal air, better seen on lung window (*C*) and scout (*D*) images (*arrows*). ERCP image (*E*) demonstrates retroperitoneal leak of contrast (*star*).

completely within the endometrial cavity, with the arms extending laterally at the fundus, approximately 3 mm from the top of the uterine cavity. Abdominal radiographs can also be helpful in suggesting an extrauterine IUD and are necessary for making a diagnosis of IUD expulsion. The IUD should be readily identified on radiographs if it has not been expelled. Expulsion occurs in up to 10% of patients, may be partial or complete, and impairs contraceptive effectiveness (**Fig. 40**).[55] CT can be used for evaluation of IUD position, but is best applied in the evaluation of complications associated with intra-abdominal IUDs, including abscess and bowel perforation. MR imaging is not typically used for IUD localization, but modern IUDs are largely MR-compatible.[54]

IUD displacement within the endometrial cavity is reported in up to 25% of patients.[57] Uterine perforation is an uncommon but serious complication, seen in about 1 in 1000 cases.[58] Perforation is variable in extent and may be seen as embedment

in the myometrium (**Fig. 41**), to complete transuterine perforation with migration into the peritoneal cavity (**Figs. 42** and **43**).[59] Complete uterine perforation and intra-abdominal migration can lead to adhesion formation, hemorrhage, bowel perforation, and abscess formation.

Ureteral stents

Indications for ureteral stent placement include relief of benign or malignant urinary tract obstruction, particularly as an adjunct to stone therapy, management of urine leak related to trauma, surgery, or fistula, or as a perioperative tool in the setting of stone disease, renal transplantation, and pelvic surgery. Most ureteral stents are made from polyurethane alone or combined with other materials and have a double-J configuration with proximal and distal pigtails to decrease migration. Complications of ureteral stents include malposition or migration, urinary tract infection, encrustation, stent occlusion, fracture and ureteral

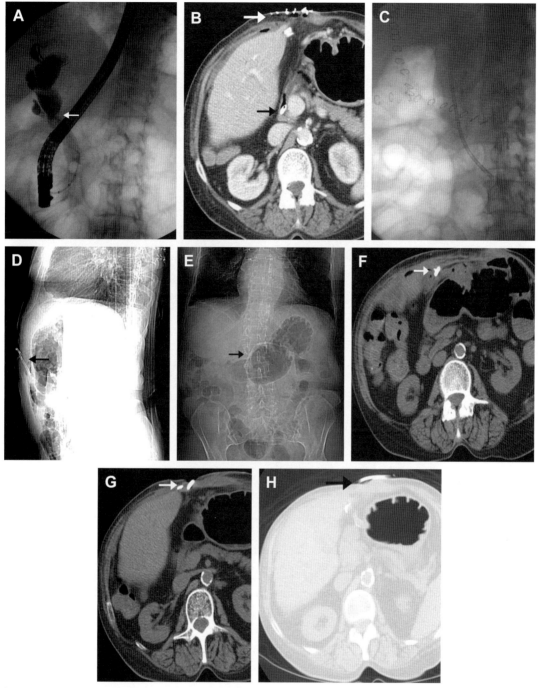

Fig. 36. Biliary stent migration, erosion, and fistulization to the skin. ERCP image (*A*) in a patient following liver transplantation demonstrates an anastomotic stricture (*arrow*). The patient was taken to the operating room for ventral hernia repair revision, removal of infected body wall mesh, and placement of a biliary stent, with postoperative changes in the body wall (*white arrow*) and biliary stent (*black arrow*) seen on CT (*B*) and ERCP (*C*). Several months later, patient noted her body wall wound had not healed and that some sort of tubing was present in the wound. Lateral (*D*) and AP scouts (*E*) from CT demonstrate a change in the position of the stent (*arrows*), now seen in the central upper abdomen extending to the skin. Axial noncontrast CT images (*F, G*) show that the stent has migrated into bowel, and fistulized with the body wall, now extending out of the skin, with the external portion of the stent (*arrow*) seen on lung window setting (*H*).

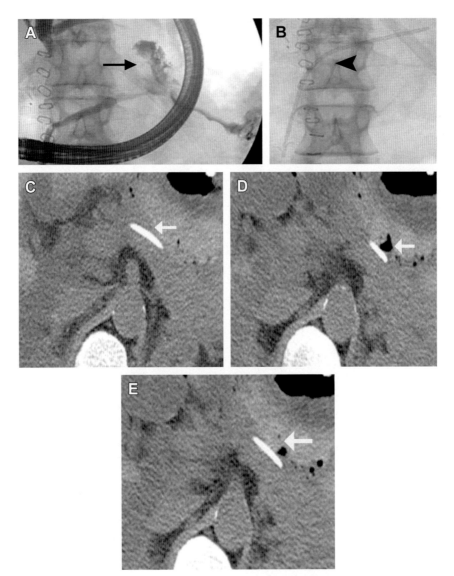

Fig. 37. Stent exposure and persistent pancreatic leak. ERCP image (*A*) demonstrates a pancreatic duct leak (*arrow*) in this patient with necrotizing pancreatitis, with subsequent stent placement (*arrowhead, B*). Progressive pancreatic necrosis led to stent exposure (*arrows*), seen on noncontrast CT images (*C–E*), with persistent pancreatic leak and pancreatic ascites. The patient ultimately underwent distal pancreatectomy.

erosion, perforation, and fistulization. Stents are often placed under fluoroscopic guidance in the operative setting. Stent position can be assessed following placement by radiography, ultrasound, or CT. The latter 2 modalities have the added capability of showing secondary signs of incomplete urinary tract decompression or leak in the setting of stent migration, occlusion, or perforation (**Fig. 44**). Ureteral erosion or fistulization is a rare but very serious complication, particularly when

the stent erodes into the adjacent arterial system, and can be assessed with CT or conventional angiography (**Fig. 45**).

Vascular Devices

Vascular devices include both arterial and venous devices. Most commonly, these include inferior vena cava (IVC) interruption filters and endovascular aortic repair (EVAR) stent grafts, the latter of

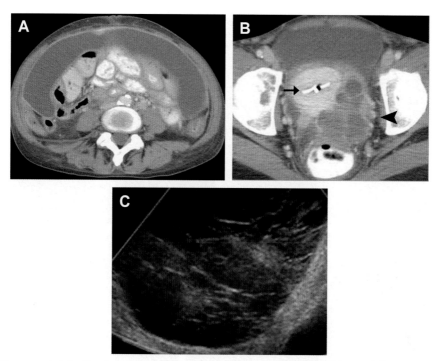

Fig. 38. Actinomycosis infection in a patient with a long-term IUD. Transverse CT image (A) demonstrates perito-neal thickening, enhancement, and ascites, indicating peritonitis. CT image of the pelvis (B) shows an IUD (arrow) in the endometrial cavity as well as a complex left adnexal collection (arrowhead). Color Doppler US image (C) shows a complex tubal collection representing a tubo-ovarian abscess.

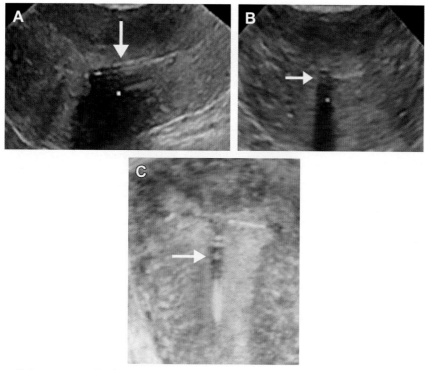

Fig. 39. Normally levonorgestrel-releasing IUD. Sagittal (A) and transverse (B) gray-scale US images demonstrate the IUD in the endometrial cavity (arrows), but the 3D US image (C) gives a more robust depiction of the IUD loca-tion (arrow).

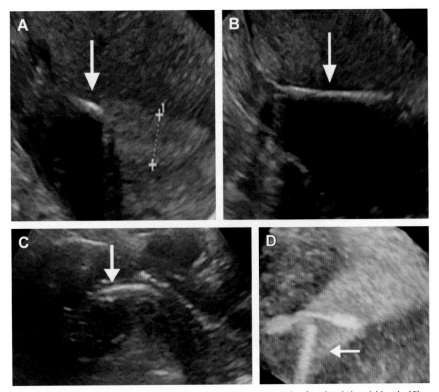

Fig. 40. Displaced, partially expelled IUD. Sagittal gray-scale images at the fundus (*A*), mid body (*B*), and cervix (*C*) demonstrate a low-lying IUD (*arrows*) extending into the cervix. Again, the 3D US image (*D*) gives a more global view of the low-lying IUD (*arrow*). A cervical location of the IUD is associated with increased incidence of unintended pregnancy.

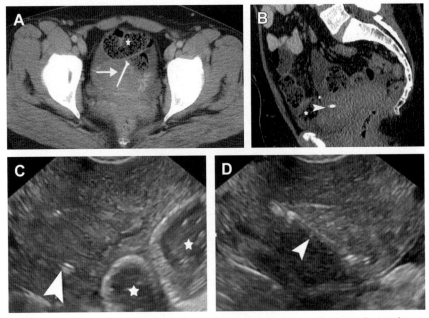

Fig. 41. Myometrial embedment. Transverse CT image (*A*) demonstrates a tilted IUD located near the uterine fundus (*arrow*). Sagittal CT image (*B*) demonstrates one of the T arms extending into the myometrium (*arrowhead*). Transverse and longitudinal gray-scale US images (*C, D*) demonstrate extension of the T arm into the myometrium (*arrowheads*). Note the dilated fecalized bowel loops seen on both CT and US (*stars*). At surgery, minimal perforation of the T arm was found with associated formation of omental adhesions.

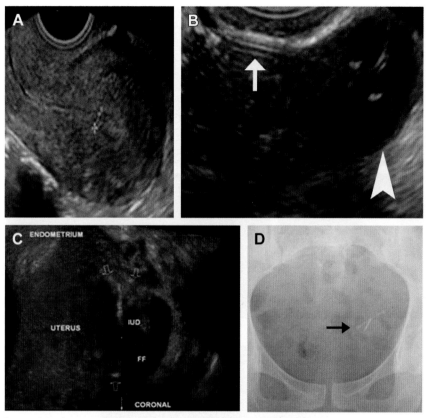

Fig. 42. Uterine perforation. Longitudinal gray-scale US image (*A*) demonstrates an empty endometrial cavity in a patient with history of IUD placement. US image of the left adnexa (*B*) demonstrates an echogenic device (*arrow*) adjacent to the left ovary (*arrowhead*). 3D US image (*C*) again demonstrates the IUD (*small arrows*) adjacent to the uterus in the left adnexa, as shown on an abdominal radiograph (*arrow, D*). FF, free fluid.

which are covered in another article in this issue by Christensen and colleagues. Radiopaque coils and smaller caliber stents may also be encountered.

IVC filters

IVC filters are usually reserved for patients with previously diagnosed thromboembolic disease who have either failed anticoagulation or are unable to receive anticoagulation (eg, recent surgery, fall risk, or intracranial metastases).[60] The recent development of retrievable filters has widened the application of IVC filters, especially in the perioperative period.[61] Imaging is rarely performed for the follow-up of IVC filters; however, they are almost always radiopaque and frequently seen incidentally on radiography and CT. IVC

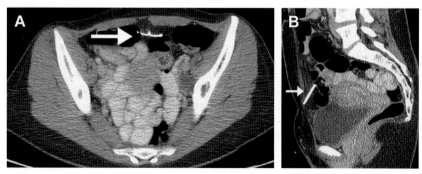

Fig. 43. Uterine perforation. Transverse (*A*) and sagittal (*B*) CT images demonstrate an empty endometrial cavity, with the IUD seen anterior to the uterus (*arrows*) abutting multiple bowel loops.

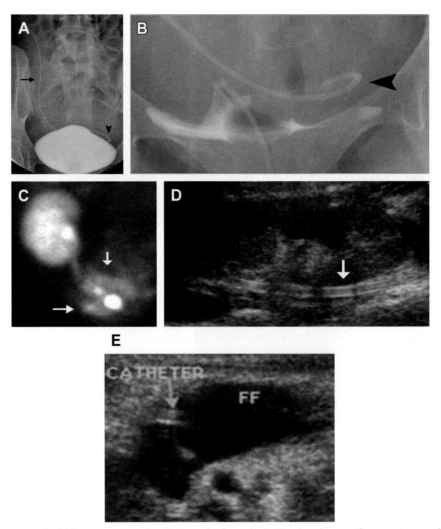

Fig. 44. Anastomotic dehiscence, stent migration, and urinary leak. Overhead image from cystogram (*A*) in a patient with a right lower quadrant renal transplant demonstrates a double-J ureteral stent (*arrow*), with the tip located along the left lateral aspect of the bladder (*arrowhead*). On the postvoid image (*B*), the catheter seems to be located slightly superior, lateral to the bladder contour (*arrowhead*). Postvoid image from technetium-99m MAG 3 renal scintigraphy (*C*) demonstrates residual radiotracer accumulating around the bladder (*arrows*). Grayscale US image of the transplant (*D*) demonstrates the stent (*arrow*) in the renal collecting system, but US image of the pelvis (*E*) demonstrates the catheter (*small arrow*) outside the bladder with surrounding free fluid (FF). Dehiscence of the ureteral anastomosis was found at surgery with the stent migrated out the dehiscence, posterior to the bladder.

filters are usually placed below the renal veins. Occasionally, a suprarenal filter may be placed (**Fig. 46**) when there is a circumaortic left renal vein, gonadal vein thrombosis, duplicated IVC, thrombus in the infrarenal IVC, or in planned pelvic surgery (because of concern for potential dislodgement).[62] Knowledge of the high purposeful location is important to prevent confusion with an embolized or migrated filter.

Overall, IVC filters are considered safe, with a major complication rate of less than 1%.[60] Complications that may be encountered on imaging include filter tilt, caval perforation, filter migration/embolization, and IVC thrombosis. When a complication is suspected, CT is usually the first line of imaging, although radiography may be used to detect unsuspected complications. Because of the artifacts associated with the metal

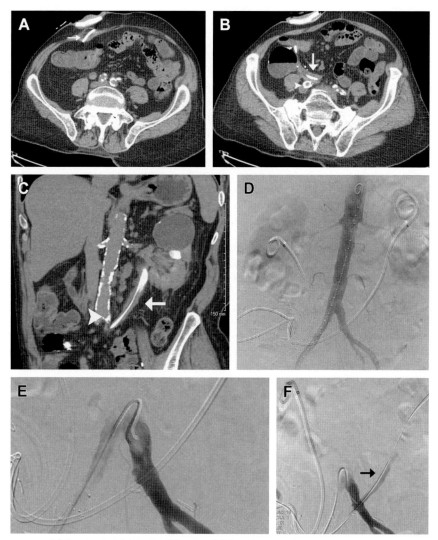

Fig. 45. Ureteroarterial fistula. Axial (*A, B*) and coronal (*C*) CT images demonstrate a right lower quadrant ileal conduit containing a left ureteral stent (*arrows*) seen crossing the left iliac artery (*arrowheads*) before exiting the urostomy in this patient with a history of bladder carcinoma, cystectomy, and radiation therapy. The patient developed hematuria and hemodynamic instability in the operating room at the time of stent change, so the stent was replaced and conventional angiography was performed. With the stent in place, DSA images obtained during injection of the aorta (*D*) and left common iliac artery (*E*) demonstrate no extravasation of contrast. However, when the stent was removed over a wire and the left iliac artery was reinjected, DSA image (*F*) demonstrates active extravasation (*arrow*), indicating a ureteroarterial fistula.

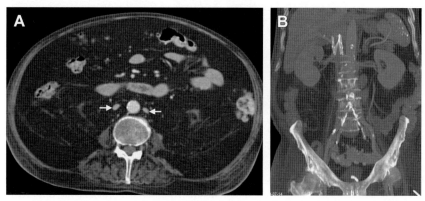

Fig. 46. Suprarenal IVC filter placement. Axial CT image (*A*) shows a duplicated infrarenal IVC (*arrows*). For this reason, an IVC filter was placed in a suprarenal location seen on coronal maximum intensity projection (MIP) image (*B*).

components of many filters, ultrasound and MR are not routinely performed to evaluate IVC filters. When CT is equivocal, the next step is usually catheter venography.

Slight tilt of the filter may be seen after deployment (**Fig. 47**). When the filter is tilted greater than 15° from vertical (parallel to the IVC long axis), it may be less effective in preventing emboli, and there is an increase in the frequency of perforation of the caval wall (see **Fig. 46**).[63] The orientation of the IVC filter can readily be appreciated on an abdominal radiograph or CT coronal reformations.

Caval perforation is defined by the extension of one or more IVC filter struts beyond 3 mm of the IVC lumen and is very common.[63] However, these perforations are usually asymptomatic and clinically insignificant. Although very rare, perforations of small bowel, aorta, and ureter have been reported, as has retroperitoneal hematoma as an IVC filter complication.[64]

Filter migration is diagnosed when the filter has moved 2 cm on imaging.[63] As with perforation, migration is usually asymptomatic and clinically inconsequential. Rarely, migration across a major venous tributary may result in visceral venous thrombosis and end organ damage. The most serious potential complication is filter embolization to another location (**Fig. 48**). Although the entire filter may embolize, usually only a portion of the filter dislodges, particularly a broken strut.[61] These embolized pieces should be reported because they usually end up in the right heart (either atrium or ventricle). Retrieval is attempted only if the risk of intervention is thought to be less than the risk to the patient from the filter fragment.

IVC thrombosis may result in about 10% of patients who receive permanent IVC filters.[64] The net effect may be extensive collateral formation in the retroperitoneum and abdominal wall. Newer materials may be less thrombogenic and decrease the incidence of this complication.[61]

Miscellaneous vascular devices

Besides TIPS and EVARs, vascular stents may be used in other veins and arteries. Accordingly, their size and orientation will vary. Complications, including infection, stenosis, and thrombosis, may be identified. Usually these are detected on radiography but are better evaluated with CT, MR, or ultrasound. Gore-Tex grafts frequently used for aortic arterial bypass may also be seen on radiography. As with the other stents, they are usually detected on radiography but are better characterized on cross-sectional imaging examinations.

Another potential vascular foreign body is an embolization coil. These embolization coils are used to achieve hemostasis and are often used in the setting of a bleeding aneurysm/pseudoaneurysm following surgery or trauma. Coils offer the advantages of ease of use, availability, and rapid deployment.[65] Their main disadvantage is that they can only be used in larger arteries, and that if deployed too proximally, may result in collateral vessel formation. Other agents used in smaller arteries, such as gelfoam, glue, and ethanol, will not be visible on imaging unless they are mixed with radiopaque contrast.

Occasionally, a central catheter will be placed into an external iliac vein or artery. Central catheters are usually temporary lines that are placed in

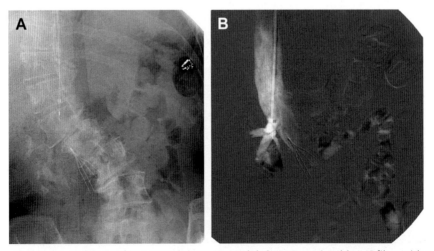

Fig. 47. Normal placement of an IVC filter. Coned-down image (*A*) shows a retrievable IVC filter with a prominent tilt. However, the patient has moderately severe scoliosis. The cavagram (*B*) confirms that the long axis of the IVC is nearly parallel to the long axis of the filter.

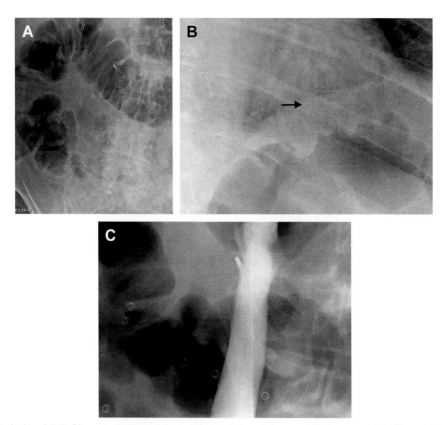

Fig. 48. Embolized IVC filter strut. Coned-down view of the abdomen (*A*) shows an IVC filter with abnormal orientation and configuration. Magnified view of the heart (*B*) confirms an embolized strut overlying the right ventricle (*arrow*). Patient went for possible percutaneous extraction. However, cavagram (*C*) showed that the filter had fractured and perforated the IVC. The patient went on to open extraction of the filter and strut.

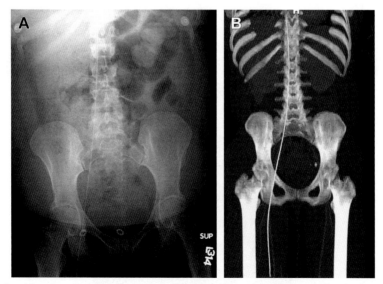

Fig. 49. Retained guide wire. Abdominal radiograph (*A*) performed for abdominal pain shows a long metallic structure in the expected location of the IVC. At first, this was thought to represent a central catheter but, on examination, no catheter was seen. Subsequent coronal MIP CT (*B*) confirms the intravascular location. This image was found to represent a retained guide wire, which was then removed percutaneously.

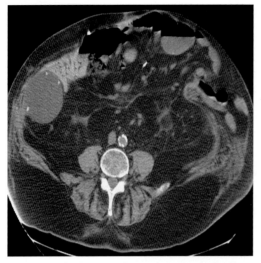

Fig. 50. Sterile peritoneal pseudocyst complicating a VP shunt. CT 2 months after VP shunt placement shows a small pseudocyst related to the intraperitoneal end of the shunt. The patient presented with altered mental status.

the groin because of a lack of access in the thorax. Understanding the role of the line can be useful in avoiding confusion with other catheters.

Almost all endovascular foreign bodies use modifications of a Seldinger technique for deployment. Knowledge of the technique is important, because complications from this technique may be encountered in imaging. Two of the most common include pseudoaneurysms at the vascular access site and retained guide wires (**Fig. 49**). The latter can look as if they belong in the patient but tend to be quite radiodense. When encountered, retained guide wires should be removed.

Neurologic Devices

Neurologic devices encountered on abdominal imaging examinations include ventriculoperitoneal (VP) shunts, epidural catheters, and a variety of stimulator and pump devices (eg, Baclofen pump). When these devices are visualized, assessment for proper positioning and physical integrity should be routinely performed. In addition to

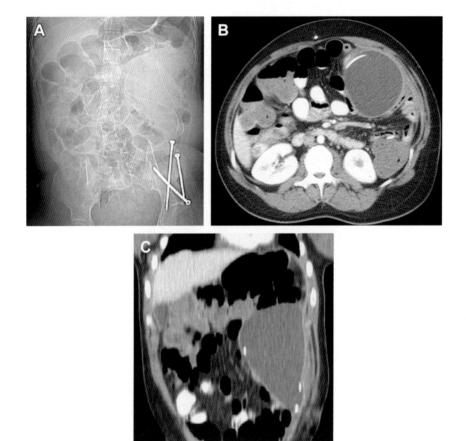

Fig. 51. Infected VP shunt pseudocyst. Abdominal radiograph (*A*) shows a paucity of bowel gas in the left hemiabdomen related to the peritoneal end of the VP shunt. Transverse (*B*) and coronal (*C*) CT images confirm formation of a peritoneal pseudocyst, which proved to be infected.

malpositioning and discontinuity, another complication of VP shunts is obstruction related to pseudocyst formation (**Figs. 50** and **51**).[66] Psuedocyst formation complicates fewer than 5% of VP shunts, with approximately 80% of cases related to infection. Predisposing factors include peritoneal adhesions, cerebrospinal fluid with high protein content, and altered peritoneal absorption. Although ultrasound may be useful for detection of peritoneal pseudocysts and for demonstrating internal septations, overall gas-filled bowel loops may limit evaluation. CT provides for better overall assessment of pseudocysts and the orientation of the associated VP shunt (see **Figs. 50** and **51**).[66]

SUMMARY

Radiologists can serve referring clinicians and patients optimally by familiarizing themselves with the imaging findings of materials used in the operating room and with devices implanted in various organ systems: GI, genitourinary, vascular, and neurologic. Possible complications should be considered and assessed carefully whenever an implanted device is encountered, because many adverse effects can only be detected on imaging. The radiologist should maintain a high index of suspicion whenever interpreting imaging examinations of a patient who had undergone prior surgery or implantation of a device.

REFERENCES

1. Gawande AA, Studdert DM, Orav EJ, et al. Risk factors for retained instruments and sponges after surgery. N Engl J Med 2003;348:229–35.
2. Kaiser CW, Friedman S, Spurling KP, et al. The retained surgical sponge. Ann Surg 1996;224:79–84.
3. Cima RR, Kollengode A, Garnatz J, et al. Incidence and characteristics of potential and actual retained foreign object events in surgical patients. J Am Coll Surg 2008;207:80–7.
4. Eggli KD, Hess MA. Imaging the Culprit's Twin: Search for the Intra-operative Retained Foreign Body. RSNA storyboard 2010. Available at: http://www.rsna.org/uploadedFiles/RSNA/Content/Science_and_Education/Quality/3057-Eggli.pdf.
5. Kernagis LY, Siegelman ES, Torigian DA. Case 145: retained sponge. Radiology 2009;251(2):608–11.
6. Bani-Hani KE, Gharaibeh KA, Yaghan RJ. Retained surgical sponges (gossypiboma). Asian J Surg 2005;28(2):109–15.
7. Kopka L, Fischer U, Gross AJ, et al. CT of retained surgical sponges (textilomas): pitfalls in detection and evaluation. J Comput Assist Tomogr 1996;20:919–23.
8. O'Connor AR, Coakley FV, Meng MV, et al. Imaging of retained surgical sponges in the abdomen and pelvis. Am J Roentgenol 2003;180:481–9.
9. Kalovidouris A, Kehagias D, Moulopoulos L, et al. Abdominal retained surgical sponges: CT appearance. Eur Radiol 1999;9:1407–10.
10. Kim CK, Park BK, Ha H. Gossypiboma in abdomen and pelvis: MRI findings in four patients. Am J Roentgenol 2007;189:814–7.
11. Agras K, Serefoglu EC, Duran E, et al. Retroperitoneal textiloma mimicking a renal tumor: case report. Int Urol Nephrol 2007;39:401–3.
12. Sahin-Akyar G, Yagci C, Aytac S. Pseudotumour due to surgical sponge: gossypiboma. Australas Radiol 1997;41:288–91.
13. Ghersin E, Keidar Z, Brook OR, et al. A new pitfall on abdominal PET/CT: a retained surgical sponge. J Comput Assist Tomogr 2004;28:839–41.
14. Yuh-Feng T, Chin-Chu W, Cheng-Tau S, et al. FDG PET CT features of an intraabdominal gossypiboma. Clin Nucl Med 2005;30:561–3.
15. Ben Meir D, Lask D, Koren R, et al. Intrarenal foreign body presenting as a solid tumor. Urology 2003;61:1035.
16. Buluş H, Şimşek G, Coşkun A, et al. Intraabdominal gossypiboma mimicking gastrointestinal stromal tumor: a case report. Turk J Gastroenterol 2011;22:534–6.
17. Justo JW, Sandler P, Cavazzola LT. Retained surgical sponge mimicking GIST: laparoscopic diagnosis and removal 34 years after original surgery. J Minim Access Surg 2013;9:29–30.
18. Yamamura N, Nakajima K, Takahashi T, et al. Intraabdominal textiloma. A retained surgical sponge mimicking a gastric gastrointestinal stromal tumor: report of a case. Surg Today 2008;38:552–4.
19. Jacobs JE, Birnbaum BA, Siegelman ES. Heterotopic ossification of midline abdominal incisions: CT and MR imaging findings. Am J Roentgenol 1996;166:579–84.
20. Gayer G, Apter S, Katz R, et al. CT findings in ten patients with failed renal allografts: comparison with findings in functional grafts. Eur J Radiol 2000;36:133–8.
21. Liao CS, Shieh MC. Laparoscopic retrieval of retained intraperitoneal drains in the immediate postoperative period. J Chin Med Assoc 2011;74:138–9.
22. Gayer G, Petrovitch I, Jeffrey RB. Foreign objects encountered in the abdominal cavity at CT. Radiographics 2011;31:409–28.
23. Gibbs VC. Retained surgical items and minimally invasive surgery. World J Surg 2011;35:1532–9.
24. Allard MA, Dondero F, Sommacale D, et al. Liver packing during elective surgery: an option that can be considered. World J Surg 2011;35:2493–8.
25. Burlew CC, Moore EE, Smith WR, et al. Preperitoneal pelvic packing/external fixation with secondary

angioembolization: optimal care for life-threatening hemorrhage from unstable pelvic fractures. J Am Coll Surg 2011;212:628–35.

26. Schiller VL, Joyce P, Sarti D. Hemostatic agent and concomitant abdominal abscess. Am J Roentgenol 1994;162:236.

27. Young ST, Paulson EK, McCann RL, et al. Appearance of oxidized cellulose (Surgicel) on postoperative CT scans: similarity to postoperative abscess. Am J Roentgenol 1993;160:275–7.

28. Parra JA, Revuelta S, Gallego T, et al. Prosthetic mesh used for inguinal and ventral hernia repair: normal appearance and complications in ultrasound and CT. Br J Radiol 2004;77:261–5.

29. Kirshtein B, Roy-Shapira A, Lantsberg L, et al. Use of the "Bogota bag" for temporary abdominal closure in patients with secondary peritonitis. Am Surg 2007;73:249–52.

30. Blachar A, Blank A, Gavert N, et al. Laparoscopic adjustable gastric banding surgery for morbid obesity: imaging of normal anatomic features and postoperative gastrointestinal complications. Am J Roentgenol 2007;188:472–9.

31. Pieroni S, Sommer EA, Hito R, et al. The "O" sign, a simple and helpful tool in the diagnosis of laparoscopic adjustable gastric band slippage. Am J Roentgenol 2010;195:137–41.

32. Woodall BH, Winfield DF, Bisset GS. Inadvertent tracheobronchial placement of feeding tubes. Radiology 1987;165:727–9.

33. Balogh GJ, Adler SJ, Vanderwoude J, et al. Pneumothorx as a complication of feeding tube placement. Am J Roentgenol 1983;141:1275–7.

34. Huang SY, Levine MS, Raper SE. Gastrocolic fistula with migration of feeding tube into transverse colon as a complication of percutaneous endoscopic gastrostomy. Am J Roentgenol 2005;184:S65–6.

35. Canon CL, Baron TH, Morgan DE, et al. Treatment of colonic obstruction with expandable metal stents: radiologic features. Am J Roentgenol 1997;168:199–205.

36. Jang JK, Song HY, Kim JH, et al. Tumor overgrowth after expandable metallic stent placement: experience in 583 patients with malignant gastroduodenal obstruction. Am J Roentgenol 2011;196:W831–6.

37. Winkelbauer FW, Schofl R, Niederle B, et al. Palliative treatment of obstructing esophageal cancer with nitinol stents: value, safety, and long-term results. Am J Roentgenol 1996;166:79–84.

38. Cura M, Cura A, Suri R, et al. Causes of TIPS dysfunction. Am J Roentgenol 2008;191:1751–7.

39. Saxon RR, Mendel-Hartvig J, Corless CL, et al. Bile duct injury as a major cause of stenosis and occlusion in transjugular intrahepatic portosystemic shunts: comparative histopathologic analysis in humans and swine. J Vasc Interv Radiol 1996;7:487–97.

40. Pokrajac B, Cejna M, Kettenbach J, et al. Intraluminal 192Ir brachytherapy following transjugular intrahepatic portosystemic shunt revision: long-term results and radiotherapy parameters. Cardiovasc Radiat Med 2001;2:133–7.

41. Clark TW, Agarwal R, Haskal ZJ, et al. The effect of initial shunt outflow position on patency of transjugular intrahepatic portosystemic shunts. J Vasc Interv Radiol 2004;15:147–52.

42. Wallace M, Swaim M. Transjugular intrahepatic portosystemic shunts through hepatic neoplasms. J Vasc Interv Radiol 2003;14:501–7.

43. Rosado B, Kamath PS. Transjugular intrahepatic portosystemic shunts: an update. Liver Transpl 2003;9:207–17.

44. Kanterman RY, Darcy MD, Middleton WD, et al. Doppler sonography findings associated with transjugular intrahepatic portosystemic shunt malfunction. Am J Roentgenol 1997;168:467–72.

45. McNaughton DA, Abu-Yousef MM. Doppler US of the liver made simple. Radiographics 2011;31:161–88.

46. Rustagi T, Aslanian HR. Endoscopic management of biliary leaks after laparoscopic cholecystectomy. J Clin Gastroenterol 2013. [Epub ahead of print].

47. Ott DJ, Gilliam JH 3rd, Zagoria RJ, et al. Interventional endoscopy of the biliary and pancreatic ducts: current indications and methods. Am J Roentgenol 1992;158:243–50.

48. Catalano O, De Bellis M, Sandomenico F, et al. Complications of biliary and gastrointestinal stents: MDCT of the cancer patient. Am J Roentgenol 2012;199:W187–96.

49. Diller R, Senninger N, Kautz G, et al. Stent migration necessitating surgical intervention. Surg Endosc 2003;17:1803–7.

50. Fiori E, Mazzoni G, Galati G, et al. Unusual breakage of a plastic biliary endoprosthesis causing an enterocutaneous fistula. Surg Endosc 2002;16:870.

51. Namdar T, Raffel AM, Topp SA, et al. Complications and treatment of migrated biliary endoprostheses: a review of the literature. World J Gastroenterol 2007;13:5397–9.

52. Gulliver DJ, Edmunds S, Baker ME, et al. Stent placement for benign pancreatic diseases: correlation between ERCP findings and clinical response. Am J Roentgenol 1992;159:751–5.

53. Lakhtakia S, Reddy DN. Pancreatic leaks: endotherapy first? J Gastroenterol Hepatol 2009;24:1158–60.

54. Boortz HE, Margolis DJ, Ragavendra N, et al. Migration of intrauterine devices: radiologic findings and implications for patient care. Radiographics 2012;32:335–52.

55. Sivin I, Schmidt F. Effectiveness of IUDs: a review. Contraception 1987;36:55–84.

56. Ha HK, Lee HJ, Kim H, et al. Abdominal actinomycosis: CT findings in 10 patients. Am J Roentgenol 1993;161:791–4.

57. Thonneau P, Goulard H, Goyaux N. Risk factors for intrauterine device failure: a review. Contraception 2001;64:33–7.

58. Harrison-Woolrych M, Ashton J, Coulter D. Uterine perforation on intrauterine device insertion: is the incidence higher than previously reported? Contraception 2003;67:53–6.

59. Zakin D, Stern WZ, Rosenblatt R. Complete and partial uterine perforation and embedding following insertion of intrauterine devices. II. Diagnostic methods, prevention, and management. Obstet Gynecol Surv 1981;36:401–17.

60. Kaufman J, Kinney T, Streiff MB, et al. Guidelines for the use of retrievable and convertible vena cava filters: report from the Society of Interventional Radiology multidisciplinary consensus conference. J Vasc Interv Radiol 2006;17:449–59.

61. Harvey J, Hopkins J, McCafferty I, et al. Inferior vena cava filters: what radiologists need to know. Clin Radiol 2013;68:721–32.

62. Kalva S, Chlapoutaki C, Wicky S, et al. Suprarenal inferior vena cava filters: a 20-year single-center experience. J Vasc Interv Radiol 2008;19:1041–7.

63. Caplin D, Nikolic B, Kalva S, et al. Quality improvement guidelines for the performance of inferior vena cava filter placement for the prevention of pulmonary embolism. J Vasc Interv Radiol 2011;22: 1499–506.

64. Streiff M. Vena caval filters: a comprehensive review. Blood 2000;15:3669–77.

65. Coldwell D, Stokes K, Yakes W. Embolotherapy: agents, clinical applications, and techniques. Radiographics 1994;14:623–43.

66. Chung JJ, Yu JS, Kim JH, et al. Intraabdominal complications secondary to ventriculoperitoneal shunts: CT findings and review of the literature. Am J Roentgenol 2009;193:1311–7.

Imaging of Chemotherapy-related Iatrogenic Abdominal and Pelvic Conditions

Chitra Viswanathan, MD[a,*], Mylene Truong, MD[b],
Tara Sagebiel, MD[a], Naveen Garg, MD[a], Priya Bhosale, MD[a]

KEYWORDS

• Toxicity • Complication • Abdomen • Pelvis • Cytotoxic chemotherapy • Targeted therapy

KEY POINTS

- It is crucial for the radiologist to know the imaging appearance of chemotherapy-related complications, to alert the clinicians and to avoid misdiagnosis.
- Complications may occur as a result of chemotherapy with conventional agents and the new molecular targeted agents and are usually related to the mechanism of action of the drug.
- Examples of chemotherapy-related complications that occur are colitis, hepatitis, cholecystitis, fluid retention, and perforation.

INTRODUCTION

Oncologic therapy is constantly evolving to improve patient outcomes, especially with regard to chemotherapy. The use of combination therapies and development and implementation of molecular targeted therapy (MTT) lead to iatrogenic conditions that the radiologist must be aware of in interpreting examinations of and caring for the oncologic patient. Understanding the drug mechanisms may provide some insight into potential toxicities. This article provides a brief overview of some of the actions of the more common cytotoxic agents and MTT. Discussed are some of the complications, such as hepatitis, pancreatitis, and enterocolitis, and their imaging presentations in the abdomen and pelvis, although there may be other toxicities present clinically which do not manifest on imaging but may provide a clue to the diagnosis. It is important to alert the clinicians to ensure rapid cessation of the agent if necessary and decrease the morbidity and mortality to the patient.

DRUG MECHANISMS

Conventional Therapy

The mode of action of conventional cytotoxic agents is to target rapidly proliferating cancer cells and interrupt their cell cycle and development. They may also inadvertently affect normal rapidly proliferating cells within the body, leading to toxicity. The typical categories used to classify cytotoxic agents are alkylating agents (which may include platinum analogues), antimetabolites, antibiotics, topoisomerase inhibitors, and mitotic inhibitors, such as vinca alkaloids and taxanes. Examples of alkylating agents are cyclophosphamide and ifosfamide, used in the treatment of leukemia and other tumors. Oxaliplatin and cisplatin are platinum analogues. Gemcitabine and 5-fluorouracil (5-FU) are antimetabolites that act as pyrimidine analogues. Doxorubicin is an example of an antitumor antibiotic. A topoisomerase inhibitor used to treat colorectal carcinoma and other malignancies is irinotecan. Examples of vinca

[a] Department of Diagnostic Radiology, UT MD Anderson Cancer Center, 1515 Holcombe Boulevard, Unit 1473, Houston, TX 77030, USA; [b] Department of Diagnostic Radiology, UT MD Anderson Cancer Center, Unit 1478, Houston, TX 77030, USA
* Corresponding author.
E-mail address: chitra.viswanathan@mdanderson.org

Radiol Clin N Am 52 (2014) 1029–1040
http://dx.doi.org/10.1016/j.rcl.2014.05.008

radiologic.theclinics.com

alkaloids are vincristine and vinblastine. Paclitaxel and docetaxel belong to the taxane family.[1,2]

Molecular-Targeted Therapies

Targeted therapies were developed to target the cell signaling proteins to inhibit cancer cell proliferation. MTT are usually small molecules or monoclonal antibodies. Tamoxifen is an example of one of the first MTT that targets the estrogen receptor in patients with breast cancer. MTT can work by a variety of mechanisms, from inhibiting signal transduction, blocking angiogenesis, inducing apoptosis, engaging the immune system to target cancer cells, and delivering toxic compounds to cancer cells. Imatinib is a small molecule multiple tyrosine kinase inhibitor (TKI) which inhibits signal transduction and is used to treat gastrointestinal stromal tumor (GIST), leukemia, and other malignancies. Temsirolimus and everolimus are small molecule drugs used to treat renal cell carcinoma that inhibit mammalian target of rapamycin (mTor) to stop cell growth. Erlotinib is used to treat lung cancer and is a small molecule TKI of epithelial growth factor receptor (EGFR). Bevacizumab is a monoclonal antibody that binds to vascular endothelial growth factor (VEGF) to interfere with angiogenesis. Sorafenib and Sunitinib are small molecule TKIs that interrupt pathways involved with activation of VEGF. Ipilimumab is a monoclonal antibody used to treat melanoma that inhibits cytotoxic T-lymphocyte associated antigen-4 (CTLA-4) to induce the immune system to attack cancer cells.[3]

Gastrointestinal Tract

Enteritis and colitis

Inflammation and/or infection of the colon and of the small bowel, including neutropenic colitis and pseudomembranous colitis, can occur as a result of chemotherapy. The cytotoxic agents 5-FU and irinotecan when used in combination with chemotherapy can also cause diarrhea and colitis. Drugs such as the EGFR inhibitors erlotinib, sorafenib, sunitinib, imatinib, and gefitinib are all associated with diarrhea and colitis as well (**Fig. 1**).[4] Patients treated with ipilimumab for metastatic melanoma may develop enterocolitis, with grade 3 adverse effects occurring in around 10% of patients (**Fig. 2**).[5]

The exact mechanism is unknown, but is thought to be due to the target and action of the drug, including the immune-modulating effect of ipilimumab, EGFR blockade of erlotinib, and the immunosuppressive effect of the mTor inhibitor temsirolimus, for example. In colitis caused by

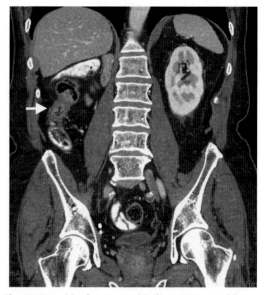

Fig. 1. Enteritis due to sunitinib. A 72-year-old man with renal cell carcinoma treated with sunitinib for 5.5 years for a metastatic sacral lesion (not shown). Coronal CT image of the abdomen for restaging shows short segment small bowel wall thickening, compatible with enteritis (*white arrow*).

ipilimumab, the development of colitis correlated with the response to therapy.[5,6]

Radiographically, there may be dilation of the bowel, bowel wall thickening, and air-fluid levels. There may be submucosal edema of the small bowel seen on computed tomography (CT).[6] In colitis, fluid-filled colonic distention and mesenteric vessel engorgement may be seen.[7] Enterocolitis can lead to obstruction and perforation, and in the case of ipilimumab, it can rapidly progress, so accurate diagnosis is essential to start the appropriate therapy.

Pneumatosis

Pneumatosis has been seen in patients treated with multikinase agents including bevacizumab, sorafenib, and sunitinib. Patients are usually asymptomatic, and pneumatosis may be an incidental finding at follow-up.[6]

Pathologically, the mechanism is thought to be disruption of the villi capillaries, possibly leading to microperforation and allowing infiltration of air.[6]

CT findings include submucosal and subserosal air cysts within the bowel wall. There may be associated pneumoperitoneum and/or portal venous gas (**Fig. 3**). The causative agent will be stopped; depending on how extensive the findings are and the status of the patient, the patient may be hospitalized.[8]

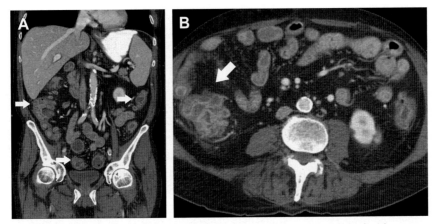

Fig. 2. Immune-related enterocolitis due to ipilimumab. A 70-year-old man with high-risk prostate cancer was treated with one dose of ipilimumab. Patient shortly thereafter developed severe diarrhea and failure to thrive. Coronal (*A*) and axial (*B*) abdominal CT images show small and large bowel wall thickening and hyperemia representing enterocolitis (*arrows*). The patient did not respond sufficiently to steroids, and was ultimately given mycophenolate and infliximab and started to improve.

Perforation

Bevacizumab has been associated with gastrointestinal perforation and anastomotic leak in patients with malignancies of the abdominal cavity, such as colorectal, pancreatic, and ovarian cancers, but also in patients with no abdominal involvement, such as lung cancer, breast cancer, and malignant glioma.[9] Perforation is most commonly seen in patients treated for metastatic colorectal cancer as part of combination chemotherapy. By

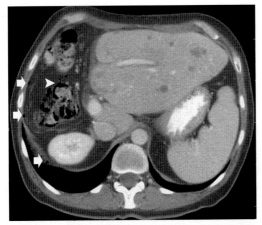

Fig. 3. Pneumatosis due to bevacizumab and sorafenib. A 47-year-old woman with metastatic cholangiocarcinoma involving the liver and the lungs was treated with 2 cycles of bevacizumab and sorafenib for progressive disease. Patient had hepatic resection before presentation at the authors' institution. Restaging CT image shows air in the bowel wall (*arrowhead*) and bubbles of free air in the abdomen (*short arrows*), along with hepatic metastases that have decreased in size. Patient was asymptomatic. Bevacizumab and sorafenib were discontinued.

inhibiting normal vascular regeneration, bevacizumab may cause ischemic bowel to develop, which may lead to perforation. In addition, antiangiogenic chemotherapy is usually not administered in the perioperative period to decrease the incidence of this condition and to allow adequate wound healing.[6] Patients may present with nausea, vomiting, abdominal pain, and fever.

Perforation can occur at the site of the tumor or at an area of serosal involvement, at the area of resection/anastomosis, or at another normal area of the colon. It may also occur in at a site of enterocolitis (**Fig. 4**). The clinicians should be notified, because a substantial number of patients are asymptomatic.

Fistula

Development of fistulae is a complication of molecular therapy. In one retrospective study of patients treated with bevacizumab who had intestinal perforation, colorectal, colovaginal, colocutaneous, rectovaginal, gastrocolic, and enterocutaneous fistulas were discovered.[10] Tumor-bowel fistulae and tumor-tracheobronchial tree fistula can also occur with treatment with targeted therapy.[11] It is thought to be due to the tumor necrosis and poor tissue healing incited because of inhibition of angiogenesis.

On CT, new air may be seen in the mass or implant, with an air track extending to the bowel. Fistulae may also be demonstrated on fluoroscopic examinations. The causative agent must be stopped.[12]

Gastrointestinal bleeding

Multikinase inhibitors, because of their antiangiogenic effect, can cause gastrointestinal bleeding.

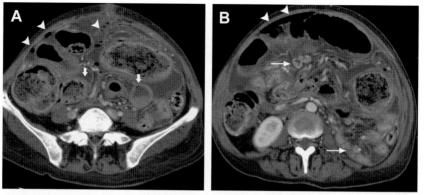

Fig. 4. Perforation due to bevacizumab. A 53-year-old woman with primary peritoneal carcinoma developed abdominal distention and pain 4 weeks after first dose of bevacizumab. (*A*) CT images (*A, B*) show free air (*arrowheads*) and enterocolitis (*small arrows*). (*B*) CT scan of the midabdomen shows peritoneal disease (*long arrows*). The exact site of perforation was not seen at CT. The patient was treated with bowel rest and bevacizumab was discontinued.

This finding has been reported in patients with hepatocellular carcinoma treated with sorafenib[13] and/or sunitinib[14,15] and in patients with GIST treated with sunitinib.[16] Other agents, including bevacizumab and gemcitabine have also been associated with high-grade hemorrhage.[17] Patients may present with hematemesis, melena, and/or bright red stool.[18]

Liver

Hypersensitivity reactions and hepatotoxicity have been noted with chemotherapeutic agents and include conditions including steatosis/steatohepatitis, sinusoidal obstruction syndrome (SOS)/veno-occlusive disease, and focal regenerative nodular hyperplasia (pseudocirrhosis).

Pseudocirrhosis
Pseudocirrhosis has been mostly seen in patients treated with chemotherapy for breast cancer, but can also occur after treatment of other cancers, such as pancreatic cancer, other gastrointestinal cancers, and medullary thyroid cancer.[19]

It is characterized pathologically by replacement of normal parenchyma by multiple regenerative nodules without bridging fibrosis, which is different from true cirrhosis. However, patients can still progress to portal hypertension.[20]

On imaging, there is decreased liver volume, enlargement of the caudate lobe, a nodular contour of the liver surface (**Fig. 5**).[21] Also, in comparison with true cirrhosis, imaging findings may progress quickly over time.

Small vessel injury
Chemotherapy can induce small vessel injury, causing entities including sclerosing cholangitis, veno-occlusive disease now better described as SOS, and peliosis. SOS has been seen with high-dose chemotherapy, with stem cell transplantation, and in patients with metastatic colorectal

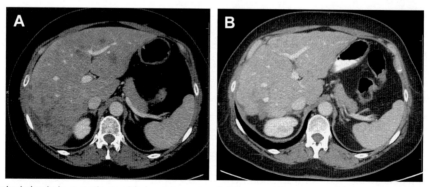

Fig. 5. Pseudocirrhosis in a patient with breast cancer. A 50-year-old woman with metastatic invasive lobular breast cancer treated with 4 cycles of 5-fluorouracil, adriamycin, and cytoxan (FAC). (*A*) Axial abdominal CT image before therapy shows multiple hypodense lesions compatible with metastatic disease. (*B*) Axial CT image after 4 cycles of FAC at the level of the portal vein shows improvement in hepatic metastatic disease, but development of a nodular contour to the liver with enlargement of the caudate lobe, representative of pseudocirrhosis.

carcinoma treated with oxaliplatin.[22,23] Nodular regenerative hyperplasia can also be caused by oxaliplatin, trastuzumab, paclitaxel, doxorubicin, and capecitabine.

On CT, nodular regenerative hyperplasia is the same attenuation as normal liver on unenhanced images, and may enhance slightly on the postcontrast images. The irregular blood-filled cavities of peliosis have low density on unenhanced images, early enhancement on arterial-phase images with the "target sign," centripetal or centrifugal flow on portal venous images, and characteristic delayed enhancement with persistent high density on delayed images.[24,25] SOS may not have findings on imaging until advanced stages, which include mosaic enhancement pattern (**Fig. 6**), periportal edema, ascites, and hepatomegaly.[24]

Steatosis and steatohepatitis

Steatosis can occur in patients with colorectal cancer treated with irinotecan, leucovorin, and 5-FU (FOLinic acid [Leucovorin], 5 FU, IRInotecan, FOLFIRI) and to a lesser extent oxaliplatin in conjunction with leucovorin and 5-FU (FOLinic acid [Leucovorin], 5 FU, OXaliplatin, FOLFOX).[26,27] There are case reports describing bevacizumab and pazopanib causing fatty liver.[28] A form of nonalcoholic steatohepatitis, known as chemotherapy-induced steatohepatitis, can also be seen due to irinotecan. It has been associated with poorer outcomes after hepatic surgery for metastatic resection.[29,30] Pathologically, the hepatocytes will show increased fat deposition in steatosis. In steatohepatitis, there is ballooning and degeneration of the hepatocytes.[27,31]

On CT, there may be focal or diffuse fatty infiltration. In the case of diffuse fatty infiltration, the liver is lower in density than the spleen (greater than 10 HU difference). At magnetic resonance (MR) imaging, the area of fatty infiltration will drop out of signal on the out-of-phase images and may be low on T2-weighted imaging (**Fig. 7**).

Hepatitis

Patients being treated with molecular-targeted therapies may develop hepatic toxicity that ranges from asymptomatic elevation in liver enzymes (transaminitis) to hepatitis to acute liver failure.[4] Immune-modulated inflammatory hepatitis may occur as a result of treatment with ipilimumab for melanoma.[32] Patients may present with abnormal liver enzymes without clinical symptoms.[33] Damage to hepatocytes may occur in the acute hepatitis pattern and damage to the biliary ducts can occur in the biliary pattern.

Imaging findings can be correlated with the elevation of liver enzymes depending on the severity of injury and include periportal edema, periportal adenopathy, and mild hepatomegaly.[32]

Gallbladder

Cholecystitis

Cholecystitis has been reported as a side effect of hepatic arterial infusion of chemotherapy and hepatic arterial embolization. Myelosuppression due to chemotherapy and bone marrow transplantation is also associated with cholecystitis. In recent years, the new agent multikinase inhibitors have been a cause of cholecystitis.[34] The underlying pathologic condition is thought to be due to gallbladder wall ischemia in the case of targeted agents. Patients with cholecystitis may present with right upper quadrant pain, nausea, and vomiting.

On imaging, the signs of chemotherapy-induced acalculus cholecystitis are similar to the other causes: pericholecystic fluid, wall thickening and edema, gallbladder enlargement, a sonographic Murphy sign. Because of the risk of cholecystitis,

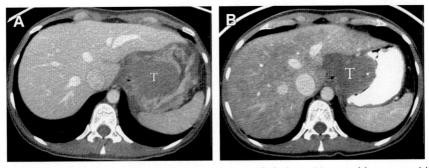

Fig. 6. Chemotherapy-induced SOS/perfusion change due to oxaliplatin. A 37-year-old woman with metastatic gastric carcinoma was treated with 8 doses of docetaxel, 5-FU, oxaliplatin, and herceptin. (*A*) Pretreatment abdominal axial CT images shows normal-appearing liver and the adjacent gastric tumor (T). (*B*) On the posttreatment CT images, the liver has a congested mottled heterogeneous appearance due to oxaliplatin (despite changes in technique). The gastric tumor (T) had slightly decreased in size, which was better seen on other images (not shown).

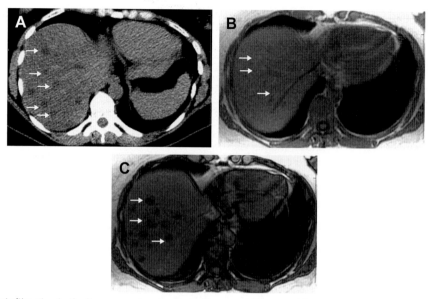

Fig. 7. Fatty infiltration in the liver secondary to chemotherapy. A 50-year-old woman with low-grade serous tumor of the ovary following 6 cycles of carboplatin and paclitaxel and 3 months of letrozole. (*A*) Noncontrast CT image from a positron-emission tomography (PET)-CT shows interval development of multiple low-density areas within the liver (*arrows*). MR imaging was ordered for further evaluation. (*B*) Axial in-phase MR imaging shows these foci to be isointense to hyperintense to liver (*arrows*). (*C*) Axial out-of-phase MR image shows these foci (*arrows*) to lose signal, representing focal fat infiltration. These findings resolved on the following PET-CT (not shown).

patients with gallstones may have prophylactic cholecystectomy before initiating therapy.[34]

However, pericholecystic fluid and gallbladder wall thickening can also be seen as a result of therapy without clinical symptoms to indicate cholecystitis (**Fig. 8**).

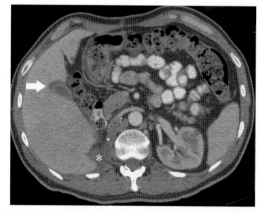

Fig. 8. Pericholecystic fluid and gallbladder wall thickening due to everolimus. A 45-year-old man with renal cell carcinoma with sarcomatoid differentiation and metastatic disease to the right pleura, bones, lungs, and lymph nodes, returned for restaging after 6 weeks of daily everolimus. Restaging axial CT image shows pericholecystic fluid and gallbladder wall thickening (*arrow*). Patient was asymptomatic and these changes were due to chemotherapy. Asterisk indicates the postnephrectomy bed.

Spleen

Splenic rupture

Splenic rupture has been reported after initiation of treatment of leukemia and also after administration of granulocyte macrophage–colony stimulating factor (GM-CSF).[35] It can be a potentially fatal condition, and there should be a high degree of suspicion for rupture when these patients present with acute abdominal pain and orthostatic abnormalities.

On CT, signs of splenic rupture include low density through the spleen, perisplenic fluid, and hemoperitoneum. There may be a high-density fluid collection or extravasation, representing active bleeding when IV contrast is administered.

Splenic infarction

Splenic infarction may occur because of arterial thrombotic events caused by chemotherapeutic drugs including cisplatin, bevacizumab, and Vascular Endothelial Growth Factor receptor (VEGF-r) TKIs sorafenib and sunitinib.[31,36,37] The underlying mechanism is due to the inhibition of VEGF, which is essential for vascular endothelial cell proliferation and survival. Inhibition of VEGF can also lead to inhibition of proliferation of the vascular smooth muscles cells and increase in erythropoietin, which may increase hematocrit and blood viscosity.

Patients may present with acute abdominal pain in the left upper quadrant. On CT, a low density in the spleen in a wedge shape is highly compatible with an infarct.

Splenomegaly

Oxaliplatin-based chemotherapy used for treatment of colorectal carcinoma can lead to splenomegaly and thrombocytopenia.[22] Three methods of oxaliplatin-induced thrombocytopenia have been postulated. One is the diffuse sinusoidal injury in the liver resulting in noncirrhotic portal hypertension, leading to splenomegaly and sequestration of platelets. The second is an oxaliplatin-induced immune thrombocytopenia. Thrombocytopenia may also occur as a result of oxaliplatin-induced overall myelosuppression.[38]

The characteristic imaging finding at CT is the slow enlargement of the spleen over the time the drug is administered. It may be insidious and is related to thrombocytopenia. It can also be seen with signs and symptoms of portal hypertension, ascites, heterogeneity of the liver, and varices.

Pancreas

Pancreatitis

Damage to the pancreas can occur as a result of drug-induced pancreatitis and pancreatic atrophy. Drugs including L-asparaginase, cytarabine, vincristine, bortezomib, doxorubicin, oxaliplatin, and methotrexate have all been associated with pancreatitis. The TKIs, sorafenib, sunitinib, and pazopanib, have also been implicated as causes of elevated pancreatic enzymes.[39] Sorafenib and sunitinib can cause acute acalculus pancreatitis.[40] Patients may present with acute abdominal pain and elevated lipase and amylase.

Imaging findings in drug-related pancreatitis do not differ from other causes of pancreatitis. Peripancreatic stranding and fluid, enlargement of the pancreas, adjacent inflammatory change of the duodenum, and low density of the pancreas are CT findings associated with pancreatitis (**Figs. 9** and **10**).

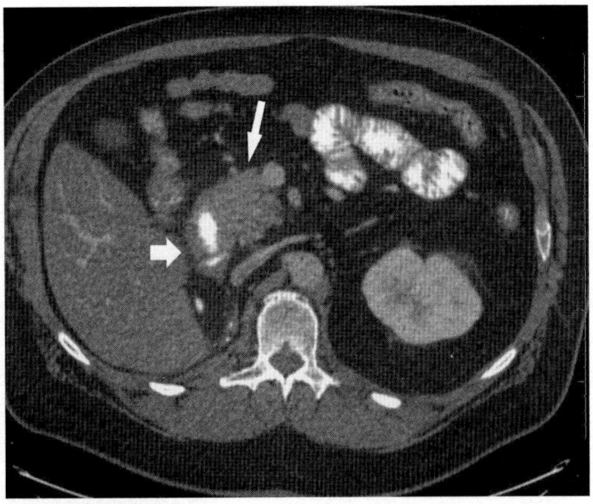

Vessels

Thromboembolism

Both arterial thromboembolism (ATE) and venous thromboembolism (VTE) are associated with chemotherapy. The anti-angiogenesis drugs including bevacizumab, sorafenib, axitinib, pazopanib, sunitinib, and ponatinib or bevacizumab or aflibercept in combination are associated with a 1% to 14% incidence of VTE. There is a slightly higher risk of VTE in combination chemotherapy than with single-agent VEGF (ie, when bevacizumab or aflibercept is used to treat colorectal cancer with other agents). The immunomodulatory

Fig. 9. Pancreatitis due to sunitinib. A 49-year-old man with renal cell carcinoma had been taking sunitinib for 4 years for right infrahilar metastatic disease. He developed hypertriglyceridemia secondary to sunitinib use and then presented with clinical signs of pancreatitis. Axial CT image through the head of the pancreas shows enlargement of the head of the pancreas (*long arrow*), mild peripancreatic stranding, and thickening of the adjacent duodenum (*short arrow*), representing pancreatitis.

agents such as thalidomide have a risk between 9% and 22%. Drugs such as bortezomib and oxaliplatin have been associated with portal vein thrombosis.

ATE is seen in patients treated with VEGF inhibitors and multikinase inhibitors. For example, ATE has been reported in patients who have received ponatinib for treatment of leukemia in phase 1 and 2 trials.[41] The ATE is associated mostly with adverse cardiac and cerebrovascular events.

Thrombosis may be seen at imaging with clots in large arteries, including the aorta, mesenteric arteries, and pelvic vessels, and also in the peripheral arteries (**Fig. 11**).[42]

Hemorrhage

Tumoral hemorrhage may occur as a result of therapy and has been reported in patients with GIST treated with imatinib.[43] The risk of hemorrhage increases with the size of the tumor. Patients may present with acute abdominal pain and a sudden decrease in their hemoglobin and hematocrit.

Findings on CT imaging include high-density or low-density fluid within the lesion or lesions, fluid-fluid levels, extralesional fluid, and hemoperitoneum (**Fig. 12**). The presence of hemorrhage within a lesion may cause it to appear larger, and this should not be confused for progression of metastatic disease.

Mesentery and Retroperitoneum

Mesenteric edema, ascites, and anasarca

Chemotherapy can cause fluid retention as a result of capillary leak syndrome. Agents such as the

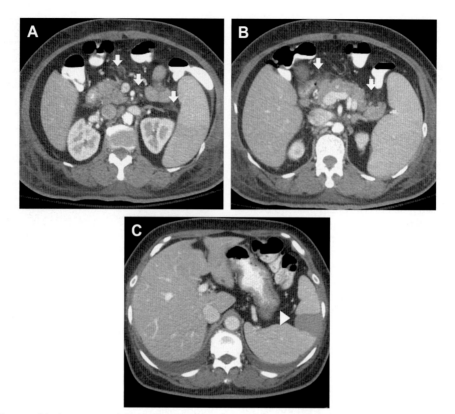

Fig. 10. Pancreatitis due to ponatinib. A 69-year-old woman with chronic myelogenous leukemia (CML) and hepatitis B received one initial dose of ponatinib of 45 mg. She then presented with shortness of breath, generalized malaise, fever, and back pain. Lipase was elevated. (*A, B*) Axial CT images of the abdomen show enlargement of the pancreas (*asterisk*) and peripancreatic stranding (*arrows*), representing acute pancreatitis. There was no sign of necrosis or pseudocyst. The patient also had pleural effusions and pneumonitis (not shown) presumably caused by the drug. Ponatinib was held. (*C*) Axial CT image obtained 1 month later shows resolution of pancreatitis (not shown) but development of a splenic infarct (*arrowhead*).

targeted therapies TKIs, dasatinib, erlotinib, imatinib, and sunitinib, may cause fluid retention.[44] In one series, fluid retention/edema was seen in 71% of patients treated with imatinib for chronic myelogenous leukemia.[45] Fluid retention may also be seen because of the increased development of congestive heart failure, such as seen with sunitinib.[46]

Patients may have weight gain and shortness of breath. Imaging findings include new pleural effusions, ascites, pericholecystic fluid, mesenteric edema, anasarca, and skin thickening. These findings should not be confused with progression of disease. In the cases of severe fluid retention, therapy may be paused or ceased.

Retroperitoneal infiltration

Patients treated with ipilimumab may develop retroperitoneal fat infiltration with lymphocytes caused by the CTLA-4 action of the drug. Patients are likely asymptomatic, and this may be seen as an incidental finding on follow-up imaging. There

will be increased opacity and stranding of the retroperitoneal fat, which may mimic findings that can be seen in lymphoma, Castleman disease, Erdheim-Chester disease, and retroperitoneal fibrosis (**Fig. 13**). In some cases, focal infiltration may mimic metastatic disease. These findings may resolve spontaneously or after cessation of therapy.[47]

URINARY TRACT
Kidneys

Nephrotoxicity has been seen with conventional agents and now with the molecular-targeted therapies. Many of the targets for molecular therapy are also expressed on the nephron. Subsequently, the drug may target the kidney, leading to proteinuria and hypertension, which is seen with VEGF and VEGF-r inhibitors such as bevacizumab, c-kit inhibitors such as imatinib, the tyrosine kinase c-MET inhibitors, and EGFR inhibitors. In the case of drugs like bevacizumab, the presence

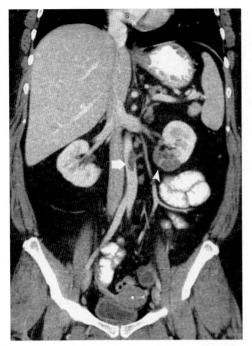

Fig. 11. Aortic thrombosis due to immune modulating agent OncoVEX GM-CSF. A 38-year-old woman with left leg cutaneous melanoma and Crohn disease presented 3 months after therapy on the OncoVEX treatment study. Coronal CT image shows a filling defect in the aorta, representing thrombus (*arrow*) and an infarct in the left kidney (*arrowhead*), due to therapy.

of hypertension is a sign of clinical efficacy. There are also case reports of patients with GIST, treated with single-agent sunitinib or sorafenib and sunitinib, who developed nephrotic syndrome due to therapy.[48,49] Nephrotoxicity is thought to be a result of glomerular nephritis, thrombotic microangiopathy, acute tubular necrosis, interstitial nephritis, and IgA nephropathy.

Bladder

Chemotherapeutic agents including cyclophosphamide and ifosfamide, as high-dose chemotherapy for the treatment of leukemia, can cause hemorrhagic cystitis.[50] Patients may have abdominal pain, dysuria, or hematuria. Imaging findings on ultrasound include thickening and increased vascularity of the bladder wall along with echogenic debris consistent with clot or active bleeding. CT findings include bladder wall thickening, perivesicular stranding, and high-density material within the bladder (**Fig. 14**).[51]

Adrenals

Adrenal insufficiency and adrenal hyperplasia have been associated with chemotherapy. Patients may have signs of adrenal crisis with

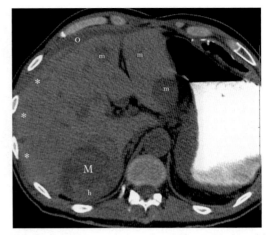

Fig. 12. Hematoma due to imatinib. A 62-year-old man with small bowel primary GIST tumor involving the stomach, liver, and peritoneal cavity was on week 2 of therapy with HSP90 inhibitor and imatinib on study. He presented to the clinic with acute abdominal pain and a decrease in his hemoglobin and hematocrit. Axial CT image with oral contrast only, shows multiple metastatic lesions (m) in the liver. There is a high-density perihepatic collection (*asterisk*), representing acute hemorrhage. The large metastasis in the right lobe (M) also has high density within it (h), representing active bleeding. There is a lower density collection (o), which may represent old blood or ascites.

chemotherapy-associated insufficiency.[52] Imaging findings of adrenal hyperplasia on CT include interval increase in the size and the enhancement of the adrenals uniformly.

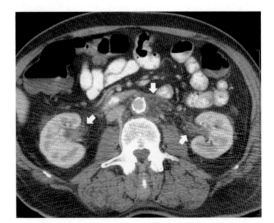

Fig. 13. Retroperitoneal infiltration due to ipilimumab. A 65-year-old man with metastatic melanoma (tumor not shown) developed hypophysitis, uveitis, and lower extremity weakness after 4 cycles of ipilimumab. Restaging studies were performed. Axial CT image through the level of the kidneys shows soft-tissue stranding around the retroperitoneum and proximal ureters (*arrows*), a finding that can be seen with ipilimumab. Findings resolved on the subsequent examination (not shown).

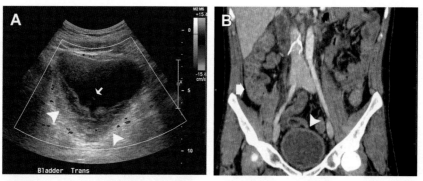

Fig. 14. Cystitis due to high-dose chemotherapy for stem cell transplant. A 24-year-old man with acute myelogenous leukemia following a second stem cell transplantation underwent induction with melphalan, antithymocyte globulin, and fludarabine. Patient complained of abdominal pain and urinating clots of blood 1 week after transplant. (*A*) Transverse ultrasound image of the bladder shows thickening of the bladder wall with increased vascularity (*arrowheads*) and debris consistent with clots (*arrow*). (*B*) Coronal CT image obtained 1 month later shows persistent bladder wall thickening (*arrowhead*). Patient had also developed neutropenic colitis with thickening of the cecum and ileum (*arrow*).

SUMMARY

The radiologist must be aware of iatrogenic conditions that may arise in the treatment of the oncologic patient. Knowledge of the chemotherapeutic agents and the imaging appearances of associated toxicities can impact patient management.

REFERENCES

1. American Cancer Society. Chemotherapy principles. Atlanta (GA): American Cancer Society; 2013 [updated February 07, 2013; cited January 5, 2014]. Available at: http://www.cancer.org/treatment/treatmentsandsideeffects/treatmenttypes/chemotherapy/chemotherapyprinciplesanin-depthdiscussionofthetechniquesanditsroleintreatment/chemotherapy-principles-types-of-chemo-drugs.

2. Chikarmane SA, Khurana B, Krajewski KM, et al. What the emergency radiologist needs to know about treatment-related complications from conventional chemotherapy and newer molecular targeted agents. Emerg Radiol 2012;19(6):535–46.

3. National Cancer Institute. Targeted cancer therapies. Bethesda (MD): National Cancer Institute; 2012 [cited January 05, 2014]. Available at: http://www.cancer.gov/cancertopics/factsheet/Therapy/targeted.

4. Boussios S, Pentheroudakis G, Katsanos K, et al. Systemic treatment-induced gastrointestinal toxicity: incidence, clinical presentation and management. Ann Gastroenterol 2012;25(2):106–18.

5. Beck KE, Blansfield JA, Tran KQ, et al. Enterocolitis in patients with cancer after antibody blockade of cytotoxic T-lymphocyte-associated antigen 4. J Clin Oncol 2006;24(15):2283–9.

6. Thornton E, Howard SA, Jagannathan J, et al. Imaging features of bowel toxicities in the setting of molecular targeted therapies in cancer patients. Br J Radiol 2012;85(1018):1420–6.

7. Kim KW, Ramaiya NH, Krajewski KM, et al. Ipilimumab-associated colitis: CT findings. AJR Am J Roentgenol 2013;200(5):W468–74.

8. Coriat R, Ropert S, Mir O, et al. Pneumatosis intestinalis associated with treatment of cancer patients with the vascular growth factor receptor tyrosine kinase inhibitors sorafenib and sunitinib. Invest New Drugs 2011;29(5):1090–3.

9. Abu-Hejleh T, Mezhir J, Goodheart M, et al. Incidence and management of gastrointestinal perforation from bevacizumab in advanced cancers. Curr Oncol Rep 2012;14(4):277–84.

10. Borofsky SE, Levine MS, Rubesin SE, et al. Bevacizumab-induced perforation of the gastrointestinal tract: clinical and radiographic findings in 11 patients. Abdom Imaging 2013;38(2):265–72.

11. Chow H, Jung A, Talbott J, et al. Tumor fistulization associated with targeted therapy: computed tomographic findings and clinical consequences. J Comput Assist Tomogr 2011;35(1):86–90.

12. Tirumani S, Baez J, Jagannathan J, et al. Tumor-bowel fistula: what radiologists should know. Abdom Imaging 2013;38(5):1014–23.

13. Zavaglia C, Airoldi A, Mancuso A, et al. Adverse events affect sorafenib efficacy in patients with recurrent hepatocellular carcinoma after liver transplantation: experience at a single center and review of the literature. Eur J Gastroenterol Hepatol 2013;25(2):180–6.

14. Je Y, Schutz FA, Choueiri TK. Risk of bleeding with vascular endothelial growth factor receptor tyrosine-kinase inhibitors sunitinib and sorafenib: a

systematic review and meta-analysis of clinical trials. Lancet Oncol 2009;10(10):967–74.

15. Han G, Zhao Y, Qi X, et al. Hepatocellular carcinoma treated with sorafenib. Aliment Pharmacol Ther 2011;34(11–12):1347–8.

16. Liu Y, Zhang HL, Zhang Y, et al. Digestive tract hemorrhage due to complications with gastrointestinal stromal tumor treated with sunitinib: a case report. Oncol Lett 2013;5(2):699–701.

17. Hu Y, Wang J, Tao H, et al. Increased risk of high-grade hemorrhage in cancer patients treated with gemcitabine: a meta-analysis of 20 randomized controlled trials. PLoS One 2013;8(9):e74872.

18. Asnacios A, Naveau S, Perlemuter G. Gastrointestinal toxicities of novel agents in cancer therapy. Eur J Cancer 2009;45(Suppl 1):332–42.

19. Jeong WK, Choi SY, Kim J. Pseudocirrhosis as a complication after chemotherapy for hepatic metastasis from breast cancer. Clin Mol Hepatol 2013;19(2):190–4.

20. Jha P, Poder L, Wang ZJ, et al. Radiologic mimics of cirrhosis. AJR Am J Roentgenol 2010;194(4): 993–9.

21. Young ST, Paulson EK, Washington K, et al. CT of the liver in patients with metastatic breast carcinoma treated by chemotherapy: findings simulating cirrhosis. AJR Am J Roentgenol 1994; 163(6):1385–8.

22. Overman MJ, Maru DM, Charnsangavej C, et al. Oxaliplatin-mediated increase in spleen size as a biomarker for the development of hepatic sinusoidal injury. J Clin Oncol 2010;28(15):2549–55.

23. Rubbia-Brandt L, Lauwers GY, Wang H, et al. Sinusoidal obstruction syndrome and nodular regenerative hyperplasia are frequent oxaliplatin-associated liver lesions and partially prevented by bevacizumab in patients with hepatic colorectal metastasis. Histopathology 2010;56(4):430–9.

24. Shanbhogue AK, Virmani V, Vikram R, et al. Spectrum of medication-induced complications in the abdomen: role of cross-sectional imaging. AJR Am J Roentgenol 2011;197(2):W286–94.

25. Iannaccone R, Federle MP, Brancatelli G, et al. Peliosis hepatis: spectrum of imaging findings. AJR Am J Roentgenol 2006;187(1):W43–52.

26. Morris-Stiff G, Tan YM, Vauthey JN. Hepatic complications following preoperative chemotherapy with oxaliplatin or irinotecan for hepatic colorectal metastases. Eur J Surg Oncol 2008; 34(6):609–14.

27. Khan AZ, Morris-Stiff G, Makuuchi M. Patterns of chemotherapy-induced hepatic injury and their implications for patients undergoing liver resection for colorectal liver metastases. J Hepatobiliary Pancreat Surg 2009;16(2):137–44.

28. Howard SA, Krajewski KM, Thornton E, et al. Decade of molecular targeted therapy: abdominal manifestations of drug toxicities–what radiologists should know. AJR Am J Roentgenol 2012;199(1): 58–64.

29. Abdalla EK, Vauthey JN. Chemotherapy prior to hepatic resection for colorectal liver metastases: helpful until harmful? Dig Surg 2008; 25(6):421–9.

30. Vauthey JN, Pawlik TM, Ribero D, et al. Chemotherapy regimen predicts steatohepatitis and an increase in 90-day mortality after surgery for hepatic colorectal metastases. J Clin Oncol 2006;24(13): 2065–72.

31. Torrisi JM, Schwartz LH, Gollub MJ, et al. CT findings of chemotherapy-induced toxicity: what radiologists need to know about the clinical and radiologic manifestations of chemotherapy toxicity. Radiology 2011;258(1):41–56.

32. Kim KW, Ramaiya NH, Krajewski KM, et al. Ipilimumab associated hepatitis: imaging and clinicopathologic findings. Invest New Drugs 2013;31(4): 1071–7.

33. Tarhini A. Immune-mediated adverse events associated with ipilimumab CTLA-4 blockade therapy: the underlying mechanisms and clinical management. Scientifica (Cairo) 2013;2013:19.

34. Jayakrishnan TT, Groeschl RT, George B, et al. Review of the impact of antineoplastic therapies on the risk for cholelithiasis and acute cholecystitis. Ann Surg Oncol 2014;21(1):240–7.

35. Veerappan R, Morrison M, Williams S, et al. Splenic rupture in a patient with plasma cell myeloma following G-CSF/GM-CSF administration for stem cell transplantation and review of the literature. Bone Marrow Transplant 2007;40(4):361–4.

36. Kim SO, Han SY, Baek YH, et al. Splenic infarction associated with sorafenib use in a hepatocellular carcinoma patient. World J Gastroenterol 2011; 17(2):267–70.

37. Malka D, Van Den Eynde M, Boige V, et al. Splenic infarction and bevacizumab. Lancet Oncol 2006; 7(12):1038.

38. Jardim DL, Rodrigues CA, Novis YA, et al. Oxaliplatin-related thrombocytopenia. Ann Oncol 2012; 23(8):1937–42.

39. Pezzilli R, Fabbri D, Imbrogno A, et al. Tyrosine kinase inhibitors, pancreatic hyperenzymemia and acute pancreatitis: a review. Recent Pat Inflamm Allergy Drug Discov 2011;5(2):165–8.

40. Amar S, Wu KJ, Tan WW. Sorafenib-induced pancreatitis. Mayo Clin Proc 2007;82(4):521.

41. Cortes JE, Kim DW, Pinilla-Ibarz J, et al. A phase 2 trial of Ponatinib in Philadelphia chromosome-positive leukemias. N Engl J Med 2013;369(19): 1783–96.

42. Dy GK, Adjei AA. Understanding, recognizing, and managing toxicities of targeted anticancer therapies. CA Cancer J Clin 2013;63(4):249–79.

43. Hecker A, Hecker B, Bassaly B, et al. Dramatic regression and bleeding of a duodenal GIST during preoperative imatinib therapy: case report and review. World J Surg Oncol 2010;8:47.

44. Masiello D, Gorospe G 3rd, Yang AS. The occurrence and management of fluid retention associated with TKI therapy in CML, with a focus on dasatinib. J Hematol Oncol 2009;2:46.

45. Guilhot F. Indications for imatinib mesylate therapy and clinical management. Oncologist 2004;9(3): 271–81.

46. Richards CJ, Je Y, Schutz FA, et al. Incidence and risk of congestive heart failure in patients with renal and nonrenal cell carcinoma treated with sunitinib. J Clin Oncol 2011;29(25):3450–6.

47. Bronstein Y, Ng CS, Hwu P, et al. Radiologic manifestations of immune-related adverse events in patients with metastatic melanoma undergoing anti–CTLA-4 antibody therapy. Am J Roentgenol 2011;197(6):W992–1000.

48. Turan N, Benekli M, Ozturk SC, et al. Sunitinib- and sorafenib-induced nephrotic syndrome in a patient with gastrointestinal stromal tumor. Ann Pharmacother 2012;46(10):e27.

49. Pallotti MC, Pantaleo MA, Nannini M, et al. Development of a nephrotic syndrome in a patient with gastrointestinal stromal tumor during a long-time treatment with sunitinib. Case Rep Oncol 2012; 5(3):651–6.

50. Ribeiro RA, Lima-Junior RC, Leite CA, et al. Chemotherapy-induced hemorrhagic cystitis: pathogenesis, pharmacological approaches and new insights. J Exp Integr Med 2012;2(2): 95–112.

51. McCarville MB, Hoffer FA, Gingrich JR, et al. Imaging findings of hemorrhagic cystitis in pediatric oncology patients. Pediatr Radiol 2000;30(3): 131–8.

52. Grenader T, Shavit L. Chemotherapy-induced adrenal crisis. Int J Oncol 2005;3(1):6.

Radiation-induced Effects to Nontarget Abdominal and Pelvic Viscera

CrossMark

Christine M. Peterson, MD[a],*, Christine O. Menias, MD[b,c],
Douglas S. Katz, MD[d,e]

KEYWORDS

• Radiation • Injury • Veno-occlusion • Fistula • Stricture • Osteopenia

KEY POINTS

• Radiation therapy is a useful tool for the treatment of some patients with cancer. However, sometimes nontarget organs are irradiated.
• Radiation therapy can have temporary or permanent effects on nontarget organs.
• It is vitally important for radiologists to recognize these effects and not mistake them for other entities, particularly tumor metastasis or recurrence.

INTRODUCTION

Radiation therapy has become a mainstay of treatment of many forms of cancer. Although this article does not discuss the specifics of radiation therapy, it is of utmost importance for the radiologist interpreting an imaging examination to recognize some of the expected and unintended consequences of treatment so that the radiologist can suggest or establish the correct diagnosis, aid in the direction of further management, and not misattribute the imaging appearance of these consequences to other entities, particularly tumor recurrence or the development of metastatic disease.

Although some newer radiation therapy delivery methods decrease the dose delivered to the targeted organs so that the amount of radiation is effective but not excessive, and deliver less radiation to adjacent tissues, neighboring tissues are still exposed to radiation to some degree. As a result, inadvertent organ damage may still occur. Familiarity with the consequences of radiation therapy and their imaging appearances makes radiologists' input more clinically relevant and useful.

Newer radiation therapy techniques, such as stereotactic body radiotherapy, deliver a precise radiation dose to a small volume of tissue. As a result, less normal adjacent tissue is exposed to radiation. When exposure and subsequent damage do occur, the underlying pathologic mechanism of tissue damage is similar between the different forms of therapy. Damage to organs usually occurs as a result of microvascular injury and endothelial damage, venous thrombosis, and tissue fibrosis.[1]

Underlying chronic systemic disease may potentiate injury to normal adjacent tissues. These diseases may be as frequently encountered as diabetes and hypertension.[2]

[a] Department of Radiology, Penn State Hershey, Hershey, PA 17033, USA; [b] Mayo Clinic LL Radiology, 13400 East Shea Blvd, Scottsdale, AZ 85259, USA; [c] Mayo Clinic Hospital, 5777 East Mayo Boulevard, Phoenix, AZ 85054, USA; [d] Department of Radiology, Winthrop-University Hospital, Mineola, NY 11501, USA; [e] State University of New York at Stony Brook, Stony Brook, NY 11794, USA
* Corresponding author.
E-mail address: cpeterson3@hmc.psu.edu

Radiol Clin N Am 52 (2014) 1041–1053
http://dx.doi.org/10.1016/j.rcl.2014.05.004

LIVER

As with other abdominopelvic radiation-related organ injury, damage to the liver, or radiation-induced liver disease, is thought to occur as the result of veno-occlusive disease at the microscopic level, to the small branches of the hepatic and portal veins. As underlying liver abnormality increases, the ability of the liver to heal and regenerate decreases. Patients with chronic underlying liver disease, particularly cirrhosis or fatty deposition, have a worse prognosis with respect to liver damage from radiation therapy, compared with those individuals with otherwise normal livers.

Acute radiation injury to the liver usually occurs 4 to 16 weeks after radiation therapy,[3] and may manifest as the classic triad of hepatomegaly, ascites, and increased alkaline phosphatase,[4] and patients may have right upper quadrant abdominal pain.[5] However, there is no definitive treatment of these patients with regard to their liver abnormalities.[4] Treatment is often supportive.

The liver typically tolerates a dose of up to 35 Gy using more conventional techniques in which much of the liver is exposed. If newer techniques are used that only expose a small portion of the liver, doses up to 70 Gy can be tolerated.[6] In high-dose radiation targeted liver therapy (stereotactic therapy), tumor treatment is maximized and the dose to surrounding tissue is minimized by precise and accurate delivery of multiple radiation beams to the targeted region.[7]

On computed tomography (CT) and magnetic resonance (MR) imaging, a characteristic geographic but nonanatomic straight line (with conventional external beam radiation therapy) of low attenuation or low T1-weighted signal intensity may be seen, respectively, demarcating the edematous affected portion of the liver from the nonaffected portion (**Figs. 1–3**).[3] If CT arterial phase imaging is obtained, increased density of the affected portions of the liver may be seen, presumably as a result of decreased portal venous flow and resultant increased hepatic arterial flow. As part of a multiphasic CT protocol, portal venous phase images again show the area of low attenuation. Delayed CT images may show abnormally persistent enhancement of the affected parenchyma, likely caused by altered venous dynamics.[8]

Patient with otherwise normal livers most often fully recover from the insult, and any radiologic abnormality of the liver resolves over time. As with other organs, concomitant chemotherapy may potentiate radiation-related liver injury.[8]

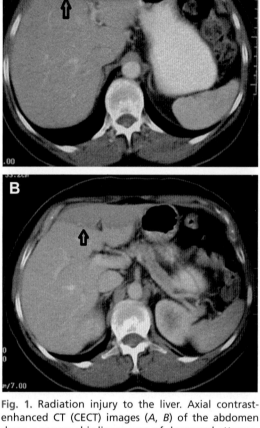

Fig. 1. Radiation injury to the liver. Axial contrast-enhanced CT (CECT) images (*A, B*) of the abdomen show a geographic linear area of decreased attenuation in the anterior aspect of the liver corresponding to the radiation port (*arrows*) in this patient who underwent radiation to the right chest wall for advanced breast carcinoma.

SPLEEN

The spleen, as with other lymphatic tissues, is exquisitely radiosensitive. However, splenic injury related to radiation is uncommon. As with the liver, radiation-related splenic injury is apparent on noncontrast CT and MR imaging as a well-defined but nonanatomic area of low attenuation or signal intensity in the parenchyma, corresponding with the radiation port. This treated area may then progress to parenchymal atrophy (**Fig. 4**).[9]

PANCREAS

The pancreas in uncommonly inadvertently injured during or after radiation injury, but, if there is injury,

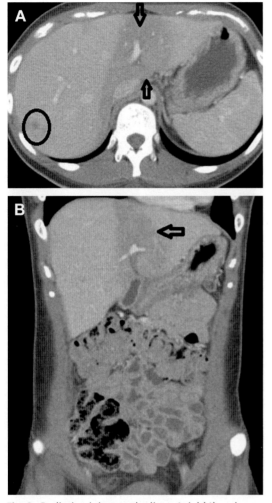

Fig. 2. Radiation injury to the liver. Axial (*A*) and coronal (*B*) CECT images in a 22-year-old woman undergoing external radiation for metastatic nasopharyngeal carcinoma to the spine and sternum shows a geographic area of decreased attenuation in the liver corresponding to the radiation port (*arrows*). Note the metastatic lesion in the liver (*circle*).

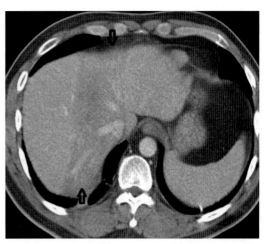

Fig. 3. Radiation injury to the liver. Axial CECT image in a different patient than demonstrated in **Fig. 2**, shows a linear geographic demarcation, with a central area of decreased attenuation in the liver corresponding to the radiation port (*arrows*).

(onset before 3 months), or chronic (onset after approximately 1 year), in which its signs and symptoms may be latent and gradual. Partly as a result of the severely deleterious effects of renal failure on lifespan and overall quality of life, the kidneys are often the dose-limiting organs for radiation therapy to the abdomen.[10]

The volume of the kidneys that is irradiated plays an important role in patient outcomes, with patients who experience injury to part of a

an appearance similar to chronic pancreatitis may ensue. Clinicians may encounter parenchymal atrophy or calcification, as well as ductal contour abnormalities as a result.[2]

KIDNEYS, URETERS, AND BLADDER

The kidneys are radiosensitive, but unlike the liver, in which there is substantial regenerative capability, injury to the kidneys tends to be permanent. Radiation-induced kidney injury may be acute

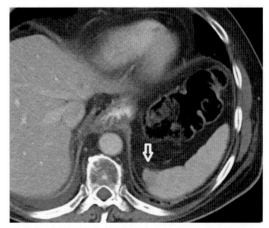

Fig. 4. Splenic injury from radiation therapy. Axial CECT image in a patient undergoing radiation therapy to the left lower lung for a peripheral lung carcinoma shows a small wedge-shaped region of decreased attenuation (*arrow*) corresponding with a region of hypoperfusion of the spleen as a result of inclusion in the radiation field.

kidney, or to a single kidney, generally faring better than patients with radiation injury to both kidneys. Patients with underlying disorders that adversely affect the kidneys, particularly diabetes and hypertension, similarly tend to have more severe injuries after radiation therapy that includes a substantial portion of each kidney in the radiation field than in patients without those conditions.[10] Doses in excess of 28 Gy over the course of 5 weeks or less may lead to renal failure. Histologic tissue damage precedes damage identifiable by imaging.[6] There is some evidence that angiotensin-converting enzyme inhibitors and/or angiotensin II receptor antagonists can be used to mitigate or treat radiation injury. However, a small subset of patients requires renal transplantation.[11]

With CT or MR imaging, typical postradiation findings after standard external beam therapy include, as in other organs, geographic but nonanatomic areas of low attenuation or T1 signal intensity corresponding with the radiation port (Fig. 5).

The ureters have some resistance to the effects of radiation, but may become damaged nonetheless, which is especially true in cases of pelvic irradiation, as may be seen in treatment of cervical or prostate carcinoma. Ureteral injury may present years after radiotherapy, and usually takes the form of a distal ureteral stricture (Fig. 6). Hydronephrosis and resultant impairment of renal function may ensue. Strictures related to radiotherapy tend to be smooth and tapering, as opposed to malignant strictures, which typically have an abrupt change in caliber, with jagged margins.[12]

Given the rapid proliferation of its epithelial cells, the bladder is the most radiosensitive organ of the urinary tract. As a result, some degree of bladder irritation often follows radiation therapy. Doses exceeding 30 Gy may produce unwanted side effects.[13] On cross-sectional imaging, nonspecific focal or diffuse bladder wall thickening with mucosal enhancement is identified, and correlation with the patient's specific history is helpful. Geographic or complete involvement of the bladder, depending on the location of the radiation therapy portal(s), strongly supports the diagnosis (Figs. 7 and 8). Hemorrhagic cystitis may occur. More chronic disease may take the form of bladder fibrosis with resultant reduced distensibility and decreased volume.[14]

There is often associated radiation change to the adjacent pelvic organs such as the rectum and pelvic ileal loops, which manifest as proctitis and radiation-related enteritis, respectively, as discussed later.

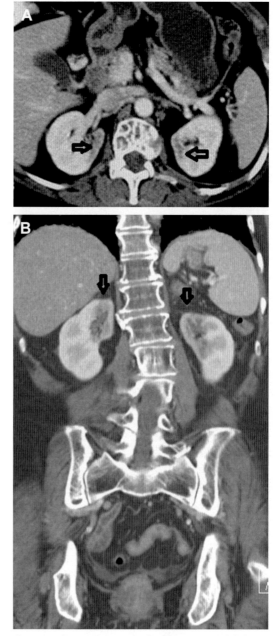

Fig. 5. Radiation injury to the kidneys. Axial (A) and coronal (B) CECT images of the abdomen show geographic areas of decreased attenuation and cortical thinning involving the superior-medial aspects of the kidneys (arrows) in this patient who underwent spinal irradiation.

BOWEL

Bowel injury as a result of radiation-related microvascular injury is an important cause of morbidity in some patients. The small bowel, in particular,

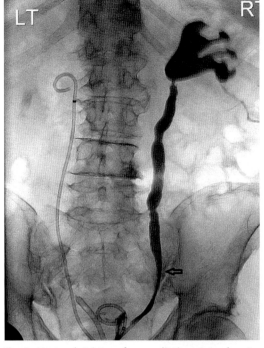

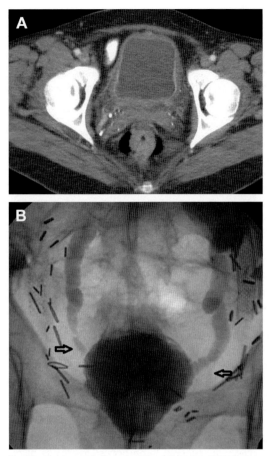

Fig. 6. Ureteral stricture from radiation. A nephrosto-gram in an elderly man treated in the distant past with radiation for prostate cancer shows smooth nar-rowing of the distal right ureter (*arrow*). There are bilateral ureteral stents and a Foley catheter in place.

is very radiosensitive and many patients treated with abdominal and/or pelvic radiation are affected with some degree of small bowel injury, also known as radiation enteritis. The small bowel mesentery may also be affected both acutely and chronically. The small bowel, similar to the kid-neys, is often the dose-limiting organ for radiation therapy in the abdomen or pelvis.[14]

Fig. 8. Acute radiation cystitis. (*A*) Axial CECT image shows circumferential thickening and mucosal hyper-enhancement of the bladder, a nonspecific appear-ance of cystitis. (*B*) Frontal image from a cystogram shows thickening of the bladder and distal ureters re-sulting in upstream ureteral dilatation caused by the radiation cystitis (*arrows*). Note the surgical clips from the patient's prostatectomy and left colonic stent placed for a synchronous colon carcinoma.

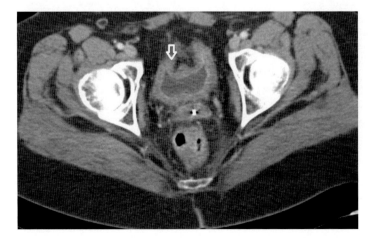

Fig. 7. Acute radiation cystitis. Axial CECT image of the pelvis in a patient receiving external beam and high-dose brachytherapy for cervical carci-noma shows a radiopaque fiducial marker within the cervix. There is associated thickening and mucosal enhancement of the urinary bladder wall representing radiation cystitis (*arrow*).

As with solid organs, chemotherapy may increase the sensitivity of the bowel to radiation injury. Patients who develop a radiation stricture may then progress to bowel obstruction. Strictures may occur months to years following the completion of radiation therapy.[12,14] If a stricture or fistula develops, the treatment is usually resection, bypass, or diversion.[15]

In the colon, lower gastrointestinal bleeding often results in the acute phase of radiation injury. The rectum, given its fixed position in the pelvis and its proximity to commonly irradiated structures, particularly the cervix and prostate gland, is most often affected. Radiation-induced tissue damage usually occurs when doses exceed 55 Gy.[13] This condition may progress to fibrosis and stricture (**Fig. 9**). In a small subset of patients, fistulae may develop.[12] Fistulae usually involve the bladder, the vagina, and/or the rectum.[13] Fistulae may occur with or without residual underlying tumor (**Figs. 10–12**).[16]

On CT, signs of radiation enteritis include mural thickening with mucosal hyperenhancement and stratification (**Figs. 13–15**), which then may result in fibrosis and develop into strictures and may lead to abscess formation (**Fig. 16**).[12]

As stated previously, the small bowel is much more radiosensitive than the colon. Nevertheless, as noted, the rectum is the most frequently injured portion of the bowel given its fixed position in the pelvis.[12] In general, large doses (fractions) given over a short period of time can be more harmful than the same dose administered in smaller

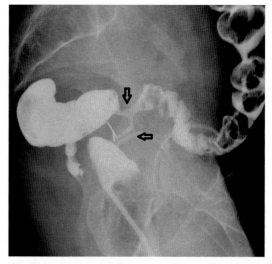

Fig. 10. Colovaginal fistula. Lateral image from a vaginogram in a 62-year-old woman following completion of radiation therapy for recurrent cervical carcinoma who presents with stool per vagina. The vaginogram shows a complex Y-shaped fistula to the adjacent rectosigmoid colon (*arrows*).

fractions over a longer period of time.[17] Radiation injury to the rectum can manifest as nonspecific proctitis on imaging, with mural edema and mucosal enhancement associated with adjacent mesorectal edema and fat stranding.

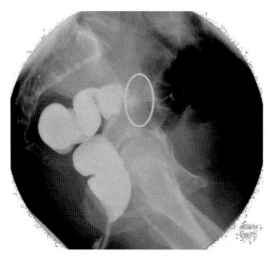

Fig. 9. Radiation-induced colonic stricture. Image from an enema examination in a patient who presents with obstipation shows marked narrowing (*circle*) of the sigmoid colon in this patient with prior pelvic radiotherapy for prostate carcinoma.

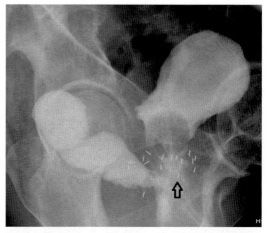

Fig. 11. Urethrorectal fistula. Lateral cystogram image in a 67-year-old man who presents with feces on voiding following completion of external beam radiotherapy and brachytherapy for high-grade prostate carcinoma. There is direct communication from the base of the bladder to the rectum from the level of the prostate (marked by brachytherapy seeds, *arrow*), corresponding to an urethrorectal fistula.

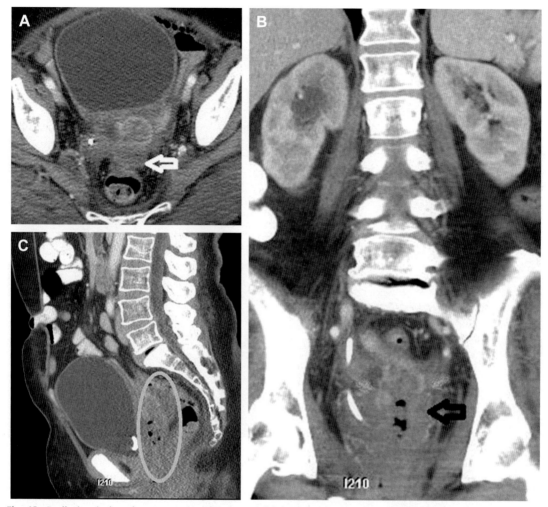

Fig. 12. Radiation-induced enterovaginal fistula. Axial (*A*), coronal reconstructed (*B*), and sagittal reconstructed (*C*) CT images in a patient with pain treated with pelvic radiation for cervical carcinoma show a gas and fluid collection (*circle* in *C*) interposed between the bladder and the rectum. Soft-tissue thickening between the vagina and the rectum is evident on the axial and coronal images (*arrows* in *A, B*).

Another common site of radiation enteritis is the terminal ileum, also given its fixed position in the right lower quadrant. However, any portion of the luminal gastrointestinal tract may be involved with radiation injury (**Figs. 17** and **18**). Complex fistulae can ensue with radiation enteritis resulting in enteroenteric, enterocolic, or enterovesical fistulae. In addition, fistulae to the adjacent vessels may follow (see **Fig. 18; Fig. 19**). Bowel perforation may rarely occur, as the result of direct injury to the bowel or bowel stricture (**Figs. 20** and **21**).

BONE

In bone, typically the thoracolumbar spine in cases of radiation therapy in the abdomen and/or pelvis, acute radiation-related injury usually takes the form of a geographic area of low density on CT

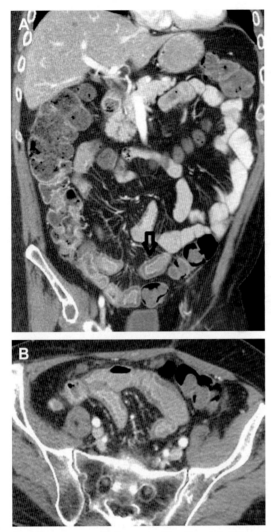

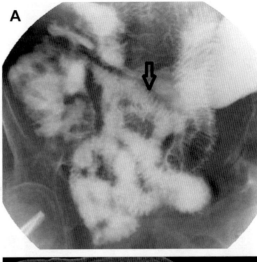

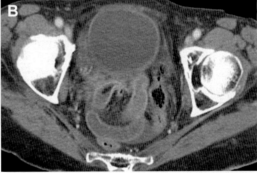

Fig. 14. Acute radiation enteritis. A small bowel follow-through examination (*A*) and axial CECT image (*B*) in a patient following completion of pelvic radiation shows several thick-walled ileal loops (*arrow* in *A*) in the pelvis.

Fig. 13. Acute radiation enteritis. Coronal (*A*) and axial (*B*) CECT images show mural thickening with stratification and mucosal hyperenhancement of a pelvic ileal loop in this patient who underwent pelvic radiation for rectal cancer (*arrow* in *A*).

or low T1 signal intensity/high T2 signal intensity on MR imaging. Imaging abnormalities tend to be long-standing or permanent. Bone that has been exposed to radiation treatment aimed at other organs is hypocellular, osteopenic, and weakened, leading to these imaging findings. Fractures that do not heal properly may result (**Fig. 22**).[16] Marrow subsequently becomes replaced by fatty tissue and thus is hyperintense on T1-weighted images.[18] These changes occur within days to weeks of exposure.[12]

Imaging abnormalities tend to be permanent, with residual abnormal bone density and, occasionally, old or healed fractures. Bone marrow is the only tissue in the body that is replaced by fat instead of fibrotic tissue after radiation-induced injury.[12] Osteopenia may then occur, resulting in insufficiency fractures of the pelvis.

Bone marrow is sometimes affected in a patchy manner, with areas of osteopenia intermixed with more normal bone, potentially simulating bone metastases.[6]

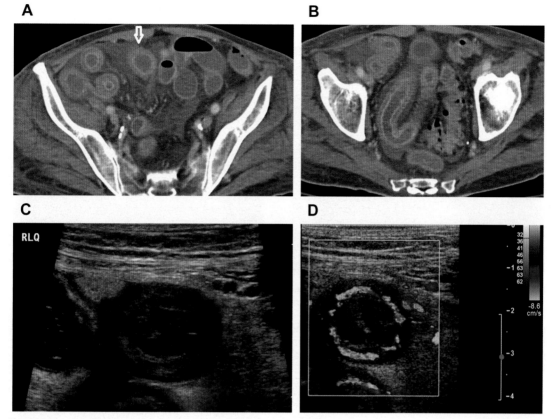

Fig. 15. Acute radiation enteritis. Axial CECT (*A, B*) in a patient who presents with an acute abdomen following pelvic radiation shows diffuse mural thickening and mucosal hyperenhancement producing a targetoid appearance of several pelvic small bowel loops (*arrow*). Ultrasonography images (*C, D*) of the inflamed small bowel in the same patient also show the mural thickening, and targetoid appearance.

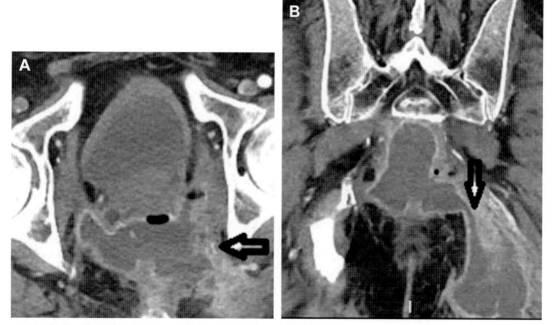

Fig. 16. Radiation-induced abscess. Axial (*A*) and coronal (*B*) CECT images in a patient who completed neoadjuvant radiation for rectal carcinoma (not shown) reveals a large gas and fluid collection (*arrow*) in the presacral space with extension of infection to the side wall.

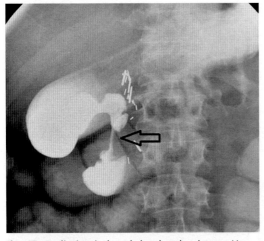

Fig. 17. Radiation-induced duodenal stricture. Upper gastrointestinal series in a patient with severe abdominal pain shows marked focal narrowing of the second portion of the duodenum (*arrow*) in this patient who had undergone radiation therapy and nephrectomy for renal cell carcinoma. The narrowing was fixed at fluoroscopic examination.

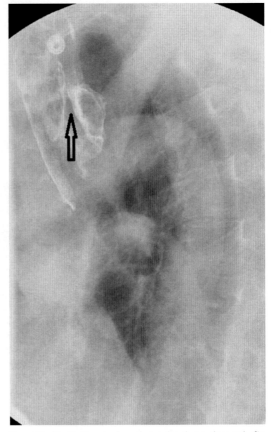

Fig. 18. Radiation-induced tracheal-esophageal fistula. Lateral image from an esophagram shows communication between the trachea and the esophagus (*arrow*) with oral contrast filling the trachea representing a tracheal-esophageal fistula in this patient presenting with recurrent pneumonia years after radiation treatment of squamous cell neck cancer.

BLOOD VESSELS

As seen with radiation to the bowel, radiation-related vascular changes usually involve the intima in the acute setting and the entire vessel wall in the chronic stage, which can lead to fibrosis. Because of inadvertent radiation injury, there is often microvascular damage as shown by endothelial damage and resultant endothelial proliferation in arterioles and thrombosis in small venules.[19–26] Secondary hypoperfusional changes can be seen at imaging, and may involve the supplied viscera. With time, this may progress to a type of endarteritis obliterans, with tissue ischemia and fibrosis. The arterial injury is termed radiation arteriopathy.[19] This same process may also occur in large vessels and, as a result, accelerated atherosclerosis in large arteries may occur, and the tissue damage with hyalinization and fibrosis ensues. Radiation arteriopathy is distinguished from other forms of atherosclerosis by focal and segmental involvement, and location in the vicinity of the radiation field (**Table 1**).

In summary, although modern radiation therapy techniques expose neighboring organs less than older techniques did, inadvertent radiation exposure, and sometimes damage, does occur, and can be an important cause of morbidity for patients. It is vitally important for the radiologist to recognize these radiation effects on imaging examinations, and to help steer the correct treatment of the patient and not to mistake this appearance with other entities, namely tumor recurrence or metastasis.

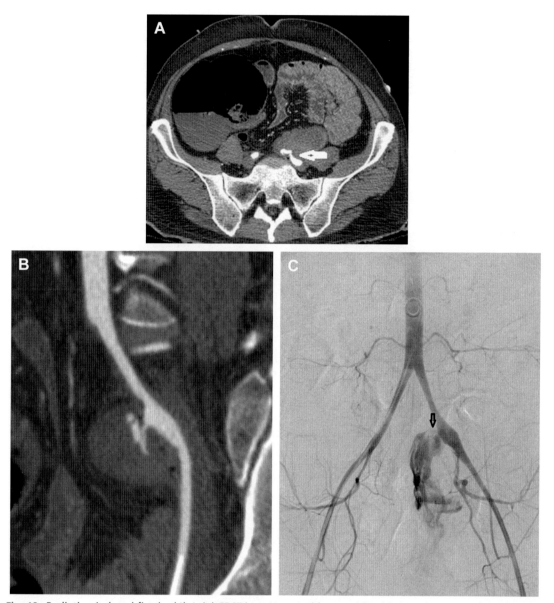

Fig. 19. Radiation-induced fistula. (*A*) Axial CECT in a 41-year-old man with a history of T3N1 rectal adenocarcinoma treated by neoadjuvant chemotherapy and radiation therapy (a total of 50.4 Gy) shows active extravasation of intravenous contrast from the left common iliac artery to the adjacent sigmoid colon (*arrow*). (*B*) Reformatted off-sagittal CT image again shows the active extravasation of contrast. (*C*) Frontal image from a catheter angiogram confirms communication of the left common iliac artery to the sigmoid colon, with pooling of contrast at the site of leakage (*arrow*).

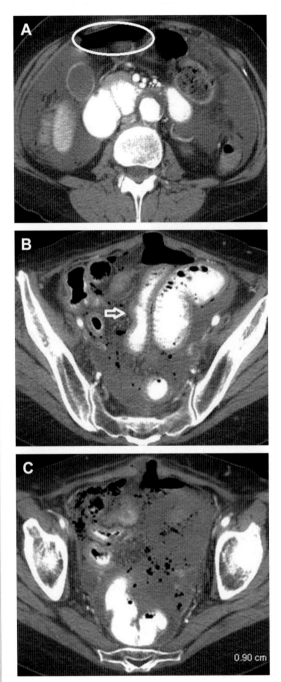

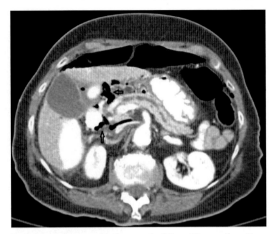

Fig. 21. Acute radiation enteritis with perforation. Axial CECT image shows pneumoperitoneum and gas around the duodenum (*arrows*).

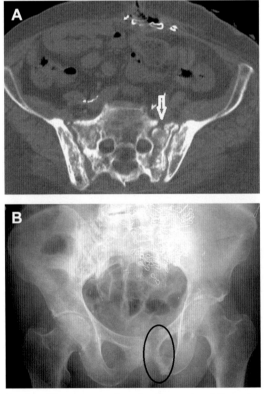

Fig. 20. Perforated radiation enteritis. Axial CECT images (*A–C*) in a 48-year-old woman following radiation therapy for cervical carcinoma (not shown) shows mural thickening of pelvic ileal small bowel loops (*arrow*) surrounded by free fluid containing foci of mottled gas, and pneumoperitoneum (*circle*). At surgery, there was diffuse peritonitis and transmural perforation of ileum caused by obliterative endarteritis related to ischemic changes from radiation.

Fig. 22. CT and conventional radiographs of the pelvis show areas of radiation-induced osteopenia intermixed with areas of osteosclerosis and fractures of the sacrum (*arrow* in *A*) and pubic rami (*circle* in *B*).

Table 1
Imaging effects of inadvertent radiation of abdominal and pelvic structures

Liver	Geographic area of low attenuation/low T1 signal intensity that usually resolves
Spleen	Geographic area of low attenuation/low T1 signal intensity that may become atrophic
Kidney	Geographic area of low attenuation/low T1 signal intensity that is usually permanent
Bowel	Mural hyperenhancement and thickening acutely that may develop into chronic strictures/fistulae
Bone	Geographic area of low attenuation/low T1 signal intensity that is usually permanent

REFERENCES

1. Cupp J, Koong A, Fisher G, et al. Tissue effects after stereotactic body radiotherapy using Cyberknife for patients with abdominal malignancies. Clin Oncol 2008;20:69–75.
2. Kwek J, Iyer R, Dunnington J, et al. Spectrum of imaging findings in the abdomen after radiotherapy. AJR Am J Roentgenol 2006;187:1204–11.
3. Khozouz R, Huq S, Perry M. Radiation-induced liver disease. J Clin Oncol 2008;26:4844–5.
4. Maor Y, Malnick S. Liver injury induced by anticancer chemotherapy and radiation therapy. Int J Hepatol 2013;2013:815105.
5. Munden R, Erasmus J, Smythe W, et al. Radiation injury to the liver after intensity-modulated radiation therapy in patients with mesothelioma: an unusual CT appearance. AJR Am J Roentgenol 2005;184:1091–5.
6. Iyer R, Jhingran A, Sawaf H, et al. Imaging findings after radiotherapy to the pelvis. AJR Am J Roentgenol 2001;177:1083–9.
7. Kirkpatrick JP, Kelsey CR, Palta M, et al. Stereotactic body radiotherapy: a critical review for non-radiation oncologists. Cancer 2014;120(7):942–54.
8. Willemart S, Nicaise N, Struyven J, et al. Acute radiation-induced hepatic injury: evaluation by triphasic contrast enhanced helical CT. Br J Radiol 2000;73:544–6.
9. Congdon C. The destructive effect of radiation on lymphatic issue. Cancer Res 1966;26:1211–20.
10. Dawson L, Kavanaugh B, Paulino A, et al. Radiation-induced kidney injury. Int J Radiat Oncol Biol Phys 2010;76:S108–15.
11. Moulder J, Cohen E. Radiation-induced multi-organ involvement and failure: the contribution of radiation effects on the renal system. Br J Radiol 2005;27:82–8.
12. Maturen K, Feng M, Wasnick A. Imaging effects of radiation therapy in the abdomen and pelvis: evaluating "innocent bystander" tissues. Radiographics 2013;33:599–619.
13. Johnson R, Carrington B. Review: pelvic radiation disease. Clin Radiol 1992;45:4–12.
14. Falconi M, Pederzoli P. The relevance of gastrointestinal fistulae in clinical practice: a review. Gut 2001;49:iv2–10.
15. Addley H, Vargas H, Moyle P, et al. Pelvic imaging following chemotherapy and radiation therapy for gynecologic malignancies. Radiographics 2010;30:1843–56.
16. Felipe de Campos-Lobato L, Vogel J. Enterocutaneous fistula associated with malignancy and prior radiation therapy. Clin Colon Rectal Surg 2010;23:176–81.
17. Yankelevitz D, Henschke C, Knapp P, et al. Effect of radiation therapy on thoracic and lumbar bone marrow: evaluation with MR imaging. AJR Am J Roentgenol 1991;157:87–92.
18. Terezakis S, Heron D, Lavigne R, et al. What the diagnostic radiologist needs to know about radiation oncology. Radiology 2011;261:30–44.
19. Katz D, Scheirey C, Bordia R, et al. Computed tomography of miscellaneous regional and diffuse small bowel disorders. Radiol Clin North Am 2013;51:45–68.
20. Hampton J. Acute radiation effects in the kidney. Radiat Res 1972;52:316–23.
21. Sheng Y, Wang Q, Li Z. Time-dependent changes in CT of radiation-induced liver injury: a preliminary study in gastric cancer patients. J Huazhong Univ Sci Technolog Med Sci 2010;30:683–6.
22. De Smet A, Kuhns A, Fayos J, et al. Effects of radiation therapy of growing long bones. AJR Am J Roentgenol 1976;127:935–9.
23. Reed G, Cox A. The human liver after radiation injury. A form of veno-occlusive disease. Am J Pathol 1966;48(4):597.
24. Iyer R, Jhingran A. Radiation injury: imaging findings in the chest, abdomen and pelvis after therapeutic radiation. Cancer Imaging 2006;6:S131–9.
25. Andreyev J. Gastrointestinal symptoms after pelvic radiotherapy: a new understanding to improve management of symptomatic patients. Lancet Oncol 2007;8:1007–17.
26. Werner-Wasik M, Rudoler S, Preston P, et al. Immediate side effects of stereotactic radiotherapy and radiosurgery. Int J Radiat Oncol Biol Phys 1999;43:299–304.

Computed Tomography of Iatrogenic Complications of Upper Gastrointestinal Endoscopy, Stenting, and Intubation

David M. Valenzuela, MD[a], Spencer C. Behr, MD[a],
Fergus V. Coakley, MD[b], Z. Jane Wang, MD[a],
Emily M. Webb, MD[a], Benjamin M. Yeh, MD[a],*

KEYWORDS

- Computed tomography • Gastrointestinal intervention • Iatrogenic complications • Iatrogenic injury
- Nasogastric tube • Endoscopic complication

KEY POINTS

- Though rare, complications of upper gastrointestinal endoscopy, stenting, and intubation occur and can be potentially life-threatening.
- On any postprocedural CT examination, careful evaluation of the path of prior instrumentation is critical in searching for extraluminal gas and fluid that may point to possible complications.
- Immediate postprocedural CT examinations may have ambiguous findings, but generally CT can be used to identify or exclude most clinically relevant iatrogenic injuries.

INTRODUCTION

The gastrointestinal tract and bile ducts are essential conduits for digestion and serve as protective barriers to toxins, corrosives, and infection. The bowel is a tubular structure which peristalses and propels material under pressure toward the anus while absorbing essential nutrients and fluid. Iatrogenic injury to these structures can lead to serious and potentially life-threatening complications. Although many diagnostic tests can be used to identify and define the extent of iatrogenic injury, computed tomography (CT) is particularly well suited for rapid evaluation of gastrointestinal iatrogenic injury because it (1) provides a rapid, large area coverage with consistently low image artifact; (2) can be used to readily distinguish amongst gas, metal clips, and calcifications; (3) is well tolerated; and (4) can be used to evaluate the abdomen through overlying monitoring equipment and dressings. This review describes common injuries that may occur with upper gastrointestinal intubation, endoscopy (including endoscopic retrograde cholangiopancreatography [ERCP]), and stenting, with an emphasis on the resultant CT findings.

CT ANATOMY OF THE UPPER GASTROINTESTINAL TRACT

The gastrointestinal system is typically divided into upper and lower portions. For the purposes of

a Department of Radiology and Biomedical Imaging, University of California, San Francisco, 505 Parnassus Avenue, San Francisco, CA 94143-0628, USA; b Department of Radiology, Oregon Health & Science University, 3181 Southwest Sam Jackson Park Road, Portland, OR 97239-3098, USA
* Corresponding author. Abdominal Imaging, University of California, San Francisco, Box 0628, 505 Parnassus Avenue, San Francisco, CA 94143-0628.
E-mail address: ben.yeh@ucsf.edu

Radiol Clin N Am 52 (2014) 1055–1070
http://dx.doi.org/10.1016/j.rcl.2014.05.011

radiologic.theclinics.com

defining the location of gastrointestinal hemorrhage, the upper gastrointestinal system is frequently described as extending from the pharynx to the duodenal-jejunal junction at the ligament of Treitz, whereas the lower gastrointestinal system has been described as extending from distal to the ligament of Treitz to the anus. In this review, as in endoscopy, the upper gastrointestinal tract refers to the esophagus, stomach, and duodenum.

At CT the esophagus appears as ovoid soft-tissue density which variably contains intraluminal air. The esophageal wall should not exceed 3 mm in thickness when the esophagus is distended. The stomach is divided into the fundus, body, antrum, and pylorus, with the gastric fundus being the most posterior. The normal gastric wall should not exceed 5 mm in thickness when the stomach is well distended. Rugal folds are commonly identified at CT. The duodenum is divided into 4 segments with the second and third portions of the duodenum being retroperitoneal. The second portion of the duodenum passes to the right of the pancreatic head and below the uncinate process, crossing anterior to the inferior vena cava and aorta. The fourth portion of the duodenum turns upward and ascends just to the left of the aorta and continues to the ligament of Treitz, where it becomes the jejunum.

CT TECHNIQUE
Oral Contrast Material Considerations

Patient preparation depends on the type of suspected injury. The use of oral contrast material is currently controversial. Positive (radiodense) contrast material has undeniable benefits, including confirming the presence and location of bowel leakage and improving the detection of fluid collections including abscesses. Unfortunately, positive contrast can also potentially obscure bowel wall hyperemia associated with inflammation or nonenhancement associated with infarction. At the authors' institutions, emergent CT scans are usually performed initially with oral water. However, oral contrast is given when there is a clinical suspicion of bowel perforation or fistula, or when evaluation of an extraluminal collection is needed. For evaluation of the esophagus (CT esophagram), an unenhanced CT of the chest is immediately followed by a scan with positive oral contrast (**Fig. 1**). If patients are able to swallow in a recumbent position, they are instructed to put contrast in their mouth, then to "hold their breath and swallow" for the scan to ensure contrast opacification of the esophageal lumen.

CT is usually performed before fluoroscopic imaging, because (1) the low concentrations of oral contrast required for CT will not interfere with a subsequent fluoroscopic examination, but the high-density fluoroscopic oral contrast material may cause substantial image artifact on subsequent CT[1]; (2) performing fluoroscopic esophagography in seriously ill patients may be technically difficult; (3) aspiration of highly concentrated hyperosmolar contrast material may result in pulmonary edema; and (4) CT is generally regarded as more sensitive for the detection of iatrogenic injuries of the abdomen in comparison with fluoroscopy, whereby false negatives may occur in 10% to 38% of cases.[2,3]

Imaging Parameters

Use of optimized technique can markedly improve the diagnostic capability of CT. Removal of as many moveable metallic objects from around the abdomen as possible will minimize streak artifact. Breath-holding or respiratory suspension minimizes motion artifact. Imaging of the chest or abdomen is generally best acquired at thin sections (1.25 mm or thinner in the authors' institutions) at high pitch for rapid coverage. Images are reconstructed in the axial, coronal, and sagittal planes. The authors use automated exposure control and iterative reconstruction for all CT imaging to minimize radiation dose.

ESOPHAGEAL INJURY FROM ENDOSCOPY
Rates of Esophageal Injury

Endoscopy of the gastrointestinal system has been performed since the mid-nineteenth century when Kussmaul developed the gastroscope. Though a relatively common procedure, endoscopy is invasive and can cause internal injuries. Iatrogenic injuries are the most common cause of esophageal trauma and include the spectrum of intramural hematoma, esophageal dissection, and perforation.[4,5] Despite the common use of upper endoscopy, the rates of complications are controversial.[6] An older survey conducted by the American Society of Gastrointestinal Endoscopy in 1974 estimated that the overall complication rate based on more than 200,000 esophagogastroduodenoscopy examinations was 0.13%, with an associated mortality of 0.004%.[7] Other published data indicate that up to 2.5% of patients required additional evaluation for complications following outpatient endoscopy.[8] Although major complications are relatively rare after esophagogastroduodenoscopy, injuries may include cardiopulmonary complications, infection, Mallory-Weiss tears, perforation, and bleeding.[6]

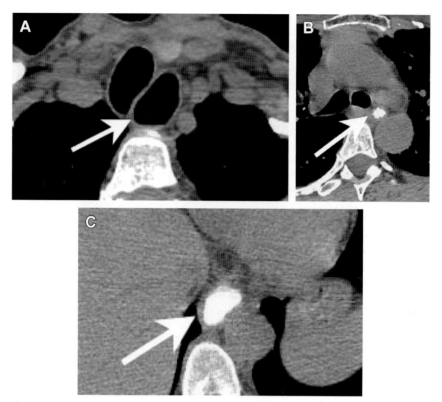

Fig. 1. Normal computed tomography (CT) esophagram. (*A*) Axial CT image of the upper thorax shows air disten-sion of the upper esophagus with a normal, thin wall (*white arrow*). (*B*) Axial image inferior to *A* shows luminal distention of the esophagus with contrast and normal-appearing esophageal mucosal folds (*white arrow*). (*C*) There is normal contrast opacification in the esophagus in the region of the gastroesophageal junction (*white arrow*).

The rate of esophageal perforation in diagnostic endoscopy ranges from 0.02% to 0.2%.[7,8] The risk of esophageal perforation increases if esoph-agogastroduodenoscopy is combined with an intervention such as biopsy, dilation, coagulation, or sclerotherapy.[9] The injection of sclerosants such as ethanol may damage adjacent normal tis-sue secondary to tracking of the agent along tissue planes, leading to perforation or fistula formation. The overall complication rate of endoscopic vari-ceal sclerotherapy has been estimated to be be-tween 35% and 78%, with a mortality rate of 1% to 5%.[6]

Complications from endoscopic variceal sclero-therapy include ulceration, perforation, esopha-geal stricture, and aspiration pneumonia. Although these complications are also seen with endoscopic band ligation of bleeding varices, the complication rates are lower and, thus, endo-scopic band ligation is the treatment of choice for esophageal varices.[6,10,11]

Esophageal perforation occurs at a higher rate in the distal one-third of the esophagus, likely because this region of the esophagus is most frequently

involved with inflammation and tumor.[12] Though rare, esophageal perforation is associated with a high mortality rate that approaches 25%.[13] The high mortality rate is related to the fact that the con-nective tissue around the esophagus provides little barrier to leakage of esophageal content. Therefore, serious sequelae, particularly mediastinitis, may develop in patients with esophageal perforation. The treatment of esophageal perforation remains broad-spectrum antibiotics, surgical drainage, and primary repair or anastomosis if possible.[14]

CT Findings of Esophageal Perforation

As suspected esophageal perforation is often evaluated with cross-sectional imaging, familiarity with the CT manifestations of esophageal perfora-tion is essential.[15] CT findings of esophageal perforation include gas and fluid collections in a periesophageal location, mediastinal fluid collec-tions/inflammation, esophageal wall thickening or a focal esophageal wall defect, and extraluminal leakage of contrast (**Fig. 2**).[16–18] In addition, most esophageal perforations occur in the distal left

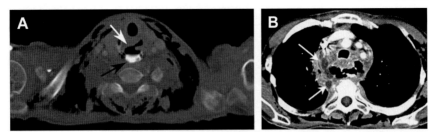

Fig. 2. Esophageal perforation after esophageal balloon dilation. (*A*) Axial image from a CT esophagram shows a defect in the posterolateral wall of the cervical esophagus (*white arrow*), with oral contrast pooling in the retro-esophageal mediastinum (*black arrow*). Note the extensive subcutaneous emphysema. (*B*) Axial image inferior to A shows extensive retroesophageal pneumomediastinum and mediastinal abscesses (*white arrows*).

posterior aspect of the esophagus, and can cause pneumomediastinum and a left pleural effusion.[5] Perforations are also more likely to occur at sites of pharyngeal or esophageal narrowing, such as an esophageal web, a diverticulum, or sites involved with tumor or inflammation.[1]

CT of Esophageal Mural Injury

Esophageal intramural hematoma and esophageal dissection are less severe injuries in the spectrum of iatrogenic esophageal trauma. A recent history of esophageal instrumentation is the most important risk factor. In the absence of such a history, clinically differentiating esophageal intramural hematoma and esophageal dissection from cardiovascular causes of chest pain, particularly myocardial infarction or aortic dissection, is extremely difficult as these disease processes may present with similar symptoms such as acute retrosternal chest pain and dysphagia. The fact that anticoagulation is contraindicated in the former but plays a central therapeutic role in the latter highlights the necessity of differentiating these disparate clinical entities. CT findings of esophageal intramural hematoma include the presence of an eccentric hyperdense mass representing blood products within the esophageal wall (**Fig. 3**). Depending on the size, an esophageal intramural hematoma will result in varying degrees of luminal narrowing and may even result in obstruction.

Esophageal dissection is typically seen as a mucosal flap with associated gas or contrast material in a submucosal distribution. Occasionally a classic double-barreled appearance of the esophagus is present, with the false lumen lying posterior to the true esophageal lumen (**Fig. 4**).

Esophageal Stents

The endoscopic placement of esophageal stents has proved to be an effective tool in treating dysphagia, anastomotic leakage after esophagectomy, and esophagorespiratory fistulas.[19] Endoscopy is also commonly used in palliation of malignancies affecting the upper gastrointestinal tract.[20,21] In fact, fewer than half the patients diagnosed with esophageal carcinoma are candidates for surgical resection. Thus, esophageal stents are commonly placed for palliation to either reestablish endoluminal patency in patients with obstructive esophageal lesions or manage esophagorespiratory fistulas. Despite the well-accepted utility of esophageal stents, several immediate and delayed complications may occur after stent placement.

Complications of Esophageal Stents

Complications of esophageal stent placement are typically categorized as early or late complications (ie, up to 7 days after stent placement and >7 days after stent placement), and include stent migration, stent fracturing, tumor ingrowth or overgrowth, and life-threatening complications include hemorrhage, perforations, fistula formation, and tracheal compression (**Figs. 5–8**). Long-term esophageal stenting is associated with high rates of migration (33%), bleeding (19%), overgrowth (36%), fistula formation (5%), and bolus impaction (23%).[22–24] Esophageal stent migration is more common when stents are placed near the gastroesophageal junction.[22,25–28] The migration rate of covered stents is higher than that of uncovered stents, likely because uncovered stents benefit from tumor ingrowth or overgrowth that helps keep the stents fixed in place. Metallic stents are preferred over plastic stents because of their lower complication rates.[29,30] Pretreatment with chemoradiotherapy has been reported to increase the incidence of complications by some investigators but not others.[31,32]

In a study of 82 patients with inoperable obstructive malignancies of the esophagus, delayed complications related to esophageal

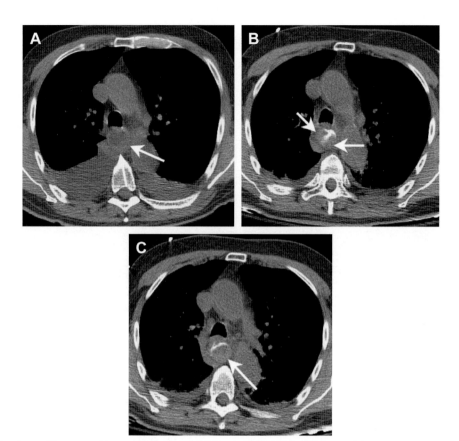

Fig. 3. Esophageal intramural hematoma after transesophageal echocardiogram. (*A*) Noncontrast CT of the chest shows an eccentric hyperdense mass (*white arrows*) representing blood products in the posterolateral aspect of the esophageal wall, resulting in partial narrowing of the fluid-filled esophagus. Bilateral pleural effusions are also present. (*B, C*) Axial images from a CT esophagram in the same patient shows narrowing and near obliteration of the oral contrast–containing mid-esophagus by the intramural hematoma (*white arrows*).

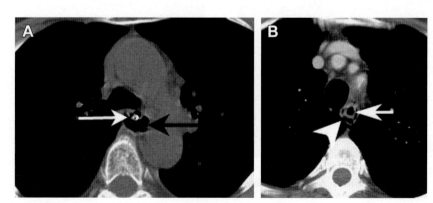

Fig. 4. Esophageal dissection after balloon dilation. (*A*) Noncontrast axial CT image of the chest shows a nasogastric (NG) tube lying dependently against the posterior wall of the esophagus (*white arrow*). The esophageal mucosa separates the true lumen containing the NG tube from the more posterior false lumen (*black arrow*). (*B*) Esophageal dissection in a different patient on a contrast-enhanced axial CT image shows the true lumen (*white arrow*) and the false lumen (*white arrowhead*) separated by the esophageal mucosa.

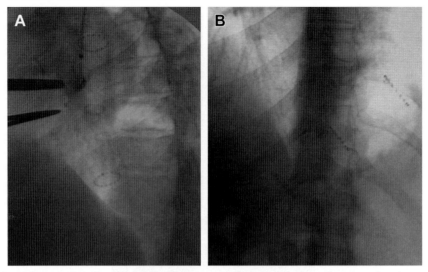

Fig. 5. Esophageal stent migration. (*A*) Lateral fluoroscopic image shows the radiopaque rings in a metallic stent in the distal esophagus. (*B*) Frontal fluoroscopic image in the same patient taken 4 months later, showing migration of the metallic stent into the stomach. Although CT may be more accurate for the detection of subtle stent complications, obvious complications such as this are readily diagnosed with radiographic and fluoroscopic images, which are quick and inexpensive.

endoprosthesis placement was reported to occur in 64% of patients, with 15.9% of patients dying from complications directly related to stent placement.[30] Life-threatening complications, defined as severe, symptomatic, stent-related injuries to the esophagus or adjacent structures, occurred in 19 patients (23.2%).[30] Irrespective of stent type, life-threatening complications occurred more frequently in patients with stent placement in the proximal third of the esophagus.[30] Dyspnea caused by stent-related tracheal compression, a rare complication with few reported cases, has occurred in 5 patients (6.1%) to our knowledge (**Fig. 9**).[30,33–35]

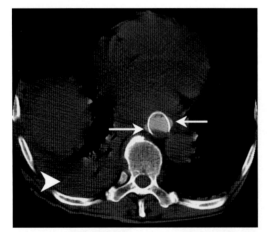

Fig. 6. Esophageal stent leak. Axial image from a CT esophagram in a patient with recurrent esophageal carcinoma and an esophageal stent. Radiodense contrast material is visible beyond the walls of the esophageal stent, consistent with a stent leak (*white arrows*). A right pleural effusion is present (*white arrowhead*). Enteric material was found in the output of the patient's chest tube (not pictured).

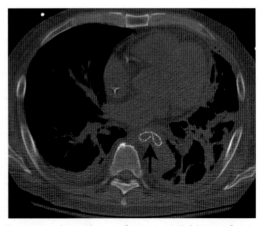

Fig. 7. Esophageal stent fracture. Axial image from a chest CT without contrast in a patient with esophageal carcinoma and recurrent dysphagia after stent placement. The posterior aspect of the stent has fractured (*black arrow*), resulting in buckling and partial luminal obstruction.

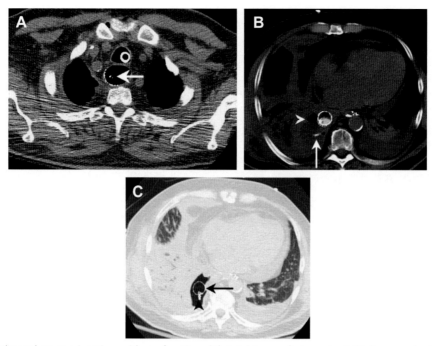

Fig. 8. Esophageal stent migration with perforation. (*A*) Axial image from a chest CT shows a stent within the esophageal lumen, with a nasogastric tube coursing through the stent (*white arrow*). (*B*) Axial CT image in the same patient obtained a few days later shows inferomedial migration of the stent and perforation outside the esophageal lumen. Note the leakage of high-density contrast material (*white arrow*) from the esophagus into the right pleural space, with associated right hydropneumothorax (*white arrowhead*). (*C*) Axial CT image with lung window obtained 6 days after *B* shows further migration of the esophageal stent into the pleural space, with the stent (*black arrow*) immediately anterior to a newly placed right chest tube (*black arrowhead*).

INJURY FROM ENDOSCOPIC GASTRODUODENAL PROCEDURES
ERCP-Related Complications

Since its introduction in 1968, ERCP has been commonly used in the diagnosis and treatment

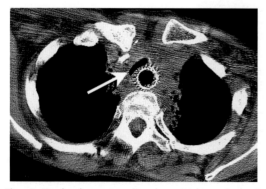

Fig. 9. Tracheal compression by esophageal stent. Noncontrast axial CT image of the chest shows narrowing of the posterior aspect of the trachea (*white arrow*) by an esophageal stent.

of biliary disease.[36] The procedure consists of an upper endoscopy followed by cannulation of the major papilla in the duodenum, at which point injection of contrast material into the biliary system and/or a sphincterotomy may be performed.[14]

The most common complication of ERCP is pancreatitis.[37,38] In a study of 2347 patients who underwent ERCP with sphincterotomy, 5.4% developed pancreatitis.[38] Factors that increase the risk of post-ERCP pancreatitis include young age (<60 years), sphincter of Oddi dysfunction, biliary balloon sphincter dilation, moderate or difficult bile duct cannulation, and more than 1 pancreatic contrast injection. Young age and sphincter of Oddi dysfunction are reported to be the most important risk factors for the development of post-ERCP pancreatitis.[38,39] The CT appearance of post-ERCP pancreatitis is identical to that of pancreatitis in general, including an enlarged and edematous pancreas with surrounding inflammatory fat stranding and fluid (**Fig. 10**).

Estimates of perforation after ERCP and sphincterotomy range from 0.3% to 0.6% after ERCP and sphincterotomy.[37–40] Perforations

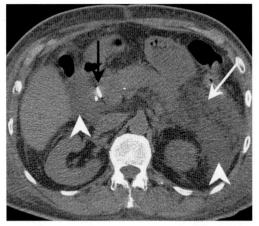

Fig. 10. Post endoscopic retrograde cholangiopan-creatography (ERCP) pancreatitis. Noncontrast axial CT image of the abdomen in a patient after ERCP placement of a biliary stent (*black arrow*) shows fat stranding around the body and tail of the pancreas (*white arrow*) and fluid adjacent to the pancreatic head and tail (*white arrowheads*).

may be intra-abdominal or retroperitoneal, and have been categorized as guide wire–induced, periampullary during sphincterotomy, and at a site remote from the papilla (**Fig. 11**).[39] The CT appearance of perforation after ERCP varies and

depends on where the perforation occurred. The most common sites of iatrogenic perforation at ERCP are the esophagus and duodenum. The appearance of esophageal perforation is depicted in **Fig. 11**. The CT findings of duodenal perforation depend on which segment of the duodenum is injured. Retroperitoneal free air is present with perforation of the second or third portion of the duodenum, while one would expect to see intra-peritoneal free air with perforation of the first or fourth portions of the duodenum (**Fig. 12**). Extra-luminal leak of contrast from the duodenum is another highly specific finding at CT. Occasionally a discrete defect in the wall of the duodenum may be seen (**Fig. 13**).

Other potential iatrogenic complications following ERCP are cholangitis, hemorrhage/he-matoma formation, infection, and complications related to therapeutic devices such as stents and stone-retrieval baskets (**Figs. 14** and **15**). The overall mortality rate after diagnostic ERCP is 0.2%, but is twice as high after therapeutic ERCP (0.4%–0.49%).[38,41]

Injuries from Endoscopic Ultrasonography

Endoscopic ultrasound-guided fine-needle aspiration (EUS-FNA) is an invaluable technique used in

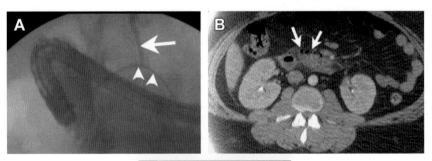

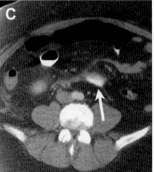

Fig. 11. Iatrogenic perforation of the pancreatic duct. (*A*) Fluoroscopic image during ERCP shows contrast opa-cification of an unusually vertically oriented pancreatic duct (*white arrow*). The guide wire (*arrowheads*) extends well beyond the confines of the pancreatic duct, indicating perforation. (*B*) Axial contrast-enhanced CT image shows small foci of gas (*white arrows*) anterior to the pancreatic neck. (*C*) A more inferior axial image shows contrast material (*white arrow*) from the ERCP that has pooled in the retroperitoneum. Findings represent perforation of the pancreatic duct.

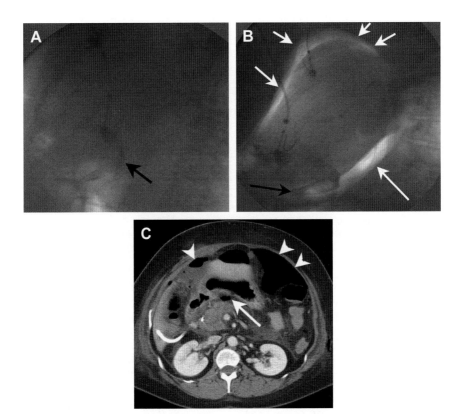

Fig. 12. Gastrointestinal perforation after ERCP. (A) Pre-ERCP fluoroscopic image shows a surgical drain in the right upper quadrant (*black arrow*, also shown in *B*). (B) Fluoroscopic image after ERCP shows new radiolucency around liver (*white arrows*), representing free intraperitoneal air and perforation. (C) Contrast-enhanced axial CT image in the same patient shows intraperitoneal gas (*white arrowheads*) and gas in the lesser sac (*white arrow*).

the diagnosis and staging of a variety of clinical entities. The utility of EUS-FNA is particularly evident in sampling pancreatic masses, where it has replaced ERCP and brush cytology as the endoscopic test of choice, owing to higher success rates combined with lower rates of procedural complications.[42] In addition, EUS-FNA is increasingly being used in sampling abdominal

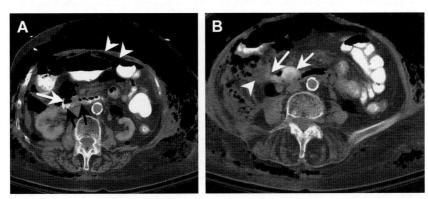

Fig. 13. Duodenal perforation after ERCP. (A) Axial CT image of the abdomen with intravenous and oral contrast shows the third portion of the duodenum (*black arrows*) with a focal defect in the anterior wall (*white arrow*). There is associated intraperitoneal free air (*white arrowheads*) and extensive subcutaneous emphysema. (B) Axial CT image inferior to A shows extraluminal leak of contrast (*white arrows*) into an amorphous fluid collection (*white arrowhead*).

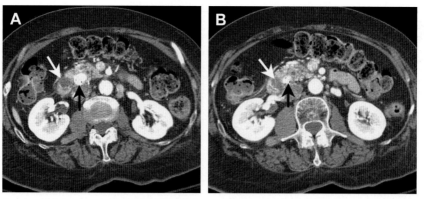

Fig. 14. Duodenal wall hematoma after ERCP. (*A, B*) Contrast-enhanced axial CT image of the abdomen in a patient with abdominal pain after ERCP for metal bile duct stent placement (*black arrows*) shows focal low density in the wall of the second portion of the duodenum (*white arrows*), representing a duodenal hematoma.

and mediastinal adenopathy when other techniques are not feasible or have failed.[43] The impact of EUS-FNA is perhaps most pronounced in the avoidance of unnecessary operative intervention in advanced lung, esophageal, and pancreatic cancers, for which resection has little clinical benefit.[43,44] Specifically, EUS-FNA can change management in a high percentage of patients

with suspected lung cancer and mediastinal adenopathy, and in patients with esophageal cancer and local regional adenopathy.[43,45,46]

The major complications of EUS-FNA include infections in cystic lesions, bleeding, pancreatitis, and perforation. Compared with ERCP, EUS-FNA has been shown to have a lower rate of iatrogenic pancreatitis. In a large study with cohort of 4909

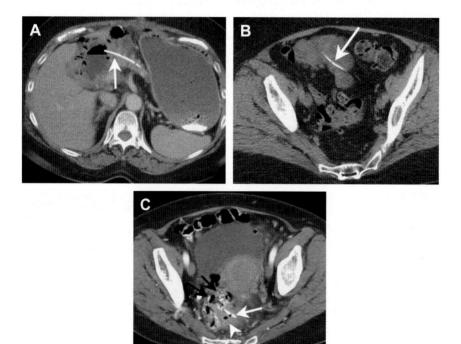

Fig. 15. Pancreatic stent migration and perforation. (*A*) Contrast-enhanced axial CT image of the abdomen shows an endoscopically placed pancreatic stent (*white arrow*) extending into the second portion of the duodenum. (*B*) Axial CT image obtained 1 year later shows that the stent (*white arrow*) has migrated into the ileum. (*C*) Axial CT image of the pelvis obtained approximately 10 months after *B* shows that the stent (*white arrow*) has migrated into and perforated through the rectum (*black arrows*). A small fluid collection with associated foci of gas (*white arrowhead*) is seen at the site of perforation.

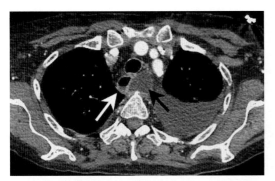

Fig. 16. Esophageal perforation after transesophageal echocardiogram. Axial chest CT image with contrast shows a fluid collection (*black arrow*) adjacent to the fluid-filled esophagus (*white arrow*) in a patient with esophageal perforation after transesophageal echocardiogram. An associated left pleural effusion is present.

patients, 0.29% developed pancreatitis.[47] In addition, EUS-FNA has a lower rate of perforation and hemorrhage compared with ERCP.[42,48,49] This lower complication rate is likely due to the less invasive nature of the procedure, as tissue sampling is commonly performed with a 22-gauge needle and the procedure does not require bile duct cannulation or sphincterotomy. Data suggest that the complication rate of EUS-FNA closely approximates that seen with diagnostic upper endoscopy.[49]

INJURIES FROM GASTROINTESTINAL INTUBATION

In addition to esophagogastroduodenoscopy, gastrointestinal instrumentation of any kind may also result in the aforementioned iatrogenic esophageal injuries. Esophageal injury has been reported after nasogastric tube placement, Sengstaken-Blakemore tube insertion, enteroclysis tube insertion, transesophageal echocardiography, and endotracheal tube placement (Figs. 16 and 17).[5]

Iatrogenic injury related to the placement of nasoenteric tubes deserves special attention because these tubes are so commonly used. Maintaining enteral nutrition increases blood flow to the gut, maintains gastrointestinal integrity, decreases stress-induced injury, helps maintain immunocompetence, and preserves normal gut flora.[50,51] Nasoenteric tubes are typically made of silicone or polyurethane. Silicone tubes are generally thinner and more pliable but have weaker walls than polyurethane tubes. By contrast, polyurethane tubes are more durable and less prone to fragmentation, and therefore are likely more suitable for long-term use (Fig. 18).[52–54] Both materials are radiodense compared with soft tissue, and are easily seen at CT.

Complications of Nasoenteric Intubation

Although relatively rare, complications related to nasoenteric tubes can be severe. Major complications related to the placement of nasoenteric tubes include perforation, pulmonary injury/pneumothorax, aspiration, and intracranial placement.[55,56] Complication rates increase with the difficulty of placing nasoenteric tubes. Difficult insertions may occur in patients with airway intubation, depressed mental status, or altered anatomy.[56] Other reported complications associated with the

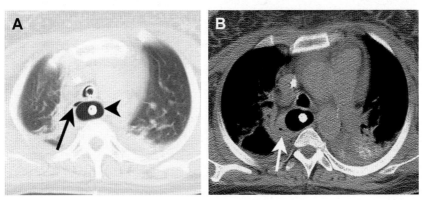

Fig. 17. Esophageal perforation after Sengstaken-Blakemore placement. (A) Axial CT image of the chest in lung windows shows an inflated Sengstaken-Blakemore tube in the mid-esophagus (*black arrowhead*). A small curvilinear focus of gas (*black arrow*) extends beyond the inflated cuff from a rent in the esophageal wall. (B) Axial CT image inferior to A shows thickening of the lateral esophageal wall, which contains a small focus of gas (*white arrow*). Findings are consistent with iatrogenic esophageal perforation.

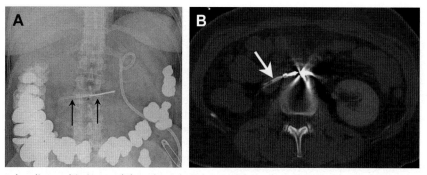

Fig. 18. Frontal radiographic image (*A*) and axial CT image (*B*) show a nasoenteric tube fragment in the duodenum (*black arrows* in *A, white arrow* in *B*).

placement of nasoenteric tubes include ulceration and bleeding, stricture formation, intrapulmonary feeding and empyema, vocal cord injury, and aortoesophageal fistula.[56,57]

Thoracic complications of nasoenteric tubes occur in up to 8% of cases, and may include bronchial placement resulting in atelectasis, pneumonia, or lung abscess; bronchial perforation and pleural cavity penetration; pneumothorax; empyema; and pulmonary hemorrhage.[51,56] Pneumothorax accounts for approximately 60% of tracheopulmonary nasoenteric tube complications (**Fig. 19**).[51] Most tracheopulmonary complications resulting from the placement of nasoenteric tubes occur in patients who are intubated.[58]

Gastrointestinal perforation is another rare complication of nasoenteric tube placement.

Perforation most often occurs in the esophagus or duodenum, although gastric perforation may also occur (**Fig. 20**). Risk factors include repeated attempts at placement, anatomic abnormalities, altered mental status, tracheal intubation, and the presence of cervical osteophytes.[56] CT findings of esophageal perforation secondary to nasoenteric tube placement consist of those already described for esophageal perforation. Cases of esophageal perforation resulting from nasoenteric tube placement are also frequently associated with pneumothorax.[56,59]

CT Pitfalls

A pitfall in the CT evaluation of nasoenteric tubes is mistaking a tube that has tented the lumen of

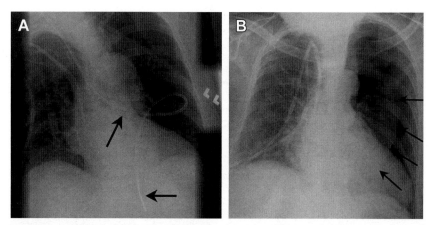

Fig. 19. Iatrogenic pneumothorax from malpositioned enteric tube. (*A*) Frontal radiograph of the chest shows an enteric tube coursing through the trachea and down the left main bronchus with the tip in the costophrenic sulcus medially (*black arrows*). (*B*) Frontal radiograph after the removal of the enteric tube shows a new left pneumothorax (*black arrows*). Radiographic examination is often the most appropriate initial imaging test to diagnose many complications resulting from esophageal intubation. CT may subsequently be used for a more complete evaluation if necessary.

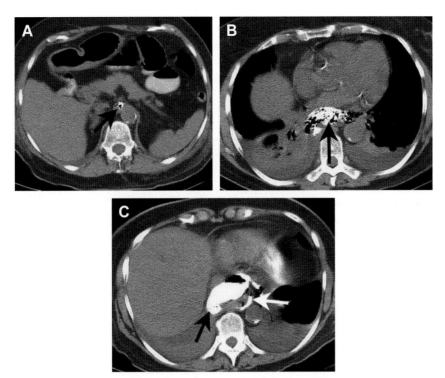

Fig. 20. Esophageal perforation by nasogastric tube. (*A*) Noncontrast axial CT image of the abdomen shows the abnormal position of an enteric tube (*black arrow*) just anteromedial to the aorta. (*B*) Axial image from a chest CT obtained after the administration of contrast through the enteric tube shows abnormal pooling of contrast in the mediastinum (*black arrow*). (*C*) Axial image more inferior to *B* shows contrast extending into the retroperitoneum (*black arrow*), resulting in mass effect on the contrast-containing gastroesophageal junction (*white arrow*).

bowel for one that has perforated through the wall. On cross-sectional imaging, a tube that tents the bowel wall can appear to be beyond the expected margin of the bowel. Absence of extraluminal gas, fluid, hematoma, or fat stranding helps differentiate a tube that has merely tented the bowel wall from one that has actually caused perforation (**Fig. 21**).

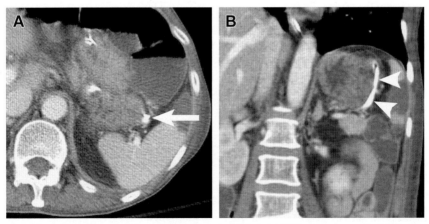

Fig. 21. Pseudoperforation of stomach by nasogastric tube. (*A*) Axial CT image shows that the nasogastric tube (*white arrow*) appears to be positioned just beyond the expected contour of the stomach's greater curvature. (*B*) The coronal CT image also does not show definite gastric wall around the nasogastric tube (*arrowheads*). However, absence of extraluminal gas, fluid, or fat stranding suggests that the tube has not actually perforated the stomach, but rather is merely tenting the stomach wall.

SUMMARY

Complications of upper gastrointestinal endoscopy, stenting, and intubation are potentially life-threatening. Although some of these complications are amenable to radiographic evaluation, examination with CT is invaluable because it provides rapid coverage of a large area, is more practical than fluoroscopy in evaluating seriously ill patients, and is very sensitive in detecting iatrogenic injuries of the upper gastrointestinal tract. The upper gastrointestinal system is subject to a variety of iatrogenic injuries. Familiarization with the different locations and types of iatrogenic injuries to this system will help the radiologist make a quicker and more accurate diagnosis.

REFERENCES

1. Rubesin SE, Levine MS. Radiologic diagnosis of gastrointestinal perforation. Radiol Clin North Am 2003;41(6):1095–115.
2. White CS, Templeton PA, Attar S. Esophageal-perforation - CT findings. Am J Roentgenol 1993; 160(4):767–70.
3. Swanson JO, Levine MS, Redfern RO, et al. Usefulness of high-density barium for detection of leaks after esophagogastrectomy, total gastrectomy, and total laryngectomy. Am J Roentgenol 2003;181(2):415–20.
4. Skinner DB, Little AG, DeMeester TR. Management of esophageal perforation. Am J Surg 1980;139(6): 760–4.
5. Younes Z, Johnson DA. The spectrum of spontaneous and iatrogenic esophageal injury: perforations, Mallory-Weiss tears, and hematomas. J Clin Gastroenterol 1999;29(4):306–17.
6. Eisen GM, Baron TH, Dominitz JA, et al. Complications of upper GI endoscopy. Gastrointest Endosc 2002;55(7):784–93.
7. Silvis SE, Nebel O, Rogers G, et al. Endoscopic complications. Results of the 1974 American Society for Gastrointestinal Endoscopy Survey. JAMA 1976;235(9):928–30.
8. Zubarik R, Eisen G, Mastropietro C, et al. Prospective analysis of complications 30 days after outpatient upper endoscopy. Am J Gastroenterol 1999; 94(6):1539–45.
9. Merchea A, Cullinane DC, Sawyer MD, et al. Esophagogastroduodenoscopy-associated gastrointestinal perforations: a single-center experience. Surgery 2010;148(4):876–80 [discussion: 881–2].
10. Stiegmann GV, Goff JS, Michaletzonody PA, et al. Endoscopic sclerotherapy as compared with endoscopic ligation for bleeding esophageal-varices. N Engl J Med 1992;326(23): 1527–32.
11. Jensen DM, Kovacs TOG, Randall GM, et al. Initial results of a randomized prospective-study of emergency banding vs sclerotherapy for bleeding gastric or esophageal-varices. Gastrointest Endosc 1993;39(2):279.
12. Berry BE, Ochsner JL. Perforation of esophagus - 30 year review. J Thorac Cardiovasc Surg 1973; 65(1):1–7.
13. Pettersson G, Larsson S, Gatzinsky P, et al. Differentiated treatment of intrathoracic oesophageal perforations. Scand J Thorac Cardiovasc Surg 1981;15(3):321–4.
14. Kavic SM, Basson MD. Complications of endoscopy. Am J Surg 2001;181(4):319–32.
15. Huber-Lang M, Henne-Bruns D, Schmitz B, et al. Esophageal perforation: principles of diagnosis and surgical management. Surg Today 2006; 36(4):332–40.
16. Young CA, Menias CO, Bhalla S, et al. CT features of esophageal emergencies. Radiographics 2008; 28(6):1541–53.
17. Lee S, Mergo PJ, Ros PR. The leaking esophagus: CT patterns of esophageal rupture, perforation, and fistulization. Crit Rev Diagn Imaging 1996; 37(6):461–90.
18. Fadoo F, Ruiz DE, Dawn SK, et al. Technical innovation - helical CT esophagography for the evaluation of suspected esophageal perforation or rupture. Am J Roentgenol 2004;182(5):1177–9.
19. Mergener K, Kozarek RA. Stenting of the gastrointestinal tract. Dig Dis 2002;20(2):173–81.
20. Vakil N, Morris AI, Marcon N, et al. A prospective, randomized, controlled trial of covered expandable metal stents in the palliation of malignant esophageal obstruction at the gastroesophageal junction. Am J Gastroenterol 2001;96(6): 1791–6.
21. Langer FB, Schoppmann SF, Prager G, et al. Temporary placement of self-expanding oesophageal stents as bridging for neo-adjuvant therapy. Ann Surg Oncol 2010;17(2):470–5.
22. Schoppmann SF, Langer FB, Prager G, et al. Outcome and complications of long-term self-expanding esophageal stenting. Dis Esophagus 2013;26(2):154–8.
23. Tuebergen D, Rijcken E, Mennigen R, et al. Treatment of thoracic esophageal anastomotic leaks and esophageal perforations with endoluminal stents: efficacy and current limitations. J Gastrointest Surg 2008;12(7):1168–76.
24. Segalin A, Bonavina I, Carazzone A, et al. Improving results of esophageal stenting: a study on 160 consecutive unselected patients. Endoscopy 1997;29(8):701–9.
25. Saxon RR, Barton RE, Rosch J. Complications of esophageal stenting and balloon dilation. Semin Intervent Radiol 1994;11(3):276–82.

26. Saxon RR, Barton RE, Katon RM, et al. Treatment of malignant esophageal obstructions with covered metallic Z stents: long-term results in 52 patients. J Vasc Interv Radiol 1995;6(5):747–54.

27. Saxon RR, Morrison KE, Lakin PC, et al. Malignant esophageal obstruction and esophagorespiratory fistula: palliation with a polyethylene-covered Z-stent. Radiology 1997;202(2):349–54.

28. Kim HC, Han JK, Kim TK, et al. Duodenal perforation as a delayed complication of placement of an esophageal stent. J Vasc Interv Radiol 2000;11(7):902–4.

29. DL CL, MS B, MI C, et al. Technology assessment status evaluation: stents for gastrointestinal strictures. May, 1997. ASGE. American Society for Gastrointestinal Endoscopy. Gastrointest Endosc 1998;47(6):588–93.

30. Wang MQ, Sze DY, Wang ZP, et al. Delayed complications after esophageal stent placement for treatment of malignant esophageal obstructions and esophagorespiratory fistulas. J Vasc Interv Radiol 2001;12(4):465–74.

31. Raijman I, Siddique I, Lynch P. Does chemoradiation therapy increase the incidence of complications with self-expanding coated stents in the management of malignant esophageal strictures? Am J Gastroenterol 1997;92(12):2192–6.

32. Kinsman K, Degregorio B, Katon R, et al. Prior radiation and chemotherapy increases the risk of life-threatening complications after insertion of metallic stents for esophagogastric malignancies. Gastrointest Endosc 1995;41(4):306.

33. Dasgupta A, Jain P, Sandur S, et al. Airway complications of esophageal self-expandable metallic stent. Gastrointest Endosc 1998;47(6):532–5.

34. Libby ED, Fawaz R, Leano AM, et al. Airway complication of expandable stents. Gastrointest Endosc 1999;49(1):136–7.

35. Farivar AS, Vallieres E, Kowdley KV, et al. Airway obstruction complicating esophageal stent placement in two post-pneumonectomy patients. Ann Thorac Surg 2004;78(2):e22–3.

36. McCune WS, Shorb PE, Moscovitz H. Endoscopic cannulation of the ampulla of Vater - a preliminary-report. Gastrointest Endosc 1968;167:752–6.

37. Sharma VK, Howden CW. Metaanalysis of randomized controlled trials of endoscopic retrograde cholangiography and endoscopic sphincterotomy for the treatment of acute biliary pancreatitis. Am J Gastroenterol 1999;94(11):3211–4.

38. Freeman ML, Nelson DB, Sherman S, et al. Complications of endoscopic biliary sphincterotomy. N Engl J Med 1996;335(13):909–18.

39. Mallery JS, Baron TH, Dominitz JA, et al. Complications of ERCP. Gastrointest Endosc 2003;57(6):633–8.

40. Howard TJ, Tan T, Lehman GA, et al. Classification and management of perforations complicating endoscopic sphincterotomy. Surgery 1999;126(4):658–63.

41. Loperfido S, Angelini G, Benedetti G, et al. Major early complications from diagnostic and therapeutic ERCP: a prospective multicenter study. Gastrointest Endosc 1998;48(1):1–10.

42. Eloubeidi MA, Tamhane A, Varadarajulu S, et al. Frequency of major complications after EUS-guided FNA of solid pancreatic masses: a prospective evaluation. Gastrointest Endosc 2006;63(4):622–9.

43. Erickson RA. EUS-guided FNA. Gastrointest Endosc 2004;60(2):267–79.

44. Harewood GC, Wiersema MJ. Endosonography-guided fine needle aspiration biopsy in the evaluation of pancreatic masses. Am J Gastroenterol 2002;97(6):1386–91.

45. Wiersema MJ, Vazquez-Sequeiros E, Wiersema LM. Evaluation of mediastinal lymphadenopathy with endoscopic US-guided fine-needle aspiration biopsy. Radiology 2001;219(1):252–7.

46. Vazquez-Sequeiros E, Wiersema MJ, Clain JE, et al. Impact of lymph node staging on therapy of esophageal carcinoma. Gastroenterology 2003;125(6):1626–35.

47. Eloubeidi MA, Gress FG, Savides TJ, et al. Acute pancreatitis after EUS-guided FNA of solid pancreatic masses: a pooled analysis from EUS centers in the United States. Gastrointest Endosc 2004;60(3):385–9.

48. Wiersema MJ, Vilmann P, Giovannini M, et al. Endosonography-guided fine-needle aspiration biopsy: diagnostic accuracy and complication assessment. Gastroenterology 1997;112(4):1087–95.

49. Eloubeidi MA, Chen VK, Eltoum IA, et al. Endoscopic ultrasound–guided fine needle aspiration biopsy of patients with suspected pancreatic cancer: diagnostic accuracy and acute and 30-day complications. Am J Gastroenterol 2003;98(12):2663–8.

50. Moore FA, Feliciano DV, Andrassy RJ, et al. Early enteral feeding, compared with parenteral, reduces postoperative septic complications - the results of a metaanalysis. Ann Surg 1992;216(2):172–83.

51. Pillai JB, Vegas A, Brister S. Thoracic complications of nasogastric tube: review of safe practice. Interact Cardiovasc Thorac Surg 2005;4(5):429–33.

52. Blacka J, Donoghue J, Sutherland M, et al. Dwell time and functional failure in percutaneous endoscopic gastrostomy tubes: a prospective randomized-controlled comparison between silicon polymer and polyurethane percutaneous endoscopic gastrostomy tubes. Aliment Pharmacol Ther 2004;20(8):875–82.

53. Sartori S, Trevisani L, Nielsen I, et al. Longevity of silicone and polyurethane catheters in long-term enteral feeding via percutaneous endoscopic gastrostomy. Aliment Pharmacol Ther 2003;17(6):853–6.

54. Van Den Hazel S, Mulder C, Den Hartog G, et al. A randomized trial of polyurethane and silicone percutaneous endoscopic gastrostomy catheters. Aliment Pharmacol Ther 2000;14(10):1273–7.

55. McWey RE, Curry NS, Schabel SI, et al. Complications of nasoenteric feeding tubes. Am J Surg 1988;155(2):253–7.

56. Prabhakaran S, Doraiswamy VA, Nagaraja V, et al. Nasoenteric tube complications. Scand J Surg 2012;101(3):147–55.

57. Sparks DA, Chase DM, Coughlin LM, et al. Pulmonary complications of 9931 narrow-bore nasoenteric tubes during blind placement: a critical review. JPEN J Parenter Enteral Nutr 2011;35(5):625–9.

58. Marderstein EL, Simmons RL, Ochoa JB. Patient safety: effect of institutional protocols on adverse events related to feeding tube placement in the critically ill. J Am Coll Surg 2004;199(1):39–47.

59. Fisman DN, Ward ME. Intrapleural placement of a nasogastric tube: an unusual complication of nasotracheal intubation. Can J Anaesth 1996;43(12):1252–6.

Imaging of Complications of Common Bariatric Surgical Procedures

CrossMark

Bruce Lehnert, MD[a], Mariam Moshiri, MD[a,*],
Sherif Osman, MD[a], Saurabh Khandelwal, MD[b],
Saeed Elojeimy, MD[a], Puneet Bhargava, MD[a,c],
Douglas S. Katz, MD[d]

KEYWORDS

- Obesity • Bariatric surgery complications • Roux en Y • Sleeve gastrectomy • Gastric banding
- Laparoscopy

KEY POINTS

- Several techniques for the surgical management of obesity are available to bariatric surgeons.
- These interventions are performed more frequently with worsening of the obesity epidemic.
- Radiologists should be familiar with the surgical techniques, normal postoperative appearances, and potential complications for which imaging may be employed to establish a diagnosis to optimize patient care.

INTRODUCTION

The prevalence of adult obesity in the United States exceeds 30% and seems to be increasing, particularly among adult men.[1] Obesity has been associated with a number of medical comorbidities that can negatively affect quality of life and life expectancy, including type 2 diabetes, cardiovascular disease, osteoarthritis, and obstructive sleep apnea, as well as an increased risk of cancer of the breast, endometrium, and colon.[2]

Bariatric surgery is an effective therapy to achieve significant, sustained weight loss in obese patients. It is cost effective and associated with improvement in associated comorbidities, particularly hypertension and type 2 diabetes, and reduces overall mortality.[3–5] In addition, improvements in minimally invasive techniques and a declining surgical mortality rate has resulted a significant increase in the number of bariatric surgeries performed in the United States (400%–450% increase from 1998–2002).[6,7] Despite this marked increase, the vast majority of eligible obese adults have not undergone treatment,[7] suggesting that the future number of bariatric surgeries in the United States will continue to increase.

The radiologist should be familiar with the imaging appearance of the most commonly performed bariatric surgeries and their associated complications to provide optimal care for this growing patient population.

We discuss the most common operative techniques, imaging appearance, and most frequently encountered complications, for laparoscopic Roux-en-Y gastric bypass (LRGB), sleeve gastrectomy (SG), and adjustable gastric band.

[a] Department of Radiology, University of Washington School of Medicine, 1959 Northeast Pacific Street, Seattle, WA 98195, USA; [b] Department of Surgery, University of Washington School of Medicine, 1959 Northeast Pacific Street, Seattle, WA 98195, USA; [c] Department of Radiology, VA Puget Sound Health Care System, 1660 South Columbian Way, Seattle, WA 98108, USA; [d] Department of Radiology, Winthrop-University Hospital, 259 First Street, Mineola, NY 11501, USA
* Corresponding author. Department of Radiology, University of Washington School of Medicine, Box 357115, 1959 Northeast Pacific Street, Seattle, WA 98195.
E-mail address: Moshiri@uw.edu

Radiol Clin N Am 52 (2014) 1071–1086
http://dx.doi.org/10.1016/j.rcl.2014.05.009
0033-8389/14/$ – see front matter © 2014 Elsevier Inc. All rights reserved.

LRGB

The Roux-en-Y gastric bypass is the most common procedure for the treatment of obesity worldwide, accounting for approximately 47% of bariatric surgeries in 2011.[8] This procedure was initially described as an open surgery in 1967; however, a laparoscopic technique was reported in 1994, and has evolved into the reference standard procedure for surgical weight management, now accounting for more than 90% of these procedures.[9–11]

Technique

The LRGB involves dividing the stomach to form a small, proximal gastric pouch, followed by manipulation of the small bowel and gastrojejunostomy to create a contiguous alimentary tract. The gastric pouch is then completely separated from the larger lower stomach, now termed the gastric remnant.[10] The resulting gastric pouch is typically 20 to 40 mL, with smaller pouches associated with greater weight loss.[12]

The alimentary and biliopancreatic limbs of the Roux-en-Y are then constructed. The jejunum is divided approximately 50 cm distal to the ligament of Treitz to create the biliopancreatic limb. The jejunum is then measured between approximately 75 and 150 cm (75 cm for a body mass index <50 kg/m², and 150 cm for a body mass index ≥50 kg/m²) distal to this division for the site of the end-to-side jejunojejunostomy connecting the biliopancreatic and Roux limbs.[13] The Roux limb is then brought up to the stomach by dividing the greater omentum at the inferior margin of the transverse colon and anastomosed to a gastrostomy created at the inferior right aspect of the gastric pouch. This can be achieved with 2 different techniques, either an antecolic/antegastric approach, where the Roux limb is brought up anterior to the stomach and transverse colon, or a retrocolic/retrogastric approach, where the Roux limb is brought up posterior to the transverse colon and stomach through a surgically created window in the transverse mesocolon. Petersen's space between the Roux limb and the transverse colon mesentery is sutured closed to prevent future small bowel herniation (Fig. 1).[10]

There are advantages and disadvantages to both the antecolic/antegastric and the retrocolic/retrogastric approaches for constructing the Roux limb. The retrocolic/retrogastric approach generally requires longer operating times and is more technically challenging.[14] This approach has been previously associated with an higher incidence of small bowel obstruction (SBO)

related to internal hernias (IH) through the transverse mesocolon defect, the jejunojejunostomy mesenteric defect, and into Petersen's space between the mesentery of the Roux limb and the transverse mesocolon.[15–17] The antecolic/antegastric technique is less technically challenging and requires less operative time[18]; however, it requires a longer Roux limb and may be prone to increased tension at the gastrojejunostomy (Fig. 2). Data thus far do not support an increased propensity for anastomotic leak owing to Roux limb tension with the antecolic/antegastric approach. The overall complication rate for this approach is at least equal to the retrocolic/retrogastric technique.[19,20]

Complications

The mortality rate for LRGB is low, at up to 0.3%. For some complications, in the postoperative period, imaging plays an important role. These include SBO from IH or adhesions, anastomotic stenosis, and anastomotic leak.

Anastomotic leak

Anastomotic leak, although relatively uncommon (approximately 1%–5.6%), is a very serious complication of LRGB, and is an independent risk factor for patient mortality in the perioperative period.[21–24] Approximately one half of anastomotic leaks occur at the gastrojejunostomy, followed by the gastric remnant site and the jejunojejunostomy.[20] The clinical presentation of this complication may be nonspecific, including tachycardia, fever, and abdominal pain. Imaging is frequently employed to clarify the clinical picture and to expedite optimal patient management, including operative reexploration if necessary.

Fluoroscopic evaluation of the upper gastrointestinal tract (UGI) is frequently the initial imaging modality of choice for evaluation of complications, including anastomotic leak and obstruction, and is routinely requested at some centers on postoperative day 1.[20] Evaluation of the biliopancreatic limb, however, is not possible with a routine UGI series.

Gastrojejunostomy leaks on UGI typically manifest as extraluminal contrast extending into the left upper quadrant. Care must be taken to carefully evaluate indwelling drains during the fluoroscopic examination, because subtle opacification of the drain tubing may be the only sign of extraluminal contrast.[25,26]

The UGI series has the advantages of being a relatively fast and inexpensive test; however, it has been demonstrated to be somewhat unreliable for the detection of anastomotic leaks, with a detection rate of just 30%, compared with 56%

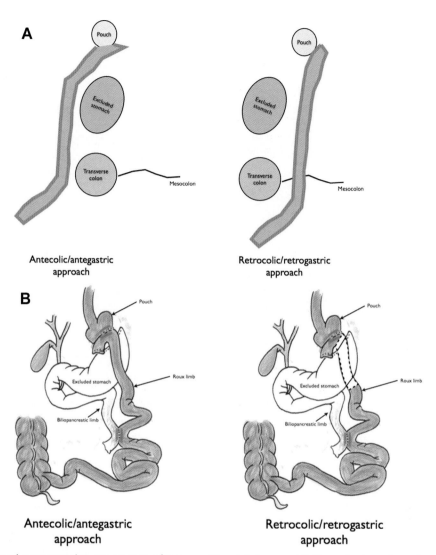

Fig. 1. Normal postoperative appearance of Roux-en-Y gastric bypass. (*A*) Normal retrocolic and antecolic approaches to anastomosis of the efferent (or Roux) jejunal limb to the gastric pouch. (*B*) Food material travels through the gastric pouch and into the Roux limb, while the biliopancreatic continuity with the alimentary tract is maintained through a jejunojejunostomy.

for computed tomography (CT). Combining the 2 tests improves detection rate to approximately 70%.[20,27]

On CT, an anastomotic leak has various manifestations, including a fluid or gas collection adjacent to the gastric pouch, a tract of enteric contrast extending through the anastomotic defect, staple line dehiscence, or diffuse peritoneal fluid (**Fig. 3**).[28]

Communication between the gastric pouch and the colon (**Fig. 4**), or the gastric pouch and gastric remnant, is often associated with an extraluminal leak in the perioperative period, or may present with suboptimal weight loss in a delayed

fashion owing to ingested material entering the biliopancreatic limb.[29] This complication is the result of staple line dehiscence in the early postoperative period, or later as a gastrogastric fistula owing to chronic overdistention of the gastric pouch.[30] On UGI, this complication manifests as contrast entering the gastric remnant to a varying degree depending on the size of the communication, and possible associated extraluminal dissemination of contrast as well. CT in the setting of gastro-gastric communication may demonstrate enteric contrast in the gastric remnant and proximal duodenum, but not in the more distal segments of the afferent

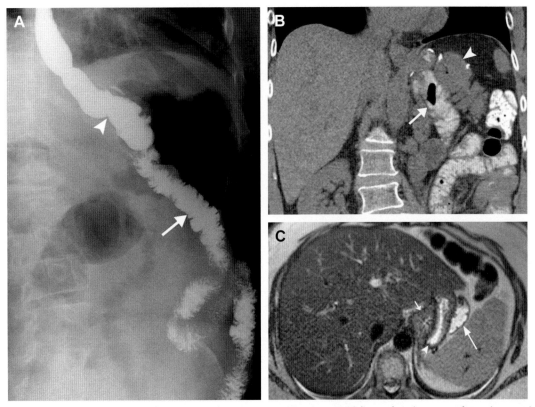

Fig. 2. (*A*) Upper gastrointestinal series in a 56-year-old man shows normal flow of oral contrast from the gastric pouch (*arrowhead*) into the Roux limb (*arrow*). The biliopancreatic limb is usually not opacified. (*B*) Coronal computed tomographic (CT) image with oral contrast only of the abdomen in a 45-year-old woman shows the normal appearance of the retrocolic anastomosis with contrast in the Roux limb (*arrow*). Note the absence of oral contrast in the excluded segment of the stomach on CT (*arrowhead*). (*C*) Axial T2-weighted magnetic resonance image of the upper abdomen in a 40-year-old man shows high signal intensity fluid in the Roux limb (*long arrow*) and in the gastric pouch (*arrowhead*). Note the collapsed gastric remnant (*short arrow*).

(biliopancreatic) limb.[28] The normal gastric remnant may contain fluid, enteric contrast, and gas related to reflux into the afferent limb from the jejunojejunostomy. In this setting, the contrast should also be found throughout the afferent limb rather than just in the stomach and/or proximal duodenum, in which case a gastro-gastric fistula should be suspected.

Anastomotic stricture

Anastomotic narrowing can be the result of self-limiting edema in the perioperative period or may manifest in a delayed fashion as a frank stricture resulting from ischemia, scar, or a circular stapled anastomosis.[31–34] These phenomena are more common at the gastrojejunostomy site (3%–9%) than at the jejunojejunostomy site (0.8%–2%).[35,36]

Narrowing at the gastrojejunal anastomosis may be visible on an UGI series, with distention and delayed emptying of the gastric pouch through the gastrojejunostomy, and persistent contrast in

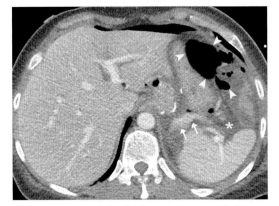

Fig. 3. Anastomotic leak of Roux-en-Y gastric bypass. Axial computed tomographic image with oral and intravenous contrast in a 43-year-old woman who presented with fever and severe abdominal pain shows free intraperitoneal gas in the left upper quadrant (*arrowheads*), and diffuse soft tissue inflammation of the surrounding omentum (*asterisk*). There is also an extraluminal leak of oral contrast adjacent to the gastrojejunal anastomosis (*small arrows*).

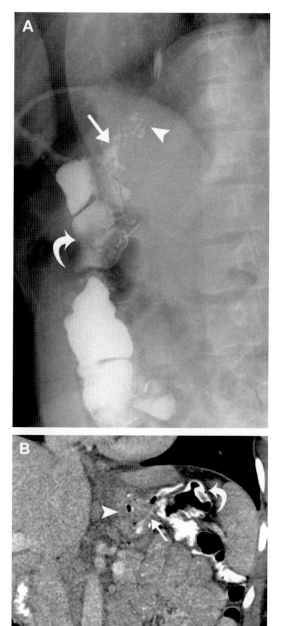

Fig. 4. Gastrocolic fistula in Roux-en-Y gastric bypass in a 35-year-old woman who presented with chronic abdominal pain. (*A*) Lateral view from an upper gastrointestinal series demonstrates flow of ingested oral contrast in a fistulous tract (*arrow*) between the stomach (*arrowhead*) and the colon (*curved arrow*). (*B*) Coronal contrast-enhanced computed tomographic image of the abdomen in the same patient demonstrates the fistulous tract (*arrow*) between the proximal stomach (*arrowhead*) and the colon (*curved arrow*), filled with oral contrast.

the esophagus.[37] Although dynamic imaging of the gastrojejunostomy is not possible with CT, findings of gastric pouch distention with contrast in the esophagus raise the possibility of anastomotic narrowing. In the case of postoperative edema, these findings should resolve on follow-up imaging. Continued distention of the gastric pouch with delayed transit across the gastrojejunostomy is concerning for anastomotic stricture (**Fig. 5**).[26]

Narrowing at the jejunojejunal anastomosis, either from postoperative edema/hematoma or delayed stricture, may manifest at imaging with distention of the Roux limb, the biliopancreatic limb, or both (**Fig. 6**).[26] CT may be particularly advantageous for evaluating the jejunojejunostomy, because it permits an excellent assessment of the biliopancreatic limb, which is not possible with fluoroscopy.

Small Bowel Obstruction

SBO may occur in up to 5% of LRGB patients. In the early postoperative period, it is typically related to edema or hematoma at the gastrojejunal or jejunojejunal anastomoses.[38] Early postoperative obstruction requires prompt evaluation and treatment owing to the potential for suture line rupture from elevated intraluminal pressure, particularly in the gastric remnant.[30] More remote SBO is often due to adhesions, IH, or intussusception (**Fig. 7**).[39]

SBO related to adhesions is more common after open Roux-en-Y gastric bypass than with LRGB (**Fig. 8**). IH resulting in SBO are more common in patients who have undergone LRGB than open Roux-en-Y gastric bypass, and in particular after significant weight loss.[15,40] As described, the risk of IH is less with an antecolic/antegastric Roux limb. The relative rarity of IH after open Roux-en-Y gastric bypass has been hypothesized to be the result of adhesions and scarring owing to peritoneal irritation associated with an open procedure preventing herniation of small bowel through mesenteric defects.[15] IH occur most commonly through a defect in the transverse mesocolon created for a retrocolic Roux limb.[41] If an antecolic Roux approach is used, IH may occur through the mesenteric defect at the jejunojejunostomy, or through a potential space between the Roux limb mesentery and the inferior aspect of transverse colon mesentery, which is known as Petersen's space.[42,43]

Tucker and colleagues[44] introduced a simple system for classifying post gastric bypass SBO based on anatomic location: *A* for the alimentary limb, *B* for the biliopancreatic limb, and *C* for the "common channel." In patients in whom there is

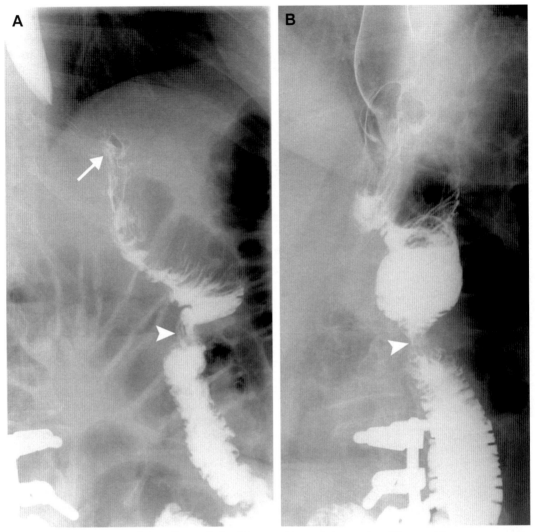

Fig. 5. Functional stricture of the efferent limb of Roux-en-Y gastric bypass in a 52-year-old woman presenting with chronic abdominal pain. (*A, B*) Oblique views from an upper gastrointestinal series demonstrate mild persistent focal narrowing of the efferent limb (*arrowheads*) a few centimeters distal to the gastrojejunal anastomosis (*arrow*), with mild proximal jejunal dilatation. This is likely owing to external compression of the efferent jejunal loop and resultant narrowing as it passes through the surgical defect in the transverse mesocolon.

a high clinical suspicion of SBO, owing to the complex postoperative anatomy, CT is the primary imaging modality of choice.[27]

Mesocolic defect herniation in the setting of a retrocolic Roux limb typically manifests with a variable length of dilated, closely approximated small bowel, including the Roux limb, positioned anterior to the gastric pouch.[35] Mass effect on and inferior displacement of the transverse colon, proportional to the degree of bowel and mesentery herniation, may also be noted. This type of herniation characteristically results in dilation of the Roux limb near the jejunojejunostomy without dilation of the biliopancreatic limb.[45]

Transmesenteric hernia refers to the herniation of small bowel and mesentery through the mesenteric defect at the jejunojejunostomy. On CT, this type of IH manifests as closely approximated, dilated loops of small bowel adjacent to the abdominal wall, typically displacing the transverse colon centrally and superiorly. Stretching and displacement of mesenteric vessels and absence of overlying omental fat may also be noted (**Fig. 9**).[46,47]

IH into Petersen's defect, as noted above, is located between the undersurface of the transverse mesocolon and the jejunal mesentery of the Roux limb. On CT, this type of IH demonstrates

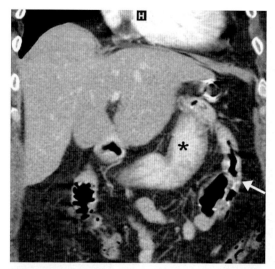

Fig. 6. Reflux in the afferent limb of a Roux-en-Y gastric bypass in a 65-year-old woman presenting with chronic mild abdominal pain. Coronal computed tomographic image with oral and intravenous contrast shows reflux of oral contrast from the proximal jejunum into the afferent limb and the gastric body (*asterisk*). *Arrow*: efferent limb.

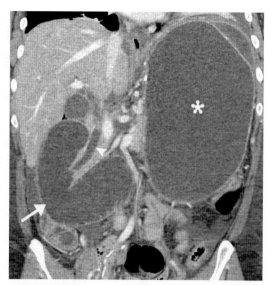

Fig. 8. Obstruction of the afferent loop in Roux-en-Y gastric bypass in a 48-year-old woman presenting with acute abdominal pain. Coronal computed tomographic image of the abdomen with intravenous contrast demonstrates marked dilatation of the excluded stomach (*asterisk*) and the afferent limb (Y-limb or biliopancreatic limb, *arrow*) with low attenuation fluid. There is abrupt transition at the level of the transverse duodenum (not shown) owing to adhesions. Note also dilatation of the common bile duct (*arrowhead*) owing to reflux of fluid from the dilated duodenum.

clustered and dilated small bowel loops located in the left upper abdomen posterior to the transverse colon and cephalad to the root of the small bowel mesentery (**Fig. 10**). Multiplanar reformations may

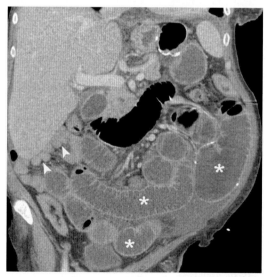

Fig. 7. Small bowel obstruction in Roux-en-Y gastric bypass in a 54-year-old woman presenting with acute abdominal pain and vomiting. Coronal computed tomographic image of the abdomen with intravenous contrast shows multiple dilated jejunal bowel loops (*asterisks*) associated with collapsed ileal loops in the right mid to lower abdomen (*arrowheads*) owing to adhesions.

be helpful to appreciate the resulting abnormal anatomic relationships.[45,48]

In the absence of CT features clearly delineating the location of the suspected IH, swirling of the mesentery has been shown to be the most sensitive finding, although the degree of swirling required to confirm reliably the presence of an IH has not yet been clearly defined to our knowledge. Nonetheless, the authors of a study that demonstrated the utility of identifying the swirling mesentery for IH detection noted that finding any amount of mesenteric swirling on CT should be considered suspicious for an IH in post LRGB patients presenting with suspected bowel obstruction.[42]

LAPAROSCOPIC SG

SG is the second most commonly performed bariatric procedure worldwide, and the frequency of its use continues to increase.[8] This procedure was initially developed as the first step before duodenal switch or Roux-en-Y gastric bypass in high-risk, high body mass index patients (>60 kg/m²). However, SG has been shown to be effective as a standalone procedure in morbidly obese patients

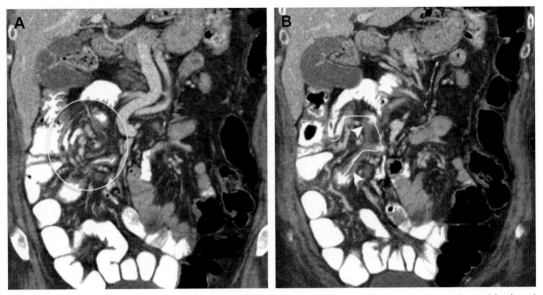

Fig. 9. Transmesenteric hernia in Roux-en-Y gastric bypass in a 61-year-old woman presenting with chronic abdominal pain. (*A*) Coronal computed tomographic (CT) image of the abdomen with oral and intravenous contrast shows swirling appearance of the mesenteric vessels (*circled*). (*B*) Coronal CT image of the abdomen at a different level demonstrates the herniated small bowel loop with associated mild wall thickening (*arrowheads*). The *white line* demarcates the herniation path.

as well. The procedure is potentially advantageous for treating high-risk patients because it can be performed quickly and requires no bowel anastomoses.[49–52]

Technique

Laparoscopic SG involves creating a narrow, tubular stomach with markedly reduced luminal volume acting as a restrictive measure for weight loss. Neurohormonal effects related to a reduction in the appetite mediator peptide ghrelin after resection of the gastric fundus also play a role in the observed weight loss in these patients.[53]

Transection of the stomach is performed laparoscopically with endostaplers extending several centimeters proximal to the pylorus to the angle of His along a path 1 to 2 cm from the border of the lesser curvature. The transected stomach, primarily consisting of the gastric body along the greater curvature, is then removed. Meticulous inspection of the staple line is then performed, including injection of the gastric lumen with methylene blue, to ensure no leak is present (**Fig. 11**).[54]

Complications

The incidence of postoperative complications after laparoscopic SG is up to 7.4%.[55] Complications primarily consist of staple line leak, staple line hemorrhage, infection, and chronic gastric strictures.[56]

Gastric leak

Staple line leak is a serious complication related to SG, occurring in approximately 2% to 3% of cases.[57] Fever, epigastric pain, and tachycardia are common clinical features of gastric leak and may be confirmed on imaging with fluoroscopy or CT.[58] Extravasation of contrast occurs most frequently along the superior one-third of the gastric staple line. It may extend into the left upper quadrant and throughout the peritoneum, or may form loculated collections (**Fig. 12**).[59] Gastric leak is frequently not visible at imaging during the early postoperative period for up to approximately 3 days, and often does not become apparent until postoperative day 4 and beyond. Over time, gastric leak may result in a loculated fluid and gas collection, associated with inflammation at the staple line, typically near the angle of His.[57,60]

Gastric stricture

Gastric luminal narrowing in the acute postoperative period is typically related to edema and is relatively uncommon. Gastric stricture presents more commonly in a delayed fashion with food intolerance, nausea, and vomiting, and may be due to a too-tight gastric remnant.[59,61] Stenosis is most common in the region of the incisura angularis.

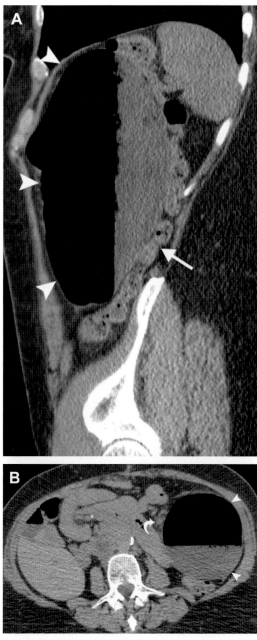

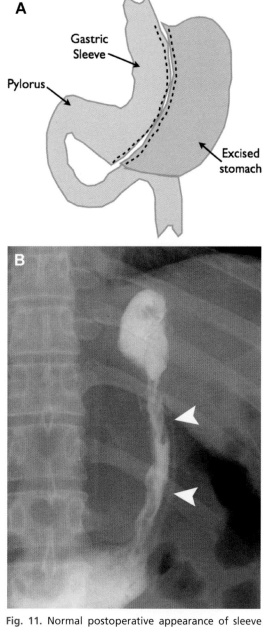

Fig. 10. Petersen hernia in Roux-en-Y gastric bypass in a 55-year-old woman presenting with acute abdominal pain. (A) Sagittal noncontrast computed tomographic image of the abdomen shows a dilated bowel loop (arrowheads) with a fluid level in the left abdomen. The descending colon posterior to the dilated bowel loop is collapsed (arrow). (B) Congested mesenteric vessels (curved arrow) are seen adjacent to the dilated bowel loop (arrowheads) on an axial CT image.

Fig. 11. Normal postoperative appearance of sleeve gastrectomy. (A) Surgically-created tubular appearance of the gastric remnant. (B) Supine frontal view from an upper gastrointestinal series in a 31-year-old-woman demonstrates expected reduced capacity of the stomach. Arrowheads: surgical suture line.

An UGI series may demonstrate a persistent contrast column in the gastric remnant associated with dilation of the distal esophagus and gastro-esophageal reflux.[51,62] Although persistent contrast may be noted in the proximal gastric remnant and esophagus on CT, this modality is not typically employed for assessment of a gastric stricture.

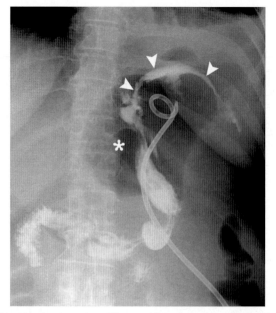

Fig. 12. Staple line leak in sleeve gastrectomy in a 56-year-old woman presenting with fever and severe abdominal pain. Supine view from an upper gastrointestinal series demonstrates leakage of oral contrast from the proximal suture line (*arrowheads*) into a large, gas-filled collection (*asterisk*). A pigtail drainage catheter was placed in the collection.

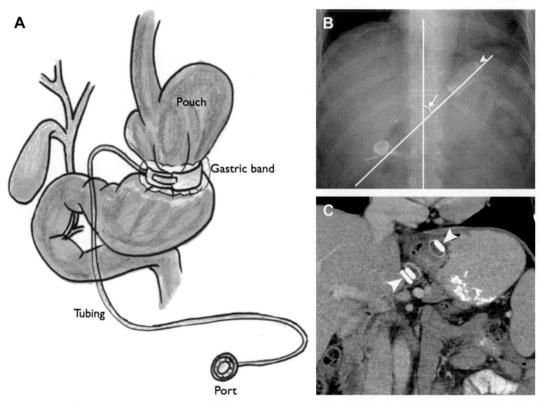

Fig. 13. Normal postoperative appearance of a laparoscopic gastric band. (*A*) Normal positioning of the band. (*B*) Supine radiograph demonstrates the normal expected position of the band a few centimeters below the diaphragm. Note the phi angle (*arrow*), measured between a line drawn along the vertical axis of the spine and a line along the axis of the gastric lap band (*arrowhead*), estimated at 55°. (*C*) Coronal computed tomographic image with intravenous and oral contrast shows the expected location of the gastric band (*arrowheads*) below the diaphragm and adequately apposed to the gastric wall.

LAPAROSCOPIC GASTRIC BANDING

Laparoscopic gastric banding involves placement of an inflatable balloon device around the proximal stomach where it acts to restrict the passage of ingested food material. The technique was first described in 1993; however, early technique resulted in a high rate of gastric herniation.[63,64] The modern approach, termed the pars flaccida technique, evolved to minimize dissection by placing the band higher on the stomach where herniation is less likely.[64]

Technique

Using laparoscopic technique, an inflatable gastric band is placed around the proximal stomach. The band is secured and covered with a permanent serosal suture approximating the stomach superior and inferior to the band (**Fig. 13**). The primary function of this suture is to prevent gastric herniation through the band. The port is then placed in the abdominal wall and connected to the gastric band, which is left empty during the 6-week postoperative recovery period.[64]

Complications

Gastric band slippage

When viewed in the anteroposterior projection, a normally placed gastric band will be inclined along its longitudinal axis at an angle from 4° to 58° to the spinal column, and will be positioned approximately 5 cm below the left hemidiaphragm. This is known as the "phi angle."[65,66] Gastric band slippage rates were as high as 22% before the development of the pars flaccida technique, which have now decreased to as low as 2%.[67]

Gastric band slippage may occur through the band anteriorly or posteriorly, resulting in eccentric dilation of the proximal gastric pouch. An anterior slippage occurs when increased pressure in the proximal gastric pouch forces the band inferiorly over the anterior stomach. This is likely owing to weakening or rupture of the serosal sutures.[68] On an UGI, an anterior band slippage manifests with eccentric dilation of the gastric pouch anteriorly and superiorly, with clockwise rotation of the gastric band beyond the normal phi angle.[66,69,70] Posterior slippage, which is rarely seen with the pars flaccida technique, occurs when the inferior and posterior stomach herniates above the gastric band with rightward, eccentric enlargement of the proximal gastric pouch and counterclockwise rotation of the gastric band to less than 4°.[66,70] In the setting of posterior slippage, the gastric band may be seen en face on frontal abdominal radiography, described as the "O sign" (**Figs. 14 and 15**).[71]

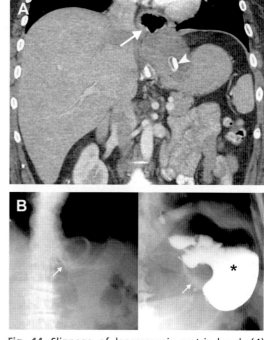

Fig. 14. Slippage of laparoscopic gastric band. (*A*) Anterior slippage. A 33-year-old woman presented with acute abdominal pain and vomiting. Coronal computed tomographic image of the abdomen with oral and intravenous contrast demonstrates inferior migration of the gastric band (*arrowhead*) along the gastric body with associated partial obstruction. There is mild dilatation of the proximal stomach with herniation of the gastric pouch above the diaphragm (*arrow*). (*B*) Posterior slippage in a 41-year-old woman. Anteroposterior scout image (*right*) and spot image (*left*) of an upper gastrointestinal series demonstrate rotation of the lap band resulting in an "O-shaped" appearance (*arrow*). There is superior herniation of the proximal stomach through the lap band (*asterisk*), with associated complete obstruction at the level of the stoma (not seen in this projection).

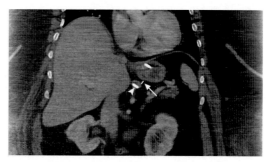

Fig. 15. Loose fit of a gastric band. A 53-year-old woman presented with failure to lose weight. Coronal computed tomographic image of the abdomen with intravenous contrast shows nonapposition of the lap band (*arrowhead*) to the gastric wall (*arrow*).

Gastric band erosion

Erosion of the gastric band through the wall of the stomach is a delayed complication, typically presenting from weeks to years after placement. In recent large case series, the incidence of this complication was approximately 0.9% to 3.4%.[72,73] Potential etiologies include gastric wall ischemia owing to extrinsic pressure from an over-distended band, infection, or chronic inflammation at the band site owing to foreign body response, or evolution of gastric injury sustained during operative placement.[74–76]

The clinical presentation of vague abdominal pain may be nonspecific. Aspiration of turbid fluid from the gastric band port or recurrent port site infections may indicate intragastric erosion.[73] A change in band position over time may be noted on abdominal radiography.[77] On fluoroscopic evaluation, extravasation of contrast around the gastric band or an open band are very likely to indicate full-thickness erosion though the gastric wall.[65] On CT, eccentric gastric wall thickening adjacent to the band or intraluminal migration of a portion of the band may be identified (**Figs. 16** and **17**).[78]

Infection and leakage

Infection of the port site may present with swelling, erythema, and fever; however, detecting signs of local infection may be difficult in patients with a large body habitus. Ultrasonography is helpful to evaluate for superficial abscess at the port reservoir. CT may be needed to visualize the entire length of the device, to assess for deeper collections.[78] As noted, recurrent infections of the port and tubing may be a sign of gastric erosion, and should prompt fluoroscopic and/or CT (**Fig. 18**).

Leakage of fluid from the band system is a potential delayed complication. It can present with insufficient or reversal of weight loss owing to lack of restriction at the banding site. A leak may occur anywhere along the system, from the access port to the gastric band. Abdominal radiography may demonstrate discontinuity of the port tubing; however, injection of the access port with water-soluble, nonionic contrast under

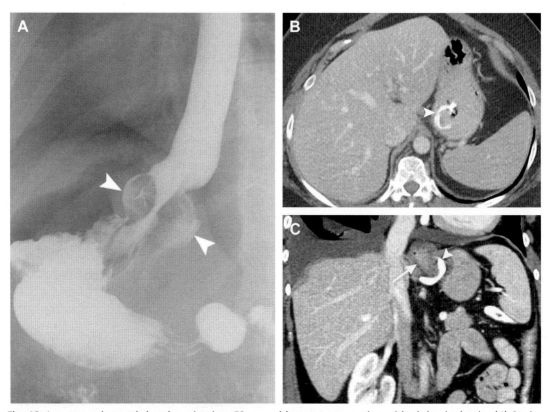

Fig. 16. Laparoscopic gastric band erosion in a 52-year-old woman presenting with abdominal pain. (*A*) Supine oblique view from an upper gastrointestinal series demonstrates contrast outlining the gastric lap band (*arrowheads*) owing to gastric lap band erosion into the lumen of the stomach. (*B*) Axial computed tomographic (CT) image in a different patient, with oral and IV contrast, shows the eroded band in the lumen of the stomach (*arrowhead*). (*C*) Coronal CT image of a different patient with intravenous and oral contrast shows erosion of the gastric band (*arrowhead*) associated with herniation of the gastric pouch superiorly (*arrow*).

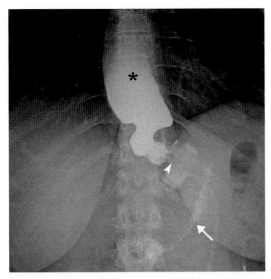

Fig. 17. Laparoscopic gastric band stomal stenosis in a 42-year-old woman presenting with acute abdominal pain and vomiting. Supine frontal view from an upper gastrointestinal series shows severe stomal stenosis of the gastric lap band (*arrowhead*) causing near-complete obstruction. There is stasis and uphold of oral contrast in the esophagus (*asterisk*) and proximal gastric pouch 30 minutes after ingestion of oral contrast. *Arrow* points to contrast in the gastric body.

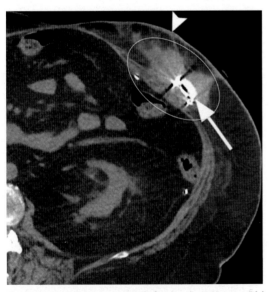

Fig. 18. Laparoscopic gastric infection in a 63-year-old woman presenting with cellulitis at the port site. Axial noncontrast computed tomographic image of the abdomen shows inflammation (*circle*) of the subcutaneous tissue around the port site (*arrow*) with overlying skin thickening (*arrowhead*).

fluoroscopy can be useful to demonstrate the site of leak in more subtle cases.[78]

SUMMARY

Several techniques for the surgical management of obesity are available to bariatric surgeons. These interventions are performed more frequently with worsening of the obesity epidemic. Radiologists should be familiar with the surgical techniques, normal postoperative appearances, and potential complications for which imaging may be employed to establish a diagnosis to optimize patient care.

REFERENCES

1. Flegal KM, Carroll MD, Ogden CL, et al. Prevalence and trends in obesity among US adults, 1999-2008. JAMA 2010;303(3):235–41.
2. Clinical guidelines on the identification, evaluation, and treatment of overweight and obesity in adults–the evidence report. National Institutes of Health. Obes Res 1998;6(Suppl 2):51S–209S.
3. Colquitt JL, Picot J, Loveman E, et al. Surgery for obesity. Cochrane Database Syst Rev 2009;(2):CD003641.
4. Picot J, Jones J, Colquitt JL, et al. The clinical effectiveness and cost-effectiveness of bariatric (weight loss) surgery for obesity: a systematic review and economic evaluation. Health Technol Assess 2009;13(41):1–190, 215–357, iii–iv.
5. Sjostrom L, Narbro K, Sjostrom CD, et al. Effects of bariatric surgery on mortality in Swedish obese subjects. N Engl J Med 2007;357(8):741–52.
6. Nguyen NT, Root J, Zainabadi K, et al. Accelerated growth of bariatric surgery with the introduction of minimally invasive surgery. Arch Surg 2005; 140(12):1198–202 [discussion: 1203].
7. Encinosa WE, Bernard DM, Steiner CA, et al. Use and costs of bariatric surgery and prescription weight-loss medications. Health Aff (Millwood) 2005;24(4):1039–46.
8. Buchwald H, Oien DM. Metabolic/bariatric surgery worldwide 2011. Obes Surg 2013;23(4):427–36.
9. Wittgrove AC, Clark GW, Tremblay LJ. Laparoscopic gastric bypass, Roux-en-Y: preliminary report of five cases. Obes Surg 1994;4(4):353–7.
10. Nguyen N, DeMaria EJ, Ikramuddin S, et al. The SAGES manual: a practical guide to bariatric surgery. New York: Springer; 2008.
11. Mason EE, Ito C. Gastric bypass in obesity. Surg Clin North Am 1967;47(6):1345–51.
12. Roberts K, Duffy A, Kaufman J, et al. Size matters: gastric pouch size correlates with weight loss after laparoscopic Roux-en-Y gastric bypass. Surg Endosc 2007;21(8):1397–402.

13. Schauer PR, Ikramuddin S, Hamad G, et al. Laparoscopic gastric bypass surgery: current technique. J Laparoendosc Adv Surg Tech A 2003; 13(4):229–39.

14. Champion JK, Williams M. Small bowel obstruction and internal hernias after laparoscopic Roux-en-Y gastric bypass. Obes Surg 2003;13(4):596–600.

15. Higa KD, Ho T, Boone KB. Internal hernias after laparoscopic Roux-en-Y gastric bypass: incidence, treatment and prevention. Obes Surg 2003;13(3):350–4.

16. Escalona A, Devaud N, Perez G, et al. Antecolic versus retrocolic alimentary limb in laparoscopic Roux-en-Y gastric bypass: a comparative study. Surg Obes Relat Dis 2007;3(4):423–7.

17. Steele KE, Prokopowicz GP, Magnuson T, et al. Laparoscopic antecolic Roux-en-Y gastric bypass with closure of internal defects leads to fewer internal hernias than the retrocolic approach. Surg Endosc 2008;22(9):2056–61.

18. Muller MK, Guber J, Wildi S, et al. Three-year follow-up study of retrocolic versus antecolic laparoscopic Roux-en-Y gastric bypass. Obes Surg 2007;17(7):889–93.

19. Bertucci W, Yadegar J, Takahashi A, et al. Antecolic laparoscopic Roux-en-Y gastric bypass is not associated with higher complication rates. Am Surg 2005;71(9):735–7.

20. Gonzalez R, Sarr MG, Smith CD, et al. Diagnosis and contemporary management of anastomotic leaks after gastric bypass for obesity. J Am Coll Surg 2007;204(1):47–55.

21. Fernandez AZ Jr, DeMaria EJ, Tichansky DS, et al. Experience with over 3,000 open and laparoscopic bariatric procedures: multivariate analysis of factors related to leak and resultant mortality. Surg Endosc 2004;18(2):193–7.

22. Schauer PR, Ikramuddin S, Gourash W, et al. Outcomes after laparoscopic Roux-en-Y gastric bypass for morbid obesity. Ann Surg 2000;232(4): 515–29.

23. Marshall JS, Srivastava A, Gupta SK, et al. Roux-en-Y gastric bypass leak complications. Arch Surg 2003;138(5):520–3 [discussion: 523–4].

24. Arteaga JR, Huerta S, Livingston EH. Management of gastrojejunal anastomotic leaks after Roux-en-Y gastric bypass. Am Surg 2002;68(12):1061–5.

25. Carucci LR, Turner MA, Conklin RC, et al. Roux-en-Y gastric bypass surgery for morbid obesity: evaluation of postoperative extraluminal leaks with upper gastrointestinal series. Radiology 2006; 238(1):119–27.

26. Shah S, Shah V, Ahmed AR, et al. Imaging in bariatric surgery: service set-up, post-operative anatomy and complications. Br J Radiol 2011;84(998):101–11.

27. Doraiswamy A, Rasmussen JJ, Pierce J, et al. The utility of routine postoperative upper GI series following laparoscopic gastric bypass. Surg Endosc 2007;21(12):2159–62.

28. Yu J, Turner MA, Cho SR, et al. Normal anatomy and complications after gastric bypass surgery: helical CT findings. Radiology 2004;231(3):753–60.

29. Carucci LR, Conklin RC, Turner MA. Roux-en-Y gastric bypass surgery for morbid obesity: evaluation of leak into excluded stomach with upper gastrointestinal examination. Radiology 2008; 248(2):504–10.

30. Carucci LR, Turner MA. Imaging after bariatric surgery for morbid obesity: Roux-en-Y gastric bypass and laparoscopic adjustable gastric banding. Semin Roentgenol 2009;44(4):283–96.

31. Nguyen NT, Stevens CM, Wolfe BM. Incidence and outcome of anastomotic stricture after laparoscopic gastric bypass. J Gastrointest Surg 2003; 7(8):997–1003 [discussion: 1003].

32. Gonzalez R, Lin E, Venkatesh KR, et al. Gastrojejunostomy during laparoscopic gastric bypass: analysis of 3 techniques. Arch Surg 2003;138(2):181–4.

33. Takata MC, Ciovica R, Cello JP, et al. Predictors, treatment, and outcomes of gastrojejunostomy stricture after gastric bypass for morbid obesity. Obes Surg 2007;17(7):878–84.

34. Herron D, Roohipour R. Complications of Roux-en-Y gastric bypass and sleeve gastrectomy. Abdom Imaging 2012;37(5):712–8.

35. Chandler RC, Srinivas G, Chintapalli KN, et al. Imaging in bariatric surgery: a guide to postsurgical anatomy and common complications. AJR Am J Roentgenol 2008;190(1):122–35.

36. Carrodeguas L, Szomstein S, Zundel N, et al. Gastrojejunal anastomotic strictures following laparoscopic Roux-en-Y gastric bypass surgery: analysis of 1291 patients. Surg Obes Relat Dis 2006;2(2):92–7.

37. Scheirey CD, Scholz FJ, Shah PC, et al. Radiology of the laparoscopic Roux-en-Y gastric bypass procedure: conceptualization and precise interpretation of results. Radiographics 2006;26(5):1355–71.

38. Carucci LR, Turner MA, Shaylor SD. Internal hernia following Roux-en-Y gastric bypass surgery for morbid obesity: evaluation of radiographic findings at small-bowel examination. Radiology 2009; 251(3):762–70.

39. Husain S, Ahmed AR, Johnson J, et al. Small-bowel obstruction after laparoscopic Roux-en-Y gastric bypass: etiology, diagnosis, and management. Arch Surg 2007;142(10):988–93.

40. Ahmed AR, Rickards G, Husain S, et al. Trends in internal hernia incidence after laparoscopic Roux-en-Y gastric bypass. Obes Surg 2007;17(12): 1563–6.

41. Garza E Jr, Kuhn J, Arnold D, et al. Internal hernias after laparoscopic Roux-en-Y gastric bypass. Am J Surg 2004;188(6):796–800.

42. Lockhart ME, Tessler FN, Canon CL, et al. Internal hernia after gastric bypass: sensitivity and specificity of seven CT signs with surgical correlation and controls. AJR Am J Roentgenol 2007;188(3): 745–50.

43. Nandipati KC, Lin E, Husain F, et al. Counterclockwise rotation of Roux-en-Y limb significantly reduces internal herniation in laparoscopic Roux-en-Y gastric bypass (LRYGB). J Gastrointest Surg 2012;16(4):675–81.

44. Tucker ON, Escalante-Tattersfield T, Szomstein S, et al. The ABC System: a simplified classification system for small bowel obstruction after laparoscopic Roux-en-Y gastric bypass. Obes Surg 2007;17(12):1549–54.

45. Sunnapwar A, Sandrasegaran K, Menias CO, et al. Taxonomy and imaging spectrum of small bowel obstruction after Roux-en-Y gastric bypass surgery. Am J Roentgenol 2010;194(1):120–8.

46. Blachar A, Federle MP, Brancatelli G, et al. Radiologist performance in the diagnosis of internal hernia by using specific CT findings with emphasis on transmesenteric hernia. Radiology 2001; 221(2):422–8.

47. Blachar A, Federle MP, Dodson SF. Internal hernia: clinical and imaging findings in 17 patients with emphasis on CT criteria. Radiology 2001;218(1): 68–74.

48. Gunabushanam G, Shankar S, Czerniach DR, et al. Small-bowel obstruction after laparoscopic Roux-en-Y gastric bypass surgery. J Comput Assist Tomogr 2009;33(3):369–75.

49. Moon Han S, Kim WW, Oh JH. Results of laparoscopic sleeve gastrectomy (LSG) at 1 year in morbidly obese Korean patients. Obes Surg 2005;15(10):1469–75.

50. Hamoui N, Anthone GJ, Kaufman HS, et al. Sleeve gastrectomy in the high-risk patient. Obes Surg 2006;16(11):1445–9.

51. Cottam D, Qureshi FG, Mattar SG, et al. Laparoscopic sleeve gastrectomy as an initial weight-loss procedure for high-risk patients with morbid obesity. Surg Endosc 2006;20(6):859–63.

52. Himpens J, Dobbeleir J, Peeters G. Long-term results of laparoscopic sleeve gastrectomy for obesity. Ann Surg 2010;252(2):319–24.

53. Langer FB, Reza Hoda MA, Bohdjalian A, et al. Sleeve gastrectomy and gastric banding: effects on plasma ghrelin levels. Obes Surg 2005;15(7): 1024–9.

54. Moy J, Pomp A, Dakin G, et al. Laparoscopic sleeve gastrectomy for morbid obesity. Am J Surg 2008;196(5):e56–9.

55. Nocca D, Krawczykowsky D, Bomans B, et al. A prospective multicenter study of 163 sleeve gastrectomies: results at 1 and 2 years. Obes Surg 2008;18(5):560–5.

56. Gumbs AA, Gagner M, Dakin G, et al. Sleeve gastrectomy for morbid obesity. Obes Surg 2007; 17(7):962–9.

57. Burgos AM, Braghetto I, Csendes A, et al. Gastric leak after laparoscopic-sleeve gastrectomy for obesity. Obes Surg 2009;19(12):1672–7.

58. Csendes A, Braghetto I, Leon P, et al. Management of leaks after laparoscopic sleeve gastrectomy in patients with obesity. J Gastrointest Surg 2010; 14(9):1343–8.

59. Barnard SA, Rahman H, Foliaki A. The postoperative radiological features of laparoscopic sleeve gastrectomy. J Med Imaging Radiat Oncol 2012; 56(4):425–31.

60. Fuks D, Verhaeghe P, Brehant O, et al. Results of laparoscopic sleeve gastrectomy: a prospective study in 135 patients with morbid obesity. Surgery 2009;145(1):106–13.

61. Sarkhosh K, Birch DW, Sharma A, et al. Complications associated with laparoscopic sleeve gastrectomy for morbid obesity: a surgeon's guide. Can J Surg 2013;56(5):347–52.

62. Triantafyllidis G, Lazoura O, Sioka E, et al. Anatomy and complications following laparoscopic sleeve gastrectomy: radiological evaluation and imaging pitfalls. Obes Surg 2011;21(4):473–8.

63. Belachew M, Jacqet P, Lardinois F, et al. Vertical banded gastroplasty vs adjustable silicone gastric banding in the treatment of morbid obesity: a preliminary report. Obes Surg 1993;3(3):275–8.

64. Fielding GA, Allen JW. A step-by-step guide to placement of the LAP-BAND adjustable gastric banding system. Am J Surg 2002;184(6B): 26S–30S.

65. Mehanna MJ, Birjawi G, Moukaddam HA, et al. Complications of adjustable gastric banding, a radiological pictorial review. AJR Am J Roentgenol 2006;186(2):522–34.

66. Peternac D, Hauser R, Weber M, et al. The effects of laparoscopic adjustable gastric banding on the proximal pouch and the esophagus. Obes Surg 2001;11(1):76–86.

67. Chevallier JM, Zinzindohoue F, Douard R, et al. Complications after laparoscopic adjustable gastric banding for morbid obesity: experience with 1,000 patients over 7 years. Obes Surg 2004;14(3):407–14.

68. Wiesner W, Weber M, Hauser RS, et al. Anterior versus posterior slippage: two different types of eccentric pouch dilatation in patients with adjustable laparoscopic gastric banding. Dig Surg 2001;18(3):182–6 [discussion: 187].

69. Blachar A, Blank A, Gavert N, et al. Laparoscopic adjustable gastric banding surgery for morbid obesity: imaging of normal anatomic features and postoperative gastrointestinal complications. AJR Am J Roentgenol 2007;188(2):472–9.

70. Prosch H, Tscherney R, Kriwanek S, et al. Radiographical imaging of the normal anatomy and complications after gastric banding. Br J Radiol 2008; 81(969):753–7.

71. Pieroni S, Sommer EA, Hito R, et al. The "O" sign, a simple and helpful tool in the diagnosis of laparoscopic adjustable gastric band slippage. Am J Roentgenol 2010;195(1):137–41.

72. Favretti F, Segato G, Ashton D, et al. Laparoscopic adjustable gastric banding in 1,791 consecutive obese patients: 12-year results. Obes Surg 2007; 17(2):168–75.

73. Chisholm J, Kitan N, Toouli J, et al. Gastric band erosion in 63 cases: endoscopic removal and rebanding evaluated. Obes Surg 2011;21(11): 1676–81.

74. Abu-Abeid S, Keidar A, Gavert N, et al. The clinical spectrum of band erosion following laparoscopic adjustable silicone gastric banding for morbid obesity. Surg Endosc 2003;17(6):861–3.

75. Niville E, Dams A, Vlasselaers J. Lap-Band erosion: incidence and treatment. Obes Surg 2001;11(6):744–7.

76. Meir E, Van Baden M. Adjustable silicone gastric banding and band erosion: personal experience and hypotheses. Obes Surg 1999;9(2):191–3.

77. Pretolesi F, Camerini G, Bonifacino E, et al. Radiology of adjustable silicone gastric banding for morbid obesity. Br J Radiol 1998;71(847):717–22.

78. Sonavane SK, Menias CO, Kantawala KP, et al. Laparoscopic adjustable gastric banding: what radiologists need to know. Radiographics 2012; 32(4):1161–78.

Complications of Optical Colonoscopy: CT Findings

Barry Daly, MD, FRCR[a],*, Minh Lu, MD[a], Perry J. Pickhardt, MD[b], Christine O. Menias, MD[c], Maher A. Abbas, MD[d], Douglas S. Katz, MD[e]

KEYWORDS

- Optical colonoscopy • Computed tomography • Complications

KEY POINTS

- The development of colorectal cancer screening programs in many countries has led to increasingly large numbers of patients undergoing optical colonoscopy.
- Although acute complications from screening optical colonoscopy are uncommon, they may occur in up to 5% or more of cases where biopsy or therapeutic procedures are performed.
- Abdominal radiographs are of value only for the detection of intraperitoneal perforation, in patients suspected of complications following optical colonoscopy.
- A wide spectrum of other important potential complications of optical colonoscopy includes extraperitoneal perforation, splenic injury, postpolypectomy syndrome, bowel obstruction, mesenteric hemorrhage, diverticulitis, appendicitis, cathartic or chemical colitis, and other less frequently encountered problems.
- Such complications are most reliably identified using abdominal and pelvic CT, which also can guide appropriate conservative, interventional, or surgical management.

INTRODUCTION

Optical colonoscopy is a common and routine procedure for screening and detection of colorectal cancer, the second leading cause of cancer-related death in the United States.[1] The expansion of federally backed colon cancer screening programs and the health needs of an aging population are contributing to a rapid increase in the number of procedures, with more than 14 million colonoscopies performed annually in the United States.[2] Similar programs are being developed in many other countries worldwide. The sheer volume of optical colonoscopy procedures means that the low overall rate of serious complications (0.1%–0.3%) still affects a considerable number of individuals and constitutes an ongoing challenge.[3,4] Moreover, acute complications may occur in up to 5% or more of those colonoscopies where biopsy or therapeutic procedures, such as stricture dilation and stent placement, are performed.[4] The most common complications of optical colonoscopy are hemorrhage and large bowel perforation, with the incidence of hemorrhage up to 2.7%, whereas the overall incidence of perforation is 0.01% to 0.7%.[5] Less commonly occurring complications include splenic injury, postpolypectomy syndrome, and acute diverticulitis. Additional rare complications are listed in **Box 1**. The clinical spectrum and management of such complications has been well described in the gastrointestinal literature[4–7] but, to the authors'

The authors have nothing to disclose.
[a] Department of Diagnostic Radiology, University of Maryland School of Medicine, 22 South Greene Street, Baltimore, MD 21201, USA; [b] Department of Radiology, University of Wisconsin School of Medicine & Public Health, 600 Highland Avenue, Madison, WI 53792, USA; [c] Department of Radiology, Mayo Clinic, 13400 East Shea Boulevard, Scottsdale, AZ 85259, USA; [d] Digestive Disease Institute, Cleveland Clinic, Al Maryah Island, Abu Dhabi, United Arab Emirates; [e] Department of Radiology, Winthrop-University Hospital, 259 First Street, Mineola, NY 11501, USA
* Corresponding author.
E-mail address: bdaly@umm.edu

Radiol Clin N Am 52 (2014) 1087–1099
http://dx.doi.org/10.1016/j.rcl.2014.05.012
0033-8389/14/$ – see front matter © 2014 Elsevier Inc. All rights reserved.

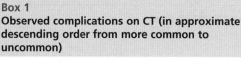

Box 1

Observed complications on CT (in approximate descending order from more common to uncommon)

Colonic perforation (intraperitoneal/extraperitoneal)

Postpolypectomy syndrome

Acute colonic diverticulitis

Splenic injury/hemorrhage

Mesenteric/retroperitoneal hemorrhage

Large bowel obstruction

Acute appendicitis

Cathartic or chemical colitis

Acute pancreatitis

Small bowel obstruction

Pneumomediastinum/pericardium, pneumothorax, subcutaneous emphysema

Ureteral obstruction

Liver abscess

Omental infarction

knowledge, only in a few studies has the spectrum of optical colonoscopy-related complications detectable on CT[8,9] been reported, as well as in a few focused articles on splenic injuries associated with optical colonoscopy.[10,11]

CASE MATERIAL AND IMAGING MODALITIES

This review is based on the authors' collective personal experiences of the clinical and CT imaging findings associated with complications of optical colonoscopy gathered at 5 medical institutions over a multiple-year period. Some of the observed cases have been previously contributed to publications[8,10] and/or presentations at major radiology conferences.[12] All of the cases included in the authors' experience had major or relatively major abdominal complications either after optical colonoscopy or associated with bowel preparation prior to the procedure. A few patients were known to have synchronous abdominal radiographs and CT at the time of presentation. The range of optical colonoscopy-related complications included is listed in **Box 1**.

Supine abdominal radiographs, obtained alone or with erect views, often comprise the imaging test of first choice in symptomatic patients with acute abdominal pain after optical colonoscopy. Arguably the only purpose of radiographs in this setting is the detection of free intraperitoneal gas signifying perforation of the colon. In contrast, CT

of the abdomen and pelvis is of considerably greater value, even where radiographs demonstrate free gas. In such cases, CT often provides additional information about the location and underlying cause of perforation, allowing for more informed surgical or other interventional planning. In cases of suspected complication where colon perforation is considered clinically unlikely, CT is the most appropriate initial imaging examination. This review describes the spectrum and diagnostic value of positive findings on CT in patients who have acute abdominal complications either after optical colonoscopy or associated with bowel preparation prior to the procedure.

COMPLICATIONS
Perforation

Although postbiopsy or therapy bleeding is the most widely recognized complication of optical colonoscopy, perforation of the colon is the most frequently encountered adverse event of radiologic importance. The incidence of perforation ranges from 0.01% to 0.6% after diagnostic colonoscopies and 5% or higher in colonoscopies performed for more challenging therapeutic purposes, such as metal stent placement and colon stricture dilation.[6,7,13–15] Perforation of the colon may be intraperitoneal and/or extraperitoneal and can be related to mechanical trauma from abrasion by the tip or shaft of the colonoscope, pneumatic insufflation, perforation of a diverticulum or area of stricture, traction injury from connecting ligaments, or therapeutic procedures. Perforation most commonly occurs in the sigmoid colon due to the acute angulation at the rectosigmoid junction, and is associated with direct mechanical forces from a slide-by or alpha maneuver of the endoscope. Intraperitoneal air often results from perforation of the transverse colon, sigmoid colon, or cecum. In some cases, perforation in these colonic segments results in atypical gas leakage confined to the mesocolon, a location typically not identified on radiographs but easily identified on CT. Signs and symptoms of free perforation into the peritoneal cavity at optical colonoscopy include persistent abdominal distention or pain, subcutaneous emphysema, fever, and leukocytosis. Perforation of the ascending colon, descending colon, or rectum is more likely to give rise to extraperitoneal air accumulation due to the retroperitoneal location of these colonic segments. In some cases, both intra- and extraperitoneal leak of gas from the colon is evident, making localization of the site of perforation more difficult (**Fig. 1**). Larger extraperitoneal gas leaks may spread to the subcutaneous tissues, leading to

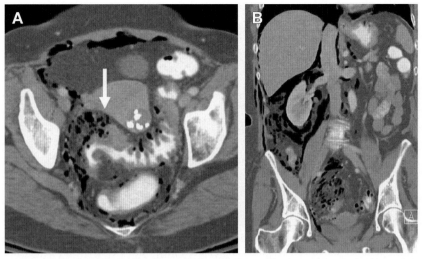

Fig. 1. Intra- and extraperitoneal leak of gas from sigmoid colon perforation at optical colonoscopy. Patient presented with abdominal pain 1 day after optical colonoscopy. There was difficulty passing the scope through the sigmoid colon. (*A*) On an axial pelvic CT image, the perforation site is noted in the midsigmoid (*arrow*), and both intra- and extraperitoneal leak of gas is seen. (*B*) Coronal CT image shows the full extent of extraperitoneal leak of gas around the inferior vena cava and the right kidney. The patient was successfully managed conservatively.

subcutaneous emphysema, and into the thorax, potentially leading to pneumomediastinum, pneumopericardium, and pneumothorax (**Fig. 2**).

As discussed previously, supine abdominal radiographs with or without erect abdominal radiographs are most often used as the initial imaging examination of first choice in patients with abdominal pain after optical colonoscopy. Supine films may be negative, however, even where the free leak of gas is large. Also, erect films may be negative where the gas is subtle, is loculated within a pericolonic mesentery, or is extraperitoneal.[8] The

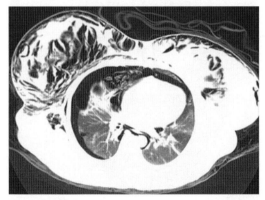

Fig. 2. Extensive subcutaneous emphysema, pneumomediastinum, and bilateral pneumothorax due to colon perforation after attempted optical colonoscopy. Axial CT image of the chest at lung window setting. Patient had a large extraperitoneal gas leak that spread across the diaphragm into the thorax, leading to extensive subcutaneous emphysema, pneumomediastinum, and pneumothorax.

development of pneumatosis coli after optical colonoscopy is also suspicious for perforation, although it may also be seen as a result of colonic overdistension or biopsy. In such settings, CT of the abdomen and pelvis demonstrates the extraperitoneal gas, and may also show focal fluid collections. This is of importance given the recent interest in nonsurgical approaches to localized colon perforation which may be amenable to colonoscopic repair with clipping devices (**Fig. 3**). When indicated, CT can be used to guide percutaneous drainage of fluid collections as an adjunct to this minimally-invasive approach.[16] Rarely, perforation of the terminal ileum may occur, typically when the ileocecal valve is traversed by the colonoscope and biopsies are obtained.

Postpolypectomy Coagulation Syndrome

Postpolypectomy coagulation syndrome most often occurs after the electrocautery of large sessile polyps at colonoscopy, and is caused by a transmural burn extending through the wall of the colon, often into the adjacent mesentery.[6,7] It is seen in 1% or fewer cases undergoing polypectomy.[17] Patients usually develop symptoms of abdominal pain that may be severe, peritoneal signs, fever, and leukocytosis, 1 to 5 days after the procedure. Abdominal radiographs are usually negative, and the diagnosis is usually made with CT. The typical findings of postpolypectomy coagulation syndrome on CT include focal wall thickening and low attenuation perilesional submucosal edema, in addition to high attenuation

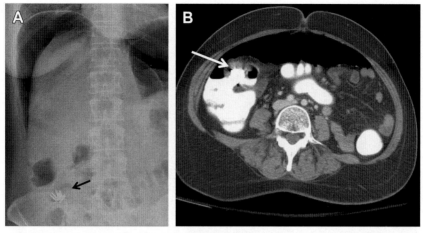

Fig. 3. Nonsurgical colonoscopic repair of ascending colon wall perforation by means of multiple endoscopic clips. (*A*) Upright abdominal radiograph obtained immediately post–optical colonoscopy demonstrates pneumoperitoneum and multiple endoclips (*arrow*) used to effectively seal a full thickness perforation of the proximal ascending colon. (*B*) Subsequently obtained abdominal CT with IV and water-soluble oral contrast demonstrates free peritoneal gas and artifact on axial image from the endoscopically-placed clips (*arrow*). No leak of contrast from the colon was seen, indicating successful repair and avoiding the need for open surgery.

infiltration of the adjacent pericolonic fat due to sterile inflammation and/or local hemorrhage (**Fig. 4**). In severe cases, symptoms of an acute abdomen may be present (**Fig. 5**). Strictly speaking, true perforation does not occur in post-polypectomy coagulation syndrome, but in some cases, there is CT evidence of limited perforation (**Fig. 6**). Recognition of this syndrome is important because it is self-limited and treatment is usually restricted to conservative management with bowel rest and antibiotics.

Splenic Injury

An unusual but under-recognized and serious complication of optical colonoscopy is splenic laceration or rupture. Several large studies of complications related to optical colonoscopy (performed without CT imaging) report no cases; however, the authors' collective experience has identified at least 21 cases on CT

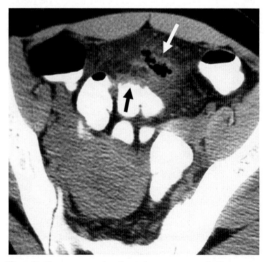

Fig. 5. Severe postpolypectomy coagulation syndrome. Pelvic CT image shows necrotic gas-containing burn extending widely into the adjacent mesenteric fat (*white arrow*) after fulguration of a sessile sigmoid polyp. Black arrow denotes polyp site. The patient had severe abdominal pain 1 day after optical colonoscopy.

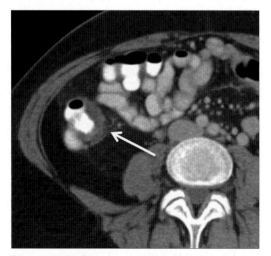

Fig. 4. Postpolypectomy coagulation syndrome. Abdominal CT image shows focal edema and inflammatory changes in the ascending colon wall in the region of the biopsy site (*arrow*).

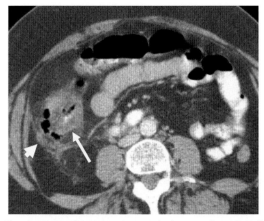

Fig. 6. Postpolypectomy coagulation syndrome and localized perforation. CT shows localized extraperitoneal perforation of the right colon (*arrowhead*), with edematous inflammatory colonic wall changes (*arrow*) after polypectomy.

examinations,[10,12] and to the authors' knowledge there are at least 66 additional cases of optical colonoscopy-related splenic injury reported in the literature.[18–20] The mechanism by which laceration occurs may be direct trauma leading to partial capsular avulsion as a result of colonoscopic maneuvers. Protracted direct compression on the spleen by the colonoscope may be more likely to develop in patients with an acutely angled splenic flexure.[10] Stretching of the colon during optical colonoscopy with consequent excessive traction or torsion on the phrenicocolic ligament is another likely precipitating cause (**Fig. 7**).

Splenic injuries also may be facilitated by adhesions from prior surgery, previous pancreatitis, or inflammatory bowel disease. This complication is also seen more often in women[10] and where the colonoscopic procedure is reported to have been technically difficult.[20] All of these factors can contribute to splenic injury, leading to subcapsular hematoma development or capsular rupture with subsequent free intraperitoneal hemorrhage.[10,19,20] Furthermore, splenomegaly and underlying splenic disease are other factors that may predispose patients to splenic injury from optical colonoscopy. A high clinical suspicion is required for the prompt diagnosis of this rare but serious and occasionally fatal complication. Such patients may present acutely after optical colonoscopy with clinical features of an acute abdomen or hemodynamic instability. More frequently, however, the presentation may be delayed for 2 to 3 days and the clinical features may include left-sided abdominal pain, sometimes with a pleural component or shoulder tip referral, leukocytosis, and/or acute anemia. CT of the abdomen demonstrates a spectrum of injury

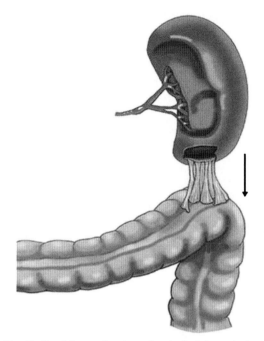

Fig. 7. Possible mechanism of splenic injury during optical colonoscopy. Diagram showing phrenicocolic ligament and a splenic capsular tear. Stretching of the colon during colonoscopy with consequent excessive traction or torsion on the splenocolic ligament is a likely precipitating cause. Arrow indicates the direction of traction most likely to cause injury. (*Modified from* Cassar K, Munro A. Iatrogenic splenic injury. J R Coll Surg Edinb 2002;47:731–41; with permission.)

from self-limiting, contained splenic subcapsular hematoma (**Fig. 8**), to small perisplenic hematoma (**Fig. 9**), to multiple lacerations with capsular rupture and free intraperitoneal hemorrhage (**Fig. 10**). Splenic artery pseudoaneurysm has also been reported in this setting.[10] Treatment may be conservative if a patient is stable, but immediate transcatheter splenic artery embolization or splenectomy may be necessary if there is persistent hypotension or bleeding.[7] Left-sided pleuritic pain may lead to suspicion of pulmonary embolic disease, and the diagnosis may be made as an unanticipated finding at CT pulmonary angiography (**Fig. 11**). When patients have persistent left-sided abdominal or pleuritic pain of undetermined origin after optical colonoscopy, CT should be obtained urgently to exclude splenic injury. As the cases illustrated in **Figs. 10** and **11** suggest, major splenic injury may result in life-threatening bleeding and may therefore require urgent interventional radiologic or surgical management.

Intraluminal and Extraluminal Hemorrhage

Intraluminal hemorrhage after optical colonoscopy is well documented and is the most frequent

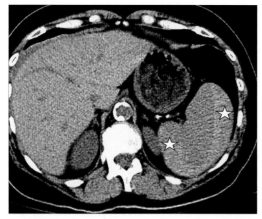

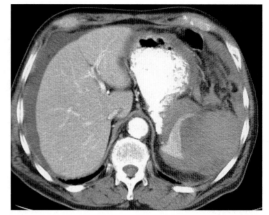

Fig. 8. Moderately large subcapsular splenic hematoma after optical colonoscopy. Patient with left upper quadrant pain 2 days after optical colonoscopy. CT image shows a moderately-large subcapsular splenic hematoma (*stars*). No splenic laceration was seen, allowing for the limitations of nonenhanced technique. The patient was admitted for observation and was successfully managed conservatively.

Fig. 10. Moderately-large splenic laceration with extensive peritoneal bleeding after optical colonoscopy. Patient presented with hypotension shortly after completion of optical colonoscopy. CT image with oral and IV contrast shows severe laceration of the spleen, with capsular rupture and extensive peritoneal bleeding. The patient underwent emergent splenectomy.

complication. It can occur in 1% to 2% of therapeutic colonoscopies.[7] This may occur from inadequate coagulation after transection of a pedunculated polyp, but large sessile polyps (>1 cm) have the greatest risk for acute hemorrhage, which may be attributed to inadequate heat seal of the blood supply after tissue transection.[21] An older study found that the bleeding rate after removal of polyps greater than 1 cm was 4.6%.[22] Intraluminal hemorrhage is usually evident clinically or can be diagnosed using a nuclear medicine tagged red blood cell scan, by CT angiography, or by repeat optical colonoscopy.

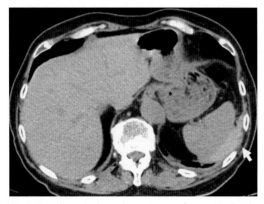

Fig. 9. Small perisplenic hematoma after optical colonoscopy. Patient with left upper quadrant pain 3 days after optical colonoscopy. Axial CT image shows small perisplenic hematoma (*arrow*). The spleen appeared normal, allowing for limitations of nonenhanced technique. Management was conservative.

Extraluminal hemorrhage is unusual and may occur as a result of peri-intestinal blood vessel injury during polyp coagulation. It may manifest as free bleeding into the peritoneal space or as bleeding into the retroperitoneal space when it involves the retroperitoneal portions of the ascending and descending colon (**Fig. 12**). Such instances of hemorrhage can result from mechanisms similar to those of splenic injury: excessive force and possible weakness of the colonic wall. This is an uncommon complication for which a high clinical suspicion is also necessary. Postpolypectomy bleeding can be managed by resnaring techniques or by injecting epinephrine at the bleeding site. Endoscopic hemoclips may also be used. Where appropriate, nonendoscopic treatment modalities include angiographic embolization and surgery.[23]

Acute Diverticulitis

There is a high prevalence of diverticular disease in the same older population, which is targeted for screening optical colonoscopy. Therefore, occasional patients are encountered who develop acute diverticulitis after colonoscopy, likely as a result of mechanical injury during the procedure.[7] It is postulated that the colonoscope may cause microperforations of the colon wall or that retained stool may be displaced into diverticula with the subsequent development of acute inflammation. Patients most often present with typical left iliac fossa pain and fever within several days of undergoing optical colonoscopy. Findings on CT are the same as those with the more typical causes of

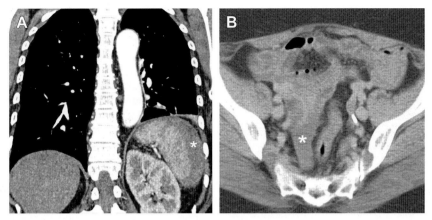

Fig. 11. Moderately large subcapsular splenic hematoma presenting with pleuritic chest pain after optical colonoscopy. Patient presented with pleuritic chest pain 2 days after optical colonoscopy. (A) CT pulmonary angiogram was negative for suspected pulmonary embolism, but on this coronal reformation shows a moderately-large subcapsular splenic hematoma (asterisk). (B) Axial image from CT venography performed at the time of CT angiography shows moderate intraperitoneal bleeding extending into the pelvis (asterisk). Splenic lacerations were noted at emergent splenectomy.

colonic diverticulitis, including colonic wall thickening, pericolic inflammatory fat infiltration, and swelling or effacement of diverticula in the affected colon segment (**Fig. 13**). Another possible factor is the uncommon subclinical or silent, smoldering variant of diverticulitis that has been recently recognized and which may be exacerbated by direct trauma from the colonoscope. This low-grade chronic variant of diverticulitis has been noted at elective surgical resection of the sigmoid colon after repeated acute diverticulitis episodes,[24] or on occasion during screening colonoscopy in asymptomatic patients,[25] as well as on CT examinations performed for reasons unrelated to the colon. In such cases, optical colonoscopy

may be incomplete due to preexisting subclinical inflammation and stricture formation, most often in the sigmoid region. Localized perforation may occur in attempts to traverse stenotic segments (**Fig. 14**). Simple diverticulitis is usually treated by rehydration, symptomatic relief, and intravenous (IV) antibiotics. Most patients with uncomplicated disease respond well to medical treatment and generally experience significant improvement in their abdominal pain, temperature, and inflammatory markers within 2 days of initiation of antibiotic treatment. Frequent complications include local perforation and abscess formation. Local perforation may proceed to open perforation necessitating urgent laparotomy. The development of

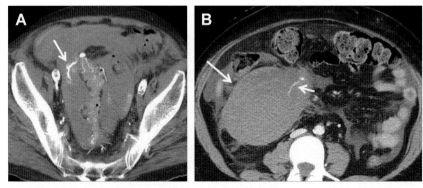

Fig. 12. Mesenteric and retroperitoneal hemorrhage after biopsy at colonoscopy (2 different patients). (A) Axial CT image of the pelvis shows active bleeding due to laceration of an inferior mesenteric artery branch (arrow), noted after sigmoid colon wall biopsy. A large volume of hemorrhagic peritoneal fluid is present. Successful transcatheter arterial embolization was performed. (B) Axial abdominal CT image in a different patient shows a large acute retroperitoneal hematoma (long arrow), from an actively bleeding superior mesenteric artery branch injury (short arrow), after biopsy of the ascending colon. Successful transcatheter arterial embolization was performed.

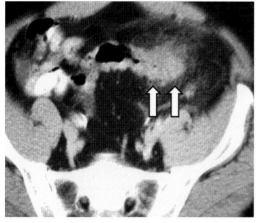

Fig. 13. Acute diverticulitis after optical colonoscopy. This patient presented with acute left lower quadrant pain and fever 3 days after optical colonoscopy. Pelvic CT image shows typical findings for acute diverticulitis in the sigmoid colon (*arrows*). Abdominal and pelvic CT (not shown) performed 2 days prior to colonoscopy demonstrated only diverticulosis.

abscess formation may require percutaneous image-guided or surgical drainage.

Bowel Obstruction

Although bowel obstruction is a rare complication associated with optical colonoscopy, a range of predisposing causes resulting in large bowel obstruction has been reported in the literature.[26–29] This has been noted in association with strictures due to colon carcinoma, cecal or sigmoid volvulus, diverticulitis, postischemia, and endometriosis. Bowel obstruction may occur immediately prior to optical colonoscopy as a result of a high-volume antegrade fluid bowel cleanser unmasking obstruction, usually of the colon, at the site of a tight stricture. Coronal and oblique 3-D CT images may be helpful to determine the exact site of obstruction and to allow planning of decompression and stent placement during optical colonoscopy (**Fig. 15**). Several mechanisms have been reported as causes for small bowel obstruction during optical colonoscopy including: (1) reflux of air through an incompetent ileocecal valve and subsequent small bowel entrapment secondary to adhesions (**Fig. 16**); (2) volvulus as a result of herniation and incarceration of a segment of small bowel; and (3) high intra-abdominal pressure causing static internal herniation of a small bowel loop.[27] These complications may be precipitated in patients who have a history of abdominal surgery, infection, or postoperative adhesions. CT may be helpful in assessing for a possible transition point and for the underlying cause. Patients with small bowel obstruction after optical colonoscopy are usually managed conservatively with bowel rest, nasogastric tube decompression, and IV fluids.

Unusual Complications

Other rare complications of diagnostic and therapeutic optical colonoscopy have been reported in the literature. They include appendicitis, cathartic or chemical colitis, acute pancreatitis, liver abscess, pneumothorax, pneumomediastinum, pneumopericardium, subcutaneous emphysema, ureteral obstruction, and omental infarction. Appendicitis resulting from optical colonoscopy may be due to several proposed mechanisms, including forcing bowel contents into the appendix

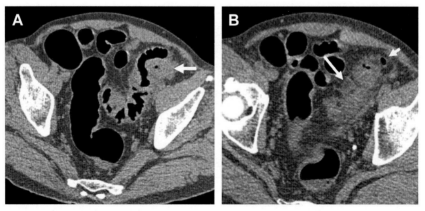

Fig. 14. Sigmoid stricture and microperforation at optical colonoscopy secondary to pre-existing subclinical diverticulitis. This patient underwent CTC immediately after incomplete colonoscopy. (*A*) Axial CT image of the pelvis shows a long sigmoid stricture with a perisigmoid inflammatory mass (*arrow*) in a region of diverticular disease. (*B*) Adjacent axial CT image shows extensive inflammatory changes representing diverticulitis (*long arrow*). Microperforation was also present (*short arrow*).

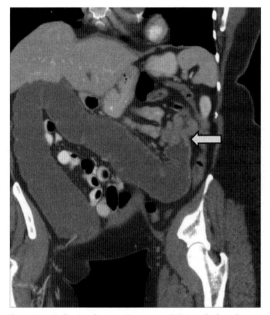

Fig. 15. Colon obstruction precipitated by large-volume antegrade bowel preparation 1 day prior to optical colonoscopy. Oblique coronal CT image shows that the distended colon is obstructed by an apple-core tumor in the distal transverse region (*arrow*). The obstruction was precipitated by large-volume antegrade bowel preparation.

from insufflation and endoscopic manipulation (**Figs. 17** and **18**), edema from mucosal trauma around the cecum, perforation at cecal biopsy sites, and barotrauma.[30]

Chemical colitis involving part or all of the colon may develop after colonoscopy if the glutaraldehyde

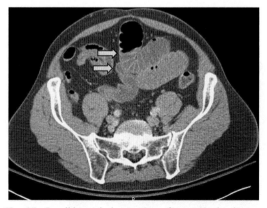

Fig. 16. Small bowel obstruction after optical colonoscopy. Axial CT image shows dilated proximal loops of small bowel and adjacent adhesions (*arrows*). Distal decompressed small bowel loops are noted in the right lower quadrant. Obstruction was probably precipitated by reflux of gas from the colon becoming trapped proximal to the low-grade preexistent adhesions.

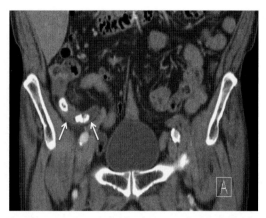

Fig. 17. Acute appendicitis after negative optical colonoscopy 48 hours earlier. Patient with right lower quadrant pain after negative optical colonoscopy 48 hours earlier. Coronal CT image shows acute appendicitis, with a fluid-filled, distended (1.4 cm) appendix and thickened wall (*arrows*). Appendicoliths are present. Suggested mechanism is bowel contents being forced into the appendix from insufflation in a patient at increased risk with multiple appendicoliths.

and/or hydrogen peroxide solutions used during disinfection have not been adequately rinsed from the colonoscope.[31] These agents induce ischemic effects on the mucosa and, on occasion, deeper layers of the colon wall (**Figs. 19** and **20**). Treatment is usually conservative, and the process is self-resolving. Chronic complications, such as colonic strictures, rarely occur.

There are a few case reports of acute pancreatitis after optical colonoscopy, although the underlying mechanism is unclear.[32] In the case of acute distal pancreatitis after colonoscopy, illustrated in **Fig. 21**, the mechanism is presumably similar to that of postcolonoscopy splenic injury—navigating the diseased left colon and splenic flexure and associated manipulations led to injury of the distal pancreas. The patient's history of Crohn disease is relevant, because inflammatory bowel disease is known to be a risk factor for splenic injury at optical colonoscopy.

As discussed previously, pneumomediastinum, pneumopericardium, and pneumothorax may occur secondary to colon perforation after optical colonoscopy (see **Fig. 2**). Extraluminal air or pneumatosis developing in the colon wall from perforation can track through the mesentery and retroperitoneum to reach the mediastinum and subsequently leak into the pleural space.[33] Snare wire entrapment can result from the snare being caught in a large polyp from therapeutic optical colonoscopy. Although liver abscess is a frequent complication of colon surgery, it is a rare development after colonoscopy. The same mechanism of

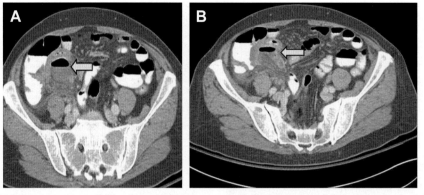

Fig. 18. Secondary acute appendicitis after cecal biopsy at optical colonoscopy. (*A*) Patient presented with short history of right lower quadrant pain and fever after colonoscopy and cecal base biopsy same day. Axial CT image shows a gas and fluid-containing cavity (*arrow*) and regional inflammation due to perforation at the biopsy site. (*B*) Axial CT image at a slightly lower level shows regional inflammation due to perforation at biopsy site. Secondary acute appendicitis was noted (*arrow*). Emergent surgery was required.

portal pyemia is believed to occur, in this case resulting from the introduction of bacteria at the biopsy site and leading to seeding of the liver (**Fig. 22**).

Ureteral inflammation and/or obstruction has been noted as a result of phlegmonous mass or abscess development in the pelvis complicating colonic perforation. Omental infarction is also rare after optical colonoscopy but likely occurs as a result of mechanical compression or torsion of the omentum during manipulation of the colonoscope (**Fig. 23**). The patient presented with localized pain and abdominal tenderness within a few days of the procedure. No other possible cause for omental infarction could be identified. To the authors' knowledge, this complication after optical colonoscopy has not been described previously.

DISCUSSION

Conventional abdominal radiography has long been considered the primary imaging modality in patients presenting with acute abdominal pain, especially after colonoscopy. Radiography has significant limitations, however, for investigation of complications related to optical colonoscopy, with the exception of detecting free pneumoperitoneum secondary to colonic perforation. As demonstrated here, colon perforation may occur into the extraperitoneal spaces (see **Figs. 1** and **6**) and may not be detectable on radiographs. There is a wide range of other complications related to optical colonoscopy, as discussed previously, for which radiographs are also unhelpful. Some of these complications are serious and potentially fatal, and require rapid and accurate diagnosis. CT has been recommended by other

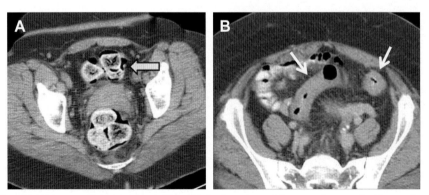

Fig. 19. Cathartic colitis secondary to aggressive colonic cleansing with purgative medications prior to colonoscopy. (*A*) Pelvic CT image shows copious inspissated stool in the sigmoid colon and rectum (*arrow*). (*B*) CT image of the pelvis 3 days later shows interval development of colitis in the descending and sigmoid colon after 48 hours of aggressive cathartic cleansing prior to colonoscopy (*arrows*).

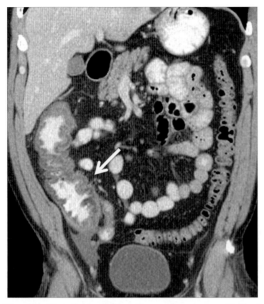

Fig. 20. Chemical colitis after colonoscopy. Patient developed abdominal pain after normal colonoscopy 2 days earlier. Coronal contrast-enhanced CT image shows development of colitis in the ascending colon (*arrow*). This was believed to be due to the cleansing agent used for the colonoscope preparation. No other cause could be determined.

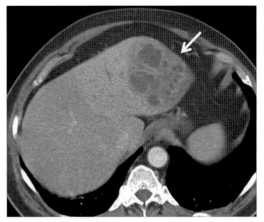

Fig. 22. Liver abscess after colon biopsy at optical colonoscopy. Abdominal CT image performed 1 week after optical colonoscopy demonstrates a large multi-loculated thick-walled fluid collection in the left lateral segment of the liver, typical for abscess (*arrow*). This was subsequently drained percutaneously.

investigators when such complications are clinically suspected,[8,10] and the authors also endorse its use in the setting of clinically concerning post-colonoscopy symptoms. With the exception of the detection of pneumoperitoneum due to gross intraperitoneal perforation, CT is superior to plain radiographs, and frequently can be used to guide appropriate conservative, interventional, or surgical management. Although the statistical risk of a serious immediate complications arising at screening optical colonoscopy is small,[3–5] most of the complications the authors have encountered in practice occurred in patients with no colonic polyps—or only diminutive lesions. If CT colonography (CTC) were used as the primary screening test for colorectal polyps,[34] this would have eliminated the need for optical colonoscopy

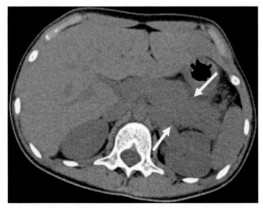

Fig. 21. Acute pancreatitis 1 day after optical colonoscopy. An 18-year-old with Crohn disease presents with acute left flank pain after colonoscopy performed the previous day. Noncontrast axial abdominal CT image shows mildly swollen pancreatic tail, and surrounding inflammatory changes with peripancreatic edema (*arrows*). Serum amylase and lipase levels were substantially elevated.

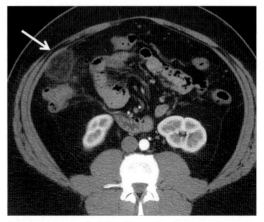

Fig. 23. Omental infarction after colonoscopy. The patient presented with right lower quadrant pain 2 days after optical colonoscopy. Abdominal CT image shows a circumscribed area of increased attenuation in the omental fat anterior to the ascending colon (*arrow*), typical for omental infarction. Treatment was conservative.

and the risk of associated complications in the vast majority of screened patients.[35] Until CTC becomes a widely accepted primary screening tool for colorectal polyps, such complications will likely be encountered more frequently with the continuing growth in colon cancer screening programs and with the increasing use of endoscopic therapies in the colon.

SUMMARY

The development of colorectal cancer screening programs in many countries has led to increasingly large numbers of patients undergoing optical colonoscopy. Although acute complications from screening optical colonoscopy are uncommon, they may occur in up to 5% or more of patients where biopsies or therapeutic procedures are performed. Abdominal radiographs are of value only for the detection of intraperitoneal perforation. A wide spectrum of other important complications potentially associated with optical colonoscopy also includes extraperitoneal perforation, splenic injury, postpolypectomy syndrome, bowel obstruction, mesenteric hemorrhage, diverticulitis, appendicitis, cathartic or chemical colitis, and other less frequently encountered problems. Such complications are most reliably identified using abdominal and pelvic CT, which also can guide appropriate conservative, interventional, or surgical management.

REFERENCES

1. Jemal A, Siegel R, Ward E, et al. Cancer statistics, 2008. CA Cancer J Clin 2008;58:71–96.
2. Seeff LC, Richards TB, Shapiro JA, et al. How many endoscopies are performed for colorectal cancer screening? Results from CDC's survey of endoscopic capacity. Gastroenterology 2004;127:1670–7.
3. Lieberman DA, Weiss D, Bond J, et al. Use of optical colonoscopy to screen asymptomatic adults for colorectal cancer. N Engl J Med 2000;343:162–8.
4. Waye JD, Lewis BS, Yessayan S. Optical colonoscopy: a prospective report of complications. Am J Gastroenterol 1993;15:347–51.
5. Pignone M, Rich M, Teutsch SM, et al. Screening for colorectal cancer in adults at average risk: a summary of the evidence for the U.S. Preventive Services Task Force. Ann Intern Med 2002;137:132–41.
6. Waye JD, Kahn O, Auerbach M. Complications of optical colonoscopy and flexible sigmoidoscopy. Gastrointest Endosc Clin N Am 1996;2:343–77.
7. ASGE Standards of Practice Committee, Fisher DA, Maple JT, Ben-Menachem T, et al. Complications of colonoscopy: guidelines. Gastrointest Endosc 2011; 74:745–52.
8. Kim DH, Pickhardt PJ, Taylor AJ, et al. Imaging evaluation of complications at optical colonoscopy. Curr Probl Diagn Radiol 2008;37:165–77.
9. Zissin R, Konikoff F, Gayer G. CT findings of Iatrogenic complications following gastrointestinal endoluminal procedures. Semin Ultrasound CT MR 2006; 27:126–38.
10. Fishback SJ, Pickhardt PJ, Bhalla S, et al. Delayed presentation of splenic rupture following optical colonoscopy: clinical and CT findings. Emerg Radiol 2011;18:539–44.
11. Galperin-Aizenberg M, Blachar A, Gayer G. Iatrogenic injury to the spleen - CT appearance. Semin Ultrasound CT MR 2007;28:52–6.
12. Lu M, Daly BD, Safdar NM, et al. Acute complications of colonoscopy: CT diagnosis. Electronic exhibit, American Roentgen Ray Society annual meeting. Chicago, IL, May 6, 2011.
13. Korman LY, Overholt BF, Box T, et al. Perforation during optical colonoscopy in endoscopic ambulatory surgical centers. Gastrointest Endosc 2003;58:554–7.
14. Avgerinos D, Llaguna O, Lo A, et al. Evolving management of colonoscopic perforations. J Gastrointest Surg 2008;12:1783–9.
15. Damore LJ 2nd, Rantis PC, Vernava AM 3rd, et al. Colonoscopic perforations. Etiology, diagnosis, and management. Dis Colon Rectum 1996;39:1308–14.
16. Trecca A, Gaj F, Gagliardi G. Our experience with endoscopic repair of large colonoscopic perforations and review of the literature. Tech Coloproctol 2008;12:315–21.
17. Cha JM, Lim KS, Lee SH, et al. Clinical outcomes and risk factors of post-polypectomy coagulation syndrome: a multicenter, retrospective, case-control study. Endoscopy 2013;45:202–7.
18. Ahmed A, Eller PM, Schiffman FJ. Splenic rupture: an unusual complication of colonoscopy. Am J Gastroenterol 1997;92:1201–4.
19. Holzer K, Thalhammer A, Bechstein WO. Splenic trauma: a rare complication during optical colonoscopy. J Gastroenterol 2004;42:509–12.
20. Saad A, Rex D. Optical colonoscopy-induced splenic injury: report of 3 cases and literature review. Dig Dis Sci 2008;53:892–8.
21. Blades E, Sivak M. Complications. In: Raskin J, Nord HJ, editors. Optical colonoscopy: principles and techniques. New York: Igaku-Shoin; 1995. p. 143–55.
22. Van Gossum A, Cozzoli A, Adler M, et al. Colonoscopic snare polypectomy: analysis of 1485 resections comparing two types of current. Gastrointest Endosc 1992;38:472–5.
23. Sorbi D, Norton I, Conio M, et al. Postpolypectomy lower GI bleeding: descriptive analysis. Gastrointest Endosc 2000;51:690–6.
24. Boostrom SY, Wolff BG, Cima RR, et al. Uncomplicated diverticulitis, more complicated than we thought. J Gastrointest Surg 2012;16:1744–9.

25. Ghorari S, Ulbright TM, Rex DK. Endoscopic findings of diverticular inflammation in colonoscopy patients without clinical acute diverticulitis: prevalence and endoscopic spectrum. Am J Gastroenterol 2003;98:802–6.

26. Raghavendran K, Novak JM, Amodeo JL, et al. Mechanical small bowel obstruction precipitated by optical colonoscopy. Available at: http://link.springer.com.proxy-hs.researchport.umd.edu/article/10.1007/s00464-002-4543-4. Accessed February 12, 2014.

27. Patterson R, Klassen G. Small bowel obstruction from internal hernia as a complication of optical colonoscopy. Can J Gastroenterol 2000;14:959–60.

28. Malki SA, Bassett ML, Pavli P. Small bowel obstruction caused by optical colonoscopy. Gastrointest Endosc 2001;53:120–1.

29. Zanati SA, Fu A, Kortan P. Routine optical colonoscopy complicated by small-bowel obstruction. Gastrointest Endosc 2005;61:781–3.

30. Chae HS, Jeon SY, Nam WS, et al. Acute appendicitis caused by optical colonoscopy. Korean J Intern Med 2007;22:308–11.

31. Sheibani S, Gerson LB. Chemical colitis. J Clin Gastroenterol 2008;42:115–21.

32. Nevins AB, Keeffe EB. Acute pancreatitis after gastrointestinal endoscopy. J Clin Gastroenterol 2002;34:94–5.

33. Ball C, Kirkpatrick A, Mackenzie S, et al. Tension pneumothorax secondary to colonic perforation during diagnostic optical colonoscopy: report of a case. Surg Today 2006;36:478–80.

34. Pickhardt PJ, Choi JR, Hwang I, et al. Computed tomographic virtual colonoscopy to screen for colorectal neoplasia in asymptomatic adults. N Engl J Med 2003;349:2191–200.

35. Pickhardt PJ, Wise SM, Kim DH. Positive predictive value for polyps detected at screening CT colonography. Eur Radiol 2010;20:1651–6.

Imaging of Iatrogenic Complications of the Urinary Tract
Kidneys, Ureters, and Bladder

Bhavik N. Patel, MD[a], Gabriela Gayer, MD[b,c],*

KEYWORDS

• Iatrogenic injury • Urinary tract • Bladder • Kidney • Ureter • Imaging

KEY POINTS

- Imaging techniques for iatrogenic injury evaluation vary depending on the type and site of injury suspected and should be tailored according to a particular patient's history.
- Anticoagulant-related suburothelial hemorrhage may mimic a neoplastic lesion in the renal pelvis.
- Pseudoaneuryms are a rare, but potentially life-threatening, postoperative complication of partial nephrectomy. Radiologists play an important role in diagnosing and embolizing these lesions.
- Ureteral injuries may present remote from surgery with nonspecific symptoms. Fluid collection and hydronephrosis on postoperative CT should raise suspicion of ureteral injury and prompt delayed scans.

INTRODUCTION

A wide spectrum of complications affecting the urinary tract may be encountered with various treatments: medical, minimally invasive, surgical, and radiation therapy.[1,2] Although most injuries require little or no intervention, some of them carry significant morbidity and mortality. Thus, it is crucial for radiologists to be familiar with iatrogenic injuries to the kidneys, ureters, and bladder. Each particular patient's medical and surgical history plays a key role in determining which injuries should be suspected, thereby allowing the radiologic evaluation to be appropriately tailored. Sometimes, however, a patient may present somewhat remote from the treatment (eg, surgical procedure) with nonspecific symptoms and signs, and the referring physician may not suspect that they reflect an iatrogenic complication. In these circumstances, the radiologist may be the first to suspect iatrogenic complication and confirm it by tailoring the imaging evaluation accordingly.

This article reviews a range of iatrogenic injuries associated with various medical and surgical interventions and the optimal imaging approach that aids in their detection.

IMAGING TECHNIQUE

Multidetector CT is the modality of choice when evaluating patients for urinary tract injury.[3] It has surpassed intravenous urography in diagnostic capability, becoming the first-line examination in

Financial Disclosures: None.
[a] Division of Abdominal Imaging, Department of Radiology, Duke University Medical Center, 3808, Durham, NC 27710, USA; [b] Division of Abdominal Imaging, Department of Radiology, Stanford University Medical Center, 300 Pasteur Drive, Stanford, CA 94304, USA; [c] Department of Radiology, Sheba Medical Center, 2 Derech Sheba, Tel-Hashomer, Ramat-Gan 52621, Israel
* Corresponding author.
E-mail address: ggayer@stanford.edu

Radiol Clin N Am 52 (2014) 1101–1116
http://dx.doi.org/10.1016/j.rcl.2014.05.013
0033-8389/14/$ – see front matter © 2014 Elsevier Inc. All rights reserved.

the imaging of patients with suspected urinary tract injuries.[4,5] Due to increased spatial resolution, CT provides precise delineation of the injury and its severity, thereby allowing appropriate management of patients and guiding possible interventions.[6] Moreover, the presence of cortical injury, vascular injury, and collecting system injury can all be elucidated.

Optimal CT imaging technique in patients suspected of injury to the urinary tract may vary according to suspicion of injury, type of injury, and upper versus lower tract involvement. Initial evaluation may begin with an unenhanced examination, which allow detection of renal hematomas.[7] Subsequently, enhanced images should be performed using a power injector to administer approximately 150 mL of intravenous contrast at a rate of at least 3 mL/s.[8] If vascular injury is suspected, enhanced images using a delay of 25 to 40 seconds should be performed to optimally opacify vascular structures and depict injury. In patients with hemodynamic disturbances, bolus tracking may be necessary rather than a standard timed-delay scanning.[3]

If a focal renal parenchymal injury is suspected, routine portal venous phase images with a delay of 60 to 70 seconds may be obtained.[9] A nephrographic phase starting no earlier than 100 seconds should be performed, however, if clear delineation of the renal medulla is required.[10,11] For suspected injuries to the renal collecting systems, a delayed acquisition to allow optimal opacification of the renal pelves and ureters is recommended. These excretory phase images obtained with a delay of at least 5 minutes after bolus injection allow detection of extravasation of urine secondary to an injury.[7,12] In an effort to reduce the number of acquisitions and reduce radiation dose, split-bolus techniques have been described, whereby the nephrographic and excretory phases are combined.[13] Although the upper renal tract and renal parenchyma may be optimally visualized with this technique, a delayed excretory phase should be performed if injury to the lower urinary tract is suspected. A triple split-bolus injection with a single acquisition combining all 3 phases (corticomedullary, nephrographic, and excretory) has also been reported.[14]

For injuries involving the bladder, a CT of the pelvis (CT cystography) should be performed after the instillation of iodinated contrast into the bladder. A minimum of 300 to 350 mL of dilute contrast material should be instilled under gravity into the bladder via a Foley catheter to achieve optimal distension of the bladder and improve sensitivity for detection of injuries.[15–17]

IATROGENIC INJURIES

Iatrogenic injuries affecting the urinary tract are discussed, focusing on the involved organs—kidneys, ureters, and bladder—and according to underlying treatment resulting in the iatrogenic complication.

Renal Injuries

Iatrogenic injuries to the kidneys may result from both medical treatment and surgical procedures. The imaging findings of complications arising from various treatments and the key role of radiologists in this setting are highlighted.

Drug-induced complications

Anticoagulant therapy is highly effective in reducing the risk of both arterial thrombosis and venous thrombosis. All anticoagulants increase the risk of bleeding, which is a common and potentially fatal complication.[18] Anticoagulant-related hematomas may occur in the perinephric space, subcapsular space, suburothelium, and renal sinus.[19–21] Patients usually present with acute flank pain and hematuria. These symptoms are indistinguishable from those of renal colic and, therefore, frequently prompt an emergent CT examination to evaluate the presumptive diagnosis of an obstructing ureteral stone. CT for this indication is performed without intravenous administration of contrast material to improve detection of stones along the collecting systems and ureters. An unenhanced scan is also optimal for revealing acute anticoagulant-related bleeding. A fresh subcapsular hematoma appears as a hyperdense crescent-shaped mass enveloping the periphery of the kidney (Fig. 1A). Its high density, relative to the renal parenchyma, and its crescentic shape are typical of a subcapsular hematoma. The high density of the hematoma is less evident on contrast-enhanced scans (see Fig. 1B). A subcapsular hematoma, particularly when large, exerts mass effect on the adjacent renal parenchyma (see Fig. 1A, B).[3,22] Follow-up CT several days later can show evolution of blood products within the hematoma, with decrease in the attenuation of the collection compared with the initial scan (see Fig. 1C).[22] Nontraumatic subcapsular hemorrhage occurs more frequently secondary to rupture of renal cell carcinoma or angiomyolipoma than due to anticoagulation.[19,21,23,24] Knowledge of anticoagulant treatment is, therefore, important to be mindful of this reversible cause of hemorrhage rather than the more common causes. Failure to consider anticoagulant-related bleeding may lead to a more exhaustive work-up to exclude the presence

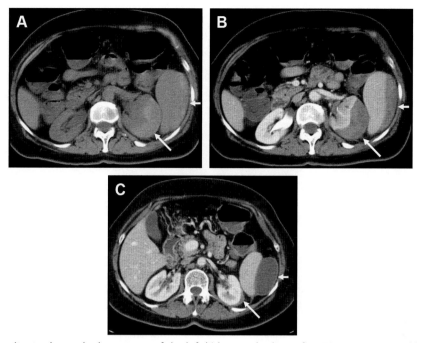

Fig. 1. Concomitant subcapsular hematoma of the left kidney and spleen after ESWL. A 60-year-old woman presented with left flank pain and a decline in hemoglobin level 2 days after ESWL treatment of a stone in the left ureter. (*A*) Unenhanced axial CT image at the level of the upper abdomen shows a crescent-like high-density mass enveloping the lateral aspect of the left kidney (*long arrow*) and another mass-like area, similar in shape and density, along the lateral aspect of the spleen (*short arrow*). The high density of these foci, relative to that of the kidney and spleen, and their crescentic shape, are typical of acute subcapsular hematomas. (*B*) On contrast-enhanced CT, these masses are considerably more conspicuous due to enhancement of only the renal parenchyma. The shape, density, and lack of enhancement of these masses are typical of subcapsular hematomas (subcapsular renal hematoma, *long arrow*; subcapsular splenic hematoma, *short arrow*). (*C*) Follow-up contrast-enhanced axial abdominal CT image obtained 6 weeks later shows marked shrinkage of the renal subcapsular hematoma (*long arrow*). The splenic subcapsular hematoma has liquefied and its density is now that of clear fluid (*short arrow*).

of an underlying renal lesion as a cause for the bleeding.

Another site of anticoagulant-related hematomas in the kidneys is the subepthelial/suburothelial space. Hemorrhage in these layers of the collecting system results in thickening of the renal pelvis and ureters. It may affect one or both kidneys. Symptoms are similar to those of subcapsular hemorrhage—acute flank pain and hematuria. Unenhanced CT images are key to establishing the diagnosis, because the hemorrhage appears hyperdense, outlining the renal pelvis (**Figs. 2**A, B and **3**A).[25] Excretory images demonstrate diffuse thickening of the collecting system (see **Fig. 2**C–E) and occasionally filling defects within the renal pelvis (see **Fig. 3**B), making differentiation from malignancy difficult, especially when unilateral.[25,26] This overlap in imaging findings has resulted in nephrectomy for presumed transitional cell carcinoma in approximately 30 cases.[25,27–29] Unenhanced CT in a patient undergoing evaluation for flank pain and hematuria

should be carefully scrutinized for high density outlining the renal pelvis, the hallmark of anticoagulant-related hemorrhage. If unenhanced CT is unavailable and filling defects are present on the excretory phase scan in patients treated with anticoagulants, follow-up CT after anticoagulant treatment withdrawal should be performed. This usually shows complete resolution within 2 to 4 weeks (see **Fig. 3**C).[20,25] Awareness of this entity and its radiologic appearance is crucial to prevent an unnecessary surgery.

Radiation-associated complications

The kidney is radiosensitive, and the risk of renal impairment increases with prior or concurrent chemotherapy. Clinical radiation damage to the kidney represents an uncommonly described toxicity of radiation that can result in considerable morbidity and/or death. Its incidence is likely under-reported owing to its long latency and because dysfunction is likely often attributed to more common causes.[30]

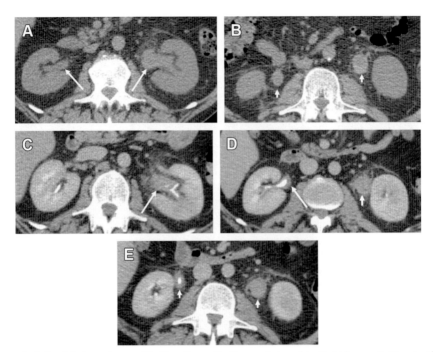

Fig. 2. Suburothelial pelvic hematoma affecting the collecting systems of both kidneys. A 49-year-old man presented with abdominal pain and macrohematuria. He had been treated with Coumadin for massive pulmonary embolism 4 months earlier. International normalized ratio (INR) on admission was 12 (therapeutic range 2.0–3.0). (*A, B*) Unenhanced axial CT images show diffuse thickening of the renal pelves (*A, long arrows*), more conspicuous on the left, and along both ureters (*B, short arrows*). Note faint peripheral high density, typical of hemorrhage, visible only on the unenhanced scan. (*C–E*) Contrast-enhanced CT images, pyelographic phase, show diffuse thickening enveloping (*C*) the left renal pelvis (*long arrow*), (*D*) the right renal pelvis (*long arrow*), and (*D, E*) both ureters (*short arrows*).

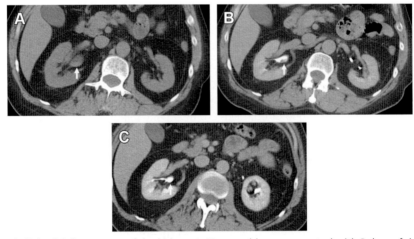

Fig. 3. Suburothelial pelvic hematoma of the kidney. A 40-year-old man presented with 3 days of right flank pain and hematuria. Patient was on Coumadin treatment of atrial fibrillation. International normalized ratio (INR) on admission was 3.6 (therapeutic range 2.0–3.0). (*A*) Unenhanced axial abdominal CT image shows a high-density focus in the dependent portion of the right renal pelvis (*arrow*). (*B*) Contrast-enhanced CT image, pyelographic phase, shows a distinct diffuse within the renal pelvis (*arrow*). Its high density, typical of hemorrhage, can no longer be appreciated due to the excretion of contrast material. This filling defect could easily be misinterpreted as transitional cell carcinoma. (*C*) Follow-up contrast-enhanced CT image, pyelographic phase, 6 weeks later, shows complete resolution of the filling defect in the right renal pelvis (*arrow*).

Radiologic changes appear months to years after treatment. If only a portion of the kidney is irradiated, only that portion is affected and appears on CT as a geographic region of decreased attenuation, which corresponds to the nonfunctioning segment of the kidney (**Fig. 4**).[31,32] This well-defined hypodense area may sometimes mimic a focal renal infarct or pyelonephritis. Ultimately, radiation changes may result in atrophic, poorly functioning but unobstructed kidneys with smooth margins.[31,32]

Complications related to minimally invasive procedure

Extracorporeal shock wave lithotripsy (ESWL) is widely used as a minimally invasive procedure in the treatment of nephrolithiasis.[33] The main aim of ESWL is the pulverization of stones and asymptomatic elimination of fragments. This procedure may not always be completely successful due to incomplete stone fragmentation. If the residual fragments are of a significant size, then ureteral blockage by fragments (*steinstrasse* [stone street]) occurs, resulting in an obstruction to the urinary flow. Obstructing stone fragments can be visualized on radiographs (**Fig. 5**) or unenhanced CT, the latter of which has the advantage of also demonstrating the degree of associated hydroureteronephrosis.[33–35] Renal injuries associated with ESWL include perinephric and subcapsular hematomas (see **Fig. 1**), renal cyst hemorrhage, and intraparenchymal hemorrhage. Although these are reported up to 30% of patients after ESWL, most are clinically insignificant (ie, requiring no intervention).[34,35]

Surgery-related complications

Iatrogenic injuries to the kidney from surgical procedures are rare but carry significant morbidity and mortality.[1] Renal hematoma is a potential complication of almost every renal intervention whereas development of arteriovenous fistula (AVF) and pseudoaneurysm tend to be more specifically associated with nephron-sparing surgery (partial nephrectomy), percutaneous interventions, and transplantation.[1,36] Although rates vary, clinically significant complications of percutaneous renal biopsies are generally less than 10%, most of which are detected in the first 24 hours post-biopsy and spontaneously resolve.[37] Rates of renal hematoma after percutaneous nephrostomy are even lower, under 5%, the majority of which are clinically insignificant.[38] Nonetheless, if there is a concern for a symptomatic (flank pain, hematuria, or decreasing hematocrit) large hematoma, an unenhanced CT shows a lenticular fluid collection in cases of hematomas; however, a quicker assessment with a renal sonogram may also be made, documenting the size of the collection as well as permitting a search for vascular complications, such as an AVF.

Partial nephrectomy (nephron-sparing surgery) has replaced, over the past 2 decades, the conventional radical nephrectomy, and indications for this more conservative approach have gradually broadened.[39,40] This technique allows maximum preservation of functioning nephrons, thereby preserving renal function. Open and laparoscopic techniques are available and although laparoscopic partial nephrectomy is less invasive, there still are associated complications.[41,42] Vascular injuries, pseudoaneurysms and AVF, after robotic or laparoscopic-assisted partial nephrectomies, have been reported to occur, with an incidence ranging from less than 2% to 12%.[43] Depending on the acuity of the situation, investigation of the vascular injury may be performed with either ultrasound (US) or CT. Pseudoaneurysms appear as a hypoechoic structure adjacent to the artery with the classic 'yin-yang sign' on color Doppler evaluation, whereas CT angiography demonstrates a contrast-opacified

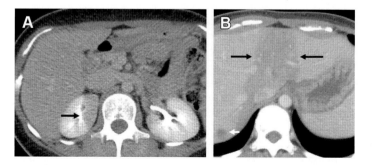

Fig. 4. Radiation injury to the right kidney and liver. A 23-year-old woman with nasopharyngeal carcinoma with sternal metastases that had been treated with radiation to the sternum. (*A*) Contrast-enhanced axial CT image shows a well-defined hypodense area (*arrow*) which enhances to a lesser degree than the normal renal parenchyma is seen in the upper pole of the right kidney. (*B*) Axial CT image at a more cranial level shows well-defined linear margins of a hypodense area of irradiated liver, conforming to radiation portals (*black arrows*). Note small hepatic metastasis (*white arrow*).

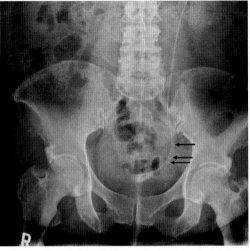

Fig. 5. Ureteral blockage by stone fragments (steinstrasse) detected on a plain abdominal film. Plain abdominal radiograph after ESWL shows multiple stone fragments (*arrows*) along the left distal ureter (steinstrasse) next to a ureteral stent inserted to drain the obstructed collecting system.

outpouching from the parent artery (**Fig. 6**).[44] AVF, however, demonstrates low-resistance, high arterial flow with pulsatile flow in the draining vein on US. Additionally, tissue reverberation artifact may be seen.[45] CT angiography demonstrates early filling of dilated renal vein(s).[46] Treatment options for renal artery pseudoaneurysms and AVFs include coil embolization (see **Fig. 6E**); less often, surgery may be needed, depending on a patient's clinical status.[47,48]

Although pseudoaneurysms and AVFs represent one spectrum of iatrogenic vascular injuries, renal infarcts represent another. Renal infarctions may also occur after various surgical procedures, such as repair of abdominal aortic aneurysm (**Fig. 7**) and retroperitoneal lymph node dissection (**Fig. 8**).[49,50] It may also occur after less invasive procedures, such as endovascular abdominal aortic aneurysm repair (**Fig. 9**). The overall rate of renal infarction after aortic stent placement is approximately 12%, with placement of an infrarenal endovascular stent resulting in iatrogenic renal infarction in 6% to 9% of the cases.[51–53] Transrenal stenting (ie, placement of a noncovered aortic stent graft with proximal portion at the level of the renal arteries) has been used because it has been reported to decrease stent migration and endoleak type I rates. The tradeoff is the potential occlusion of an accessory renal artery, however, leading to renal infarction. Although renal function may not always be compromised by occlusion, a renal

artery larger than 3 mm in diameter and supplying more than 30% of the renal parenchyma should be a contraindication to transrenal stenting.[54]

On contrast-enhanced CT, a renal infarct appears as an area of nonenhancement (see **Figs. 7–9**).[19] A cortical rim sign may or may not be present in which there is persistent enhancement of the renal cortex peripherally in cases of total renal infarction. This is due to the differences in arterial supply to this region of cortex compared with the remainder of the renal parenchyma.[55] Segmental infarcts appear as discrete wedge-shaped areas of nonenhancement compared with the remainder of the normally perfused renal parenchyma. Arterial-phase CT images can demonstrate occluded main or segmental renal arteries but are often not necessary for diagnosis compared with routine portal venous-phase images.[19,40,55,56]

Ureteral Injuries

Most ureteral injuries are iatrogenic. These usually occur during various surgical procedures, including obstetric, gynecologic, colorectal, and urologic surgeries.[1,57] In general, hysterectomies are associated with the highest incidence of ureteral injury, in up to 6% in some reports.[1,58] Most commonly, the lower third of the ureters are more likely to be injured compared with the middle and upper thirds.[59] Injury to the ureter can occur by way of ligation, transection, clamp crush injury, thermal energy injury, or devascularization.[1,60] Approximately 50% of ureteral injuries are recognized and repaired during the primary operation.[61] The remaining injuries may remain undetected for weeks and even months after the surgery.[1,57] Patients present with nonspecific symptoms, including abdominal/flank pain, fever, urinary incontinence, and hematuria. The possibility of ureteral injury is seldom entertained prior to imaging and it is important, therefore, that radiologists be aware of the recent surgery and of the often subtle CT findings of ureteral injuries. The main findings of ureteral injury are either free fluid or a localized fluid collection. Free fluid, representing extravasated urine, may dissect through fascial planes and, therefore, be seen close to or remote from the area of the ureteral injury.[62,63] It may also become loculated and may easily be mistaken for a seroma or lymphocele.[64] Another important indirect finding that should raise suspicion of a possible ureteral injury is ipsilateral hydronephrosis. Dilation of the collecting system often develops rapidly, within days, from ureteral injury (**Figs. 10** and **11**). This is likely due to periureteral fibrosis, which develops adjacent to the injured portion.[65]

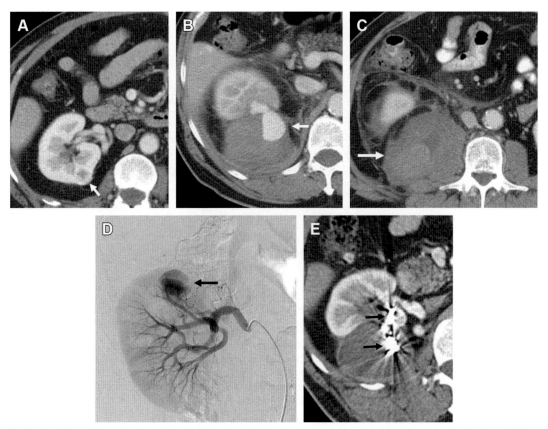

Fig. 6. Renal pseudoaneurysm after nephron-sparing surgery. Patient presented with abdominal pain and fever 15 days after resection of a small incidentally discovered renal cell carcinoma. (*A*) Preoperative contrast-enhanced axial CT image, corticomedullary phase, shows a small exophytic renal cell carcinoma (*arrow*) arising from the midpolar region of the right kidney. (*B*) Postoperative contrast-enhanced axial CT image, nephrographic phase, shows a well-circumscribed bilobed collection of contrast material with a density similar to that of the adjacent blood vessels, representing a pseudoaneurysm (*arrow*). (*C*) A large hematoma extends into the left retroperitoneal space (*arrow*). (*D*) Selective angiogram of the right renal artery shows the pseudoaneurysm (*arrow*), which was successfully coil embolized. (*E*) Follow-up axial CT image obtained several weeks later shows embolization coils with associated beam-hardening artifacts (*arrows*). Note interval decrease in density of the perinephric hematoma.

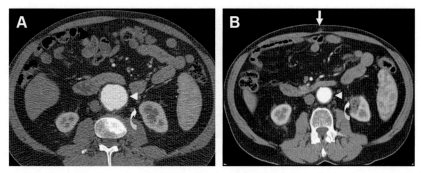

Fig. 7. Segmental renal infarct after open aortic aneurysm repair. (*A*) Preoperative contrast-enhanced axial CT image shows an aneurysm involving the infrarenal abdominal aorta (*arrowhead*). Note intact left kidney (*curved arrow*). (*B*) Postoperative contrast-enhanced axial CT image shows a segmental infarct affecting the lower pole of the left kidney (*curved arrow*). Note interval repair of the aortic aneurysm (*arrowhead*) and a midline scar in the anterior abdominal wall (*arrow*).

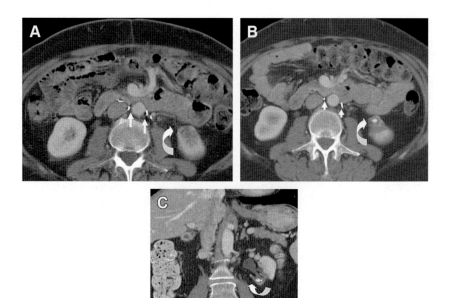

Fig. 8. Segmental renal infarct after retroperitoneal lymph node dissection in a 61-year-old woman with ovarian cancer. (*A*) Contrast-enhanced axial CT image obtained 6 months after surgery shows an ill-defined hypodense area in the lower pole of the left kidney (*curved arrow*), raising concern for a small space-occupying lesion. Arrows point to surgical clips. (*B*) Follow-up contrast-enhanced axial CT image obtained 2 years after surgery shows a small calcification within the infarcted hypodense area (*curved arrow*), with a clearer demarcation between the viable and infarcted parenchyma. (*C*) Coronal follow-up contrast-enhanced CT image obtained 5 years after surgery shows evolution of the infarct with additional tiny calcification within the shrunken infarcted parenchyma of the left lower pole (*curved arrow*).

Enhanced CT during the excretory phase may initially not demonstrate any extravasation of contrast-enhanced urine, mainly because of delayed excretion from the hydronephrotic kidney. In such an instance, it is crucial to obtain an additionally delayed phase scan (sometimes hours after the injection of intravenous contrast material) to opacify the entire collecting system and the entire ureter (see **Figs. 10** and **11**; **Fig. 12**). CT findings of concomitant fluid collection and new-onset hydronephrosis should prompt scans with longer than usual delays (up to several hours) to

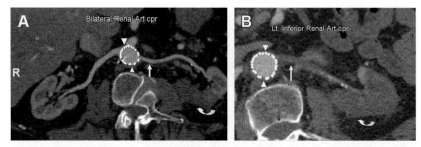

Fig. 9. Segmental renal infarct after endovascular stenting of an abdominal aortic aneurysm. (*A*) Postprocedural curved planar reformat contrast-enhanced CT image, arterial phase, shows patent left superior renal artery (*arrow*). At this level, the proximal stent (*arrowheads*) has anchor pins but is not covered with graft fabric, accounting for the normal flow into both renal arteries. A segmental infarct in the left kidney is seen (*curved arrow*). (*B*) Curved planar reformat CT image at a slightly more caudal level, corresponding to the covered portion of the stent graft (*arrowheads*), shows no contrast material in the occluded left inferior renal artery (*arrow*), and an associated lower pole infarct (*curved arrow*).

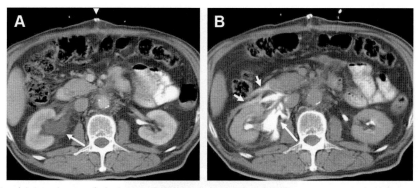

Fig. 10. Ureteral injury incurred during vascular surgery. A 68-year-old man presented with acute abdominal pain, 12 days after aorto-right femoral artery bypass. CT performed to evaluate for acute appendicitis. (*A*) Contrast-enhanced axial CT image, pyelographic phase, shows right hydronephrosis (*arrow*), a new finding compared with preoperative imaging. The left kidney shows normal excretion of contrast material. Surgical clips are still present in the anterior abdominal wall (*arrowhead*) and serve as a clue that the dilated renal pelvis may reflect a complication incurred at surgery. This prompted a repeat scan after an additional 2 hours delay. (*B*) Delayed scan 2 hours later shows extravasation of opacified urine from the right proximal ureter (*long arrow*), confirming injury to the proximal right collecting system. Extravasated opacified urine dissects into fascial plains in the retroperitoneum (*short arrows*).

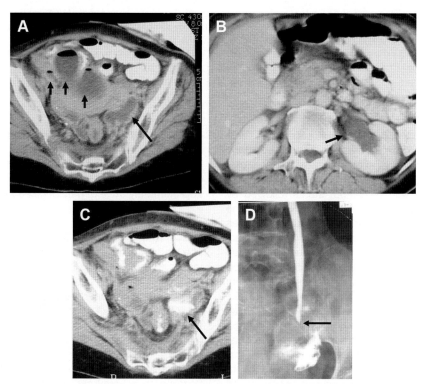

Fig. 11. Ureteral injury incurred during colostomy. A 70-year-old woman with colon cancer presenting with fever and abdominal pain 1 week after laparoscopic colostomy. (*A*) Axial CT image of the pelvis shows several fluid collections in the pelvis, 2 of which are round and contain air-fluid levels (*short arrows*). A collection in the left pelvis contains no air (*long arrow*). (*B*) Note left hydronephrosis. This was not present on the preoperative CT 10 days earlier (*arrow*). (*C*) Delayed scanning at the same level as (*A*): all fluid collections have opacified and all but one (*arrow*) appears to be bowel loops. (*D*) Antegrade pyelography confirms left ureteral injury resulting in a pelvic urinoma (*arrow*).

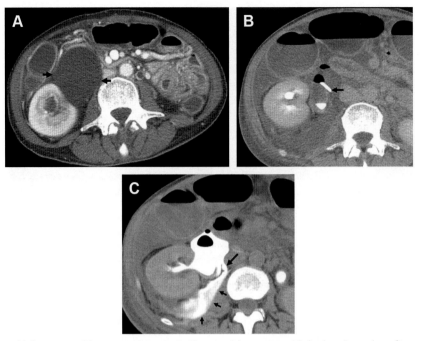

Fig. 12. Ureteral injury caused by ureteral stent. A 42-year-old woman with leukemia and graft-versus-host disease (*A*) Contrast-enhanced axial CT image shows a severely dilated right collecting system (*arrows*) prior to stent insertion. Note absence of fluid in the perinephric space (*B*) Contrast-enhanced axial CT image in the pyelographic phase after ureteral stent insertion reveals interval decompression of the right collecting system by the stent (*arrow*). There is no evidence of extravasation but new infiltration of retroperitoneum is seen. (*C*) Delayed scan after 5 hours shows extravasation of opacified urine from the extrarenal pelvis (*long arrow*) into the retroperitoneum (*short arrows*), indicating perforation of ureter by the stent.

demonstrate opacification of extravasated urine. If there has been only a laceration, and not complete ureteral transection, then the most distal ureter may be seen.[57] Treatment consists initially of nephrostomy with or without stents followed by reconstructive surgery—reanastomosis of the transected ends, ureteroneocystostomy, psoas hitch, or ureterocutaneostomy with ileal loop.[1,66,67] Prophylactic stent placement to ease identification of ureters during the aforementioned at-risk surgeries has resulted in a mixed impact on the rate of injuries.[68–70]

Ureterovaginal fistulas may develop as a result of ureteral injury, mainly after hysterectomy (**Figs. 13** and **14**). This results from urine that has collected in the pelvis dissecting into the vaginal suture line. Patients present with urinary incontinence per the vagina, sometimes accompanied by fever and chills usually within 2 to 4 weeks after surgery. The diagnosis may be established radiographically with various imaging modalities, including vaginography, CT, and MR imaging.[71] CT urography has replaced the traditional excretory urography and may reveal extravasation of contrast material in a collection outside the ureter, eventually draining into the vaginal cavity (see **Fig. 14**). Percutaneous nephrostomy and ureteral stent placement may obviate surgical repair in approximately 50% of patients (see **Fig. 13**).[71]

Bladder Injuries

The bladder is the urologic organ most often subject to iatrogenic injury. Similar to ureteral injuries, iatrogenic bladder injuries may occur during various surgical procedures, most commonly during obstetric/gynecologic interventions followed by abdominal and urologic surgeries.[1,72] Most iatrogenic injuries to the bladder are intraperitoneal.[73] If a bladder injury is detected intraoperatively, surgical repair is usually performed, with postoperative Foley catheter placement for 1 to 2 weeks.[1] For injuries suspected postoperatively, CT cystography should be performed to delineate the site of injury and to classify it as an intraperitoneal or extraperitoneal rupture, the former requiring surgical management (**Fig. 15**).[1,16] When bladder injury is not recognized

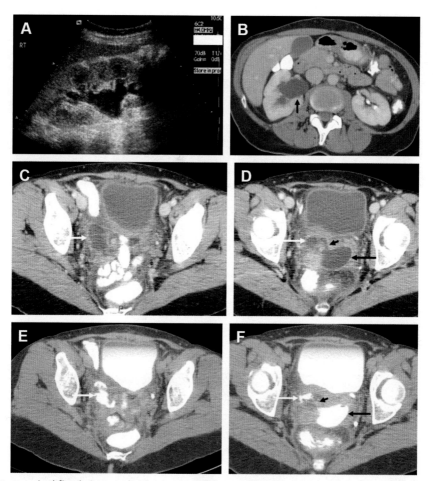

Fig. 13. Ureterovaginal fistula incurred at hysterectomy for a myomatous uterus. A 49-year-old woman with right flank pain and fever 9 days after surgery. (*A*) Longitudinal US image shows a markedly dilated right renal pelvis. (*B*) Contrast-enhanced CT confirms right hydronephrosis (*arrow*), and shows edematous right renal parenchyma. The right ureter was also dilated (not shown). The left kidney already excretes contrast material. (*C*) Contrast-enhanced axial CT image shows a well-defined pelvic fluid collection (*white arrow*) that appears to connect via a fistulous tract (*short black arrow*) with a dilated fluid-filled vagina (*long black arrow*), on a slightly more caudal level (*D*). (*E, F*) Delayed scan after 10 minutes at the same level of (*C*) and (*D*) shows contrast material within the fluid collection (*white arrow*) and within the vagina (*long black arrow*). The fistulous connection between the 2 structures (*F, short black arrow*) is also seen. The standard 5-minute delay scan did not reveal excretion from the right hydronephrotic kidney and, therefore, this scan was performed with a longer delay. (*G, H*) Antegrade pyelography shows a dilated right collecting system, an abrupt termination of a dilated right ureter at the level of the sacrum and extravasation of contrast material (*H, arrow*). (*I, J*) Follow-up antegrade pyelography 8 days later shows decrease in hydroureteronephrosis and contrast material extravasating from the distal right ureter (*J, arrow*). Conservative treatment failed and the patient subsequently underwent reimplantation of the right ureter.

intraoperatively during hysterectomy, a vesicovaginal fistula can develop due to urine leaking and following the path of least resistance and drain through the vaginal cuff suture line.[71] In this setting, several imaging modalities may be useful in establishing the diagnosis of vesicovaginal fistula. Delayed contrast-enhanced CT is a particularly useful tool. Excretion of intravenous contrast material into the vagina strongly suggests the diagnosis (**Fig. 16**).[74] Air or fluid in the vagina may also be present. Sonography and color Doppler US with a microbubble contrast agent and MRI have also shown to be useful in detection of fistulous tracts.[75–77]

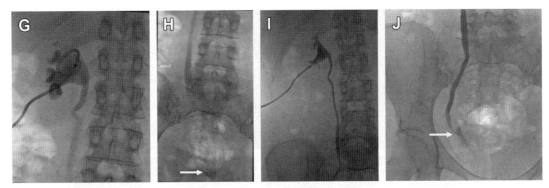

Fig. 13. (*continued*)

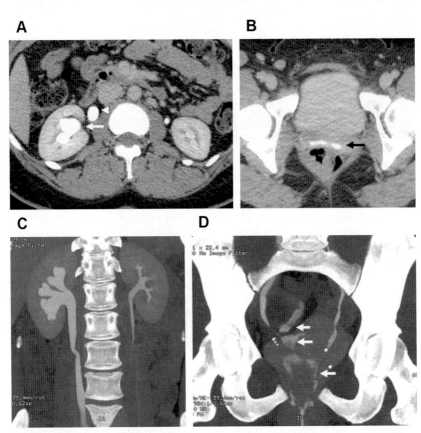

Fig. 14. Ureterovaginal fistula presenting 3 months after surgery. A 35-year-old woman with watery vaginal discharge 3 months after laparoscopic hysterectomy. (*A*) Contrast-enhanced axial CT image, pyelographic phase, shows a dilated right renal pelvis (*arrow*) and proximal right ureter (*arrowhead*). The collecting system was un-remarkable preoperatively. (*B*) Contrast-enhanced axial CT image, pyelographic phase, at the level of the pelvis, shows high-density fluid, which is opacified urine (*arrow*) within the vagina. (*C*) Right hydroureteronephrosis and (*D*) urine leak (*arrows*) into the pelvis are better appreciated on volumetric coronal reconstructions.

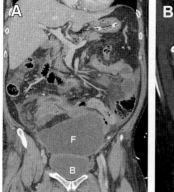
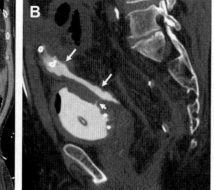

Fig. 15. Inadvertent bladder injury incurred at surgery diagnosed on CT cystography. Patient after low anterior resection of rectum and reoperation for small bowel perforation. (*A*) Coronal CT image shows a very large simple fluid (F) cranial to bladder (B). There are no findings to suggest leakage of urine from the bladder. (*B*) CT cystography, sagittal reformat, shows leak of urine into peritoneal cavity (*long arrows*), confirming bladder injury. Note the small size of the fistula (*short arrow*).

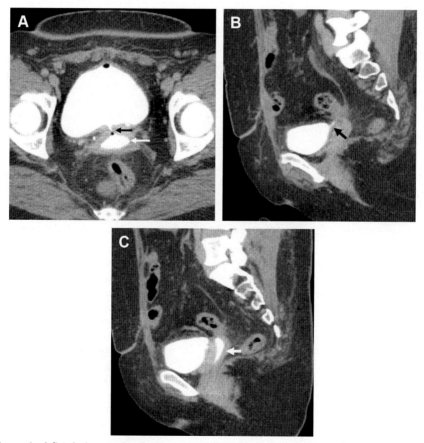

Fig. 16. Vesicovaginal fistula incurred at hysterectomy diagnosed on CT cystography 3 months after surgery. A 43-year-old woman with incontinence without sensation since hysterectomy 3 months earlier. A bladder laceration observed during hysterectomy had been repaired. (*A*) Axial image from CT cystography shows contrast material within the bladder and the vagina (*white arrow*), and a small fistulous tract (*black arrow*) between them. (*B*) Sagittal reformat shows the small size of fistula (*arrow*). (*C*). Sagittal reformat shows high-density fluid filling both the bladder and the vagina (*arrow*). Cystoscopy confirmed an obvious fistula opening posterior to the trigone.

SUMMARY

It is crucial for radiologists to be familiar with the spectrum of iatrogenic injuries to the kidneys, ureters, and bladder. Often, radiologists are relied on to determine which imaging technique to use in evaluating the suspected injury. In many cases, however, the injury may present remote from surgery and not be suspected clinically. A high index of suspicion and awareness of patient medical and surgical history are vital in these instances for radiologists to suggest the correct diagnosis. Accurate diagnosis is crucial because many iatrogenic injuries (eg, vascular and ureteral) require prompt treatment.

REFERENCES

1. Summerton DJ, Kitrey ND, Lumen N, et al. EAU guidelines on iatrogenic trauma. Eur Urol 2012; 62(4):628–39.

2. Lynch TH, Martinez-Pineiro L, Plas E, et al. EAU guidelines on urological trauma. Eur Urol 2005; 47(1):1–15.

3. Park SJ, Kim JK, Kim KW, et al. MDCT findings of renal trauma. Am J Roentgenol 2006;187(2):541–7.

4. Kawashima A, Sandler CM, Corl FM, et al. Imaging of renal trauma: a comprehensive review. Radiographics 2001;21(3):557–74.

5. Santucci RA, Wessells H, Bartsch G, et al. Evaluation and management of renal injuries: consensus statement of the renal trauma subcommittee. BJU Int 2004;93(7):937–54.

6. McAninch JW, Federle MP. Evaluation of renal injuries with computerized tomography. J Urol 1982;128(3):456–60.

7. Alonso RC, Nacenta SB, Martinez PD, et al. Kidney in danger: CT findings of blunt and penetrating renal trauma. Radiographics 2009;29(7): 2033–53.

8. Israel GM, Bosniak MA. How I do it: evaluating renal masses. Radiology 2005;236(2):441–50.

9. Daly KP, Ho CP, Persson DL, et al. Traumatic retroperitoneal injuries: Review of multidetector CT findings. Radiographics 2008;28(6):1571–90.

10. Sheth S, Scatarige JC, Horton KM, et al. Current concepts in the diagnosis and management of renal cell carcinoma: role of multidetector CT and three-dimensional CT. Radiographics 2001; 21(Spec No):S237–54.

11. Kawashima A, Vrtiska TJ, LeRoy AJ, et al. CT urography. Radiographics 2004;24(Suppl 1):S35–54 [discussion: S55–8].

12. Soto JA, Anderson SW. Multidetector CT of blunt abdominal trauma. Radiology 2012;265(3):678–93.

13. Chow LC, Kwan SW, Olcott EW, et al. Split-bolus MDCT urography with synchronous nephrographic and excretory phase enhancement. Am J Roentgenol 2007;189(2):314–22.

14. Kekelidze M, Dwarkasing RS, Dijkshoorn ML, et al. Kidney and urinary tract imaging: triple-bolus multidetector CT urography as a one-stop shop–protocol design, opacification, and image quality analysis. Radiology 2010;255(2):508–16.

15. Chan DP, Abujudeh HH, Cushing GL Jr, et al. CT cystography with multiplanar reformation for suspected bladder rupture: experience in 234 cases. Am J Roentgenol 2006;187(5):1296–302.

16. Vaccaro JP, Brody JM. CT cystography in the evaluation of major bladder trauma. Radiographics 2000;20(5):1373–81.

17. Morgan DE, Nallamala LK, Kenney PJ, et al. CT cystography: radiographic and clinical predictors of bladder rupture. Am J Roentgenol 2000;174(1): 89–95.

18. Goy J, Crowther M. Approaches to diagnosing and managing anticoagulant-related bleeding. Semin Thromb Hemost 2012;38(7):702–10.

19. Kawashima A, Sandler CM, Ernst RD, et al. CT evaluation of renovascular disease. Radiographics 2000;20(5):1321–40.

20. Fishman MC, Pollack HM, Arger PH, et al. Radiographic manifestations of spontaneous renal sinus hemorrhage. Am J Roentgenol 1984;142(6):1161–4.

21. Daskalopoulos G, Karyotis I, Heretis I, et al. Spontaneous perirenal hemorrhage: a 10-year experience at our institution. Int Urol Nephrol 2004; 36(1):15–9.

22. Schaner EG, Balow JE, Doppman JL. Computed tomography in the diagnosis of subcapsular and perirenal hematoma. Am J Roentgenol 1977; 129(1):83–8.

23. Furlan A, Fakhran S, Federle MP. Spontaneous abdominal hemorrhage: causes, CT findings, and clinical implications. Am J Roentgenol 2009; 193(4):1077–87.

24. Belville JS, Morgentaler A, Loughlin KR, et al. Spontaneous perinephric and subcapsular renal hemorrhage: evaluation with CT, US, and angiography. Radiology 1989;172(3):733–8.

25. Gayer G, Desser TS, Hertz M, et al. Spontaneous suburothelial hemorrhage in coagulopathic patients: CT diagnosis. Am J Roentgenol 2011; 197(5):W887–90.

26. Phinney A, Hanson J, Talner LB. Diagnosis of renal pelvis subepithelial hemorrhage using unenhanced helical CT. Am J Roentgenol 2000;174(4):1023–4.

27. Antopol W, Goldman L. Subepithelial hemorrhage of renal pelvis simulating neoplasm. Urol Cutaneous Rev 1948;52(4):189–95.

28. Bhatt S, MacLennan G, Dogra V. Renal pseudotumors. Am J Roentgenol 2007;188(5):1380–7.

29. Eccher A, Brunelli M, Gobbo S, et al. Subepithelial pelvic hematoma (Antopol–Goldman lesion)

simulating renal neoplasm: report of a case and review of the literature. Int J Surg Pathol 2009;17(3): 264–7.

30. Dawson LA, Kavanagh BD, Paulino AC, et al. Radiation-associated kidney injury. Int J Radiat Oncol Biol Phys 2010;76(Suppl 3):S108–15.

31. Bluemke DA, Fishman EK, Kuhlman JE, et al. Complications of radiation therapy: CT evaluation. Radiographics 1991;11(4):581–600.

32. Kwek JW, Iyer RB, Dunnington J, et al. Spectrum of imaging findings in the abdomen after radiotherapy. Am J Roentgenol 2006;187(5):1204–11.

33. D'Addessi A, Vittori M, Racioppi M, et al. Complications of extracorporeal shock wave lithotripsy for urinary stones: to know and to manage them-a review. ScientificWorldJournal 2012;2012:619820.

34. Krysiewicz S. Complications of renal extracorporeal shock wave lithotripsy reviewed. Urol Radiol 1992;13(3):139–45.

35. Gayer G, Hertz M, Stav K, et al. Minimally invasive management of urolithiasis. Semin Ultrasound CT MR 2006;27(2):139–51.

36. Cohenpour M, Strauss S, Gottlieb P, et al. Pseudoaneurysm of the renal artery following partial nephrectomy: imaging findings and coil embolization. Clin Radiol 2007;62(11):1104–9.

37. Whittier WL, Korbet SM. Timing of complications in percutaneous renal biopsy. J Am Soc Nephrol 2004;15(1):142–7.

38. Patel U, Hussain FF. Percutaneous nephrostomy of nondilated renal collecting systems with fluoroscopic guidance: technique and results. Radiology 2004;233(1):226–33.

39. Matin SF, Gill IS, Worley S, et al. Outcome of laparoscopic radical and open partial nephrectomy for the sporadic 4 cm. or less renal tumor with a normal contralateral kidney. J Urol 2002;168(4 Pt 1):1356–9 [discussion: 1359–60].

40. Rogers CG. Expanding the indications of partial nephrectomy. Eur Urol 2011;59(6):938–9.

41. Lane BR, Novick AC, Babineau D, et al. Comparison of laparoscopic and open partial nephrectomy for tumor in a solitary kidney. J Urol 2008;179(3): 847–51 [discussion: 852].

42. Novick AC. Laparoscopic and partial nephrectomy. Clin Cancer Res 2004;10(18 Pt 2):6322S–7S.

43. Hyams ES, Pierorazio P, Proteek O, et al. Iatrogenic vascular lesions after minimally invasive partial nephrectomy: a multi-institutional study of clinical and renal functional outcomes. Urology 2011;78(4): 820–6.

44. Saad NE, Saad WE, Davies MG, et al. Pseudoaneurysms and the role of minimally invasive techniques in their management. Radiographics 2005; 25(Suppl 1):S173–89.

45. Middleton WD, Kellman GM, Melson GL, et al. Postbiopsy renal transplant arteriovenous fistulas: color Doppler US characteristics. Radiology 1989; 171(1):253–7.

46. Rha SE, Byun JY, Jung SE, et al. The renal sinus: pathologic spectrum and multimodality imaging approach. Radiographics 2004;24(Suppl 1): S117–31.

47. Yang HK, Koh ES, Shin SJ, et al. Incidental renal artery pseudoaneurysm after percutaneous native renal biopsy. BMJ Case Rep 2013; February 25, 2013. http://dx.doi.org/10.1136/bcr-2012-006537.

48. Loffroy R, Guiu B, Lambert A, et al. Management of post-biopsy renal allograft arteriovenous fistulas with selective arterial embolization: immediate and long-term outcomes. Clin Radiol 2008;63(6): 657–65.

49. Zissin R, Hertz M, Apter S, et al. Focal renal infarction after retroperitoneal lymph-node dissection: CT diagnosis. Am J Roentgenol 1989;153(2): 325–6.

50. Pearce JD, Edwards MS, Stafford JM, et al. Open repair of aortic aneurysms involving the renal vessels. Ann Vasc Surg 2007;21(6):676–86.

51. Bockler D, Krauss M, Mansmann U, et al. Incidence of renal infarctions after endovascular AAA repair: relationship to infrarenal versus suprarenal fixation. J Endovasc Ther 2003;10(6):1054–60.

52. Kramer SC, Seifarth H, Pamler R, et al. Renal infarction following endovascular aortic aneurysm repair: incidence and clinical consequences. J Endovasc Ther 2002;9(1):98–102.

53. Walsh SR, Tang TY, Boyle JR. Renal consequences of endovascular abdominal aortic aneurysm repair. J Endovasc Ther 2008;15(1):73–82.

54. Sun Z, Stevenson G. Transrenal fixation of aortic stent-grafts: short- to midterm effects on renal function-a systematic review. Radiology 2006;240(1): 65–72.

55. Frank PH, Nuttall J, Brander WL, et al. The cortical rim sign of renal infarction. Br J Radiol 1974; 47(564):875–8.

56. Glazer GM, Francis IR, Brady TM, et al. Computed tomography of renal infarction: clinical and experimental observations. Am J Roentgenol 1983; 140(4):721–7.

57. Ramchandani P, Buckler PM. Imaging of genitourinary trauma. Am J Roentgenol 2009;192(6): 1514–23.

58. Hwang JH, Lim MC, Joung JY, et al. Urologic complications of laparoscopic radical hysterectomy and lymphadenectomy. Int Urogynecol J 2012; 23(11):1605–11.

59. Selzman AA, Spirnak JP. Iatrogenic ureteral injuries: a 20-year experience in treating 165 injuries. J Urol 1996;155(3):878–81.

60. Delacroix SE Jr, Winters JC. Urinary tract injures: recognition and management. Clin Colon Rectal Surg 2010;23(2):104–12.

61. Liapis A, Bakas P, Sykiotis K, et al. Urinomas as a complication of iatrogenic ureteric injuries in gynecological surgery. Eur J Obstet Gynecol Reprod Biol 2000;91(1):83–5.

62. Gayer G, Zissin R, Apter S, et al. Urinomas caused by ureteral injuries: CT appearance. Abdom Imaging 2002;27(1):88–92.

63. Gayer G, Caspi I, Garniek A, et al. Perirectal urinoma from ureteral injury incurred during spinal surgery mimicking rectal perforation on computed tomography scan. Spine 2002;27(20):E451–3.

64. Gayer G, Halperin R, Vasserman M, et al. Bilateral pelvic urinomas following ureteral injury from surgery: lymphocele look-alikes on computed tomography. Emerg Radiol 2005;11(3):167–9.

65. Gayer G, Hertz M, Zissin R. Ureteral injuries: CT diagnosis. Semin Ultrasound CT MR 2004;25(3):277–85.

66. Berkmen F, Peker AE, Alagol H, et al. Treatment of iatrogenic ureteral injuries during various operations for malignant conditions. J Exp Clin Cancer Res 2000;19(4):441–5.

67. Paick JS, Hong SK, Park MS, et al. Management of postoperatively detected iatrogenic lower ureteral injury: should ureteroureterostomy really be abandoned? Urology 2006;67(2):237–41.

68. Al-Awadi K, Kehinde EO, Al-Hunayan A, et al. Iatrogenic ureteric injuries: incidence, aetiological factors and the effect of early management on subsequent outcome. Int Urol Nephrol 2005;37(2):235–41.

69. Kuno K, Menzin A, Kauder HH, et al. Prophylactic ureteral catheterization in gynecologic surgery. Urology 1998;52(6):1004–8.

70. Bothwell WN, Bleicher RJ, Dent TL. Prophylactic ureteral catheterization in colon surgery. A five-year review. Dis Colon Rectum 1994;37(4):330–4.

71. Yu NC, Raman SS, Patel M, et al. Fistulas of the genitourinary tract: a radiologic review. Radiographics 2004;24(5):1331–52.

72. Armenakas NA, Pareek G, Fracchia JA. Iatrogenic bladder perforations: longterm followup of 65 patients. J Am Coll Surg 2004;198(1):78–82.

73. Titton RL, Gervais DA, Hahn PF, et al. Urine leaks and urinomas: diagnosis and imaging-guided intervention. Radiographics 2003;23(5):1133–47.

74. Kuhlman JE, Fishman EK. CT evaluation of entero-vaginal and vesicovaginal fistulas. J Comput Assist Tomogr 1990;14(3):390–4.

75. Yang JM, Su TH, Wang KG. Transvaginal sonographic findings in vesicovaginal fistula. J Clin Ultrasound 1994;22(3):201–3.

76. Volkmer BG, Kuefer R, Nesslauer T, et al. Colour doppler ultrasound in vesicovaginal fistulas. Ultrasound Med Biol 2000;26(5):771–5.

77. Semelka RC, Hricak H, Kim B, et al. Pelvic fistulas: appearances on MR images. Abdom Imaging 1997;22(1):91–5.

Imaging Evaluation of Maternal Complications Associated with Repeat Cesarean Deliveries

Mariam Moshiri, MD[a,*], Sherif Osman, MD[a],
Puneet Bhargava, MD[a,b], Suresh Maximin, MD[a,b],
Tracy J. Robinson, MD[c], Douglas S. Katz, MD[d]

KEYWORDS

- Cesarean delivery • Cesarean complications • Repeat cesarean • Uterine rupture • Scar pregnancy
- Uterine dehiscence • Scar niche

KEY POINTS

- The rate of cesarean deliveries continues to rise, while the rate of vaginal delivery after cesarean birth continues to decline.
- Many women now tend to undergo multiple CDs, and therefore the associated chronic maternal morbidities are of growing concern.
- Accurate diagnosis of these conditions is crucial for maternal and fetal well-being.
- Many of these complications are diagnosed by imaging, and radiologists should be aware of the type and imaging appearances of these conditions.

INTRODUCTION

The rate of cesarean deliveries (CDs) in the United States has been steadily increasing. According to National Vital Statistics Data, cesarean rates increased by 60% from 1996 to 2009, and have been steadily holding at approximately 32% of all deliveries since 2010. In 2012, approximately 1.3 million births were via CD.[1]

The increased CD rate is thought to be a result of several factors, including the relatively safety of the procedure, reduced rate of breech vaginal deliveries, increased maternal obesity, increased maternal age, unwillingness of obstetricians and women to attempt vaginal labor trials after CDs, increased rates of labor induction, and medical-legal issues.[2] More than 90% of women with a prior cesarean choose to have a repeat CD. After 2 cesareans, most women are only offered a repeat CD.[3]

Most women with a history of a previous CD are counseled for complications associated with vaginal delivery, particularly risk of uterine rupture. Multiple repeat CDs also are associated with several short-term and long-term maternal and perinatal morbidities (Table 1), which are less often discussed with the patient at the time

[a] Department of Radiology, University of Washington School of Medicine, 1959 Northeast Pacific Street, Seattle, WA 98195, USA; [b] Department of Radiology, VA Puget Sound Health Care System, 1660 South Columbian Way, Seattle, WA 98108, USA; [c] Seattle Radiologists P.S., Nordstrom Tower, 1229 Madison Street, Suite 900, Seattle, WA 98104, USA; [d] Department of Radiology, Winthrop-University Hospital, 259 First Street, Mineola, NY 11501, USA
* Corresponding author. Department of Radiology, University of Washington School of Medicine, Box 357115, 1959 Northeast Pacific Street, Seattle, WA 98195.
E-mail address: Moshiri@uw.edu

Radiol Clin N Am 52 (2014) 1117–1135
http://dx.doi.org/10.1016/j.rcl.2014.05.010

Table 1
Increased maternal and fetal complications associated with repeated cesarean deliveries

Acute Maternal Complications	Chronic Maternal Complications	Fetal Complications
Placentation abnormalities	Chronic pelvic pain	Placentation abnormalities
Uterine rupture or dehiscence	Chronic incision site pain	Still birth
Uterine atony	Cesarean scar dehiscence	Preterm birth
Excessive bleeding	Dysmenorrhea	Intrauterine growth restriction
Bladder/bowel/urethral injury	Abnormal vaginal bleeding	Small for gestation fetus
Postoperative ileus/bowel obstruction	Pelvic adhesions/scar niche	Increased need for neonatal resuscitation
Postoperative infections	Endometriosis	
Increased intensive care unit/ hospital stay	Uterine synechiae	
	Ectopic pregnancy	
	Reduced future fertility	

of delivery planning.[4] Silver and colleagues,[5] in their review of a 30,132-patient cohort with CDs, found no absolute threshold number of CD after which future pregnancies should be avoided. However, they noted a significantly increased rate of several serious postsurgical morbidities, including the need for the need for cystotomy, hysterectomy, and intensive care unit admissions.

In this article, we review the utility of ultrasound, computed tomography (CT), and magnetic resonance imaging (MRI) in imaging of various complications associated with multiple CDs, and will briefly touch on treatment options.

IMAGING TECHNIQUES

Imaging can assist in diagnosis of both acute and chronic complications of CD. The choice of imaging modality usually depends on the type and acuity of symptoms, severity of symptoms, and the anatomic site of interest. Symptoms, including heavy bleeding, fever, and other clinical signs of postoperative infection, prompt an investigation via imaging. Ultrasound is usually the first imaging modality of choice; however, CT is used relatively liberally after ultrasound for evaluation of common and/or serious postoperative complications. MRI may be used as a problem-solving tool.

POST-CESAREAN COMPLICATIONS
Uterine Dehiscence and Rupture

Uterine dehiscence refers to disruption of the myometrium at the hysterotomy site with an intact

serosal layer. Disruption or tear in the myometrium, which extends through the serosa, is defined as uterine rupture.[6] The reported incidence of a myometrial cesarean scar defect is between 1.9% and 3.8%.[7]

Women with more than one previous CD, and those attempting vaginal birth after CD, are at increased risk of uterine dehiscence and rupture. The risk of rupture is lower with a Pfannenstiel incision, at 0.2% to 1.5%. With vertical or T-shaped incisions, the risk rises to approximately 4% to 9%.[8]

Several investigators have attempted to evaluate the integrity and thickness of the cesarean scar and the lower uterine segment by 2-dimensional and 3-dimensional (3D) ultrasound, so as to predict possible obstetric complications of future pregnancies.[9] No conclusive data are yet available to our knowledge; however, Vikhareva Osser and Valentin,[10] in a recent study, suggested an association between large defects in the cesarean scar after CD detected on transvaginal ultrasound in nonpregnant women, and uterine dehiscence or rupture in subsequent pregnancy. Gizzo and colleagues[11] suggest a significant difference in the lower uterine segment size and myometrial thickness between women with multiple CDs and those without. Some investigators suggest a critical cutoff thickness of 2.5 mm or thicker for the lower uterine segment, for those women choosing to attempt a vaginal delivery after CD.[12]

In most nonpregnant women, cesarean scar dehiscence is asymptomatic, but may occasionally cause symptoms such as dysmenorrhea,

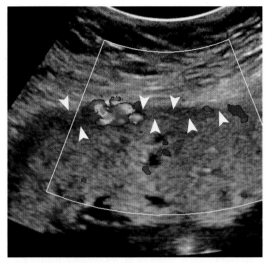

Fig. 1. Uterine dehiscence. A woman with a history of 4 CDs presents with abdominal pain at 30 weeks' gestation. Transverse color Doppler image of the lower uterine segment shows gradual thinning and subsequent disruption of the hypoechoic myometrium (*arrowheads*).

chronic pelvic pain, dyspareunia, and intermenstrual spotting.[7]

Overall, the diagnosis of uterine dehiscence and rupture is difficult to establish by imaging alone, and requires close correlation with clinical presentation. Clinically, intrapartum uterine dehiscence and rupture are diagnosed by observation of fetal heart decelerations, maternal bleeding, intrapartum fever, and severe abdominal pain.[13,14] Ultrasound can reveal intra-amniotic hemorrhage, extrauterine hematoma, extrauterine fetal parts, and bulging of membranes at the site of dehiscence. In the postpartum period, ultrasound findings are nonspecific and may depict intrauterine or pelvic hematoma. However, myometrial and serosal disruptions are not readily detectable (**Fig. 1**).[15]

On CT, there is an overlap of findings with the expected post-cesarean characteristics. Uterine dehiscence may present with nonspecific imaging features, including free pelvic fluid or gas, pleural effusion, bowel dilation, or abscess. Discontinuity of the myometrium seen on CT is also a normal finding in the immediate post-cesarean period. Low attenuation within the incision could be due to edema rather than disruption of the myometrium. A bladder flap hematoma larger than 5 cm, a large pelvic hematoma, and extension of gas or a fluid collection from the endometrium into the peritoneum should be highly suspicious for uterine dehiscence in the proper clinical setting (**Fig. 2**).[16]

Multiplanar MRI, including imaging perpendicular to the cesarean scar, is the best imaging modality for the assessment of uterine dehiscence and rupture. Because of its superior soft-tissue differentiation, myometrial and serosal disruption is readily visible (**Fig. 3**).[17]

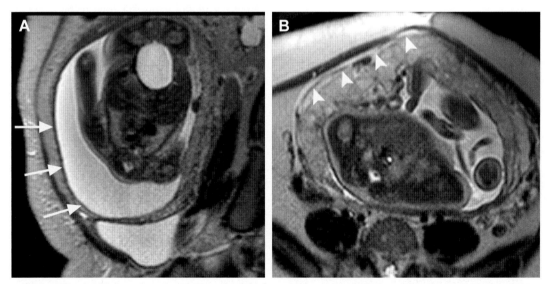

Fig. 2. Uterine dehiscence. A woman with a history of 2 CDs presents with lower abdominal pain in the mid second trimester. (*A*) Sagittal and (*B*) axial T2-weighted MR images show gradual thinning and subsequent interruption of the low signal intensity myometrium (*arrows* in *A*, *arrowheads* in *B*).

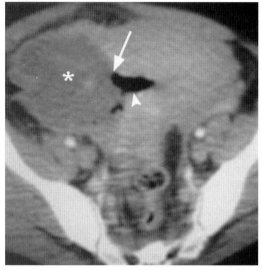

Fig. 3. Uterine rupture. A woman presents with progressively worsening fever and pelvic pain 13 days after CD. Axial contrast-enhanced CT image of the pelvis shows a relatively large amount of gas in the uterine cavity (*arrowhead*) and the site of uterine rupture (*arrow*), with an adjacent fluid pocket (*asterisk*) communicating with the uterine cavity. The findings were proven at subsequent surgical repair.

A vaginal or laparoscopic approach can be used to repair a suspected cesarean scar dehiscence in a symptomatic nonpregnant patient. During pregnancy, uterine dehiscence can be managed expectantly; however, uterine rupture requires immediate surgical intervention.[12]

Scar Pregnancy

Implantation of a gestational sac within the myometrial cesarean scar occurs in approximately 0.15% of those with history of a previous CD. Scar pregnancy had been considered a rare form of ectopic pregnancy; however, the more accurate term may be cesarean scar pregnancy (CSP).[18] Its occurrence rate has risen in the past years secondary to a growing rate of CDs.[19] Scar pregnancy is a potentially life-threatening condition, and can lead to complications, including placental implantation abnormalities, uterine arteriovenous malformation, uterine rupture, and massive maternal hemorrhage. Presenting symptoms usually include vaginal bleeding in the first trimester of pregnancy with some degree of abdominal pain. Severe abdominal pain and heavy vaginal bleeding can herald impending uterine rupture.[20,21] Early diagnosis enables clinicians to use conservative treatment methods, allowing for preservation of

the uterus and future fertility, as well as reducing the risk of maternal morbidity and mortality.[22]

The mechanism of development of CSP is not well understood. Researchers hypothesize a communication tract between the myometrium and the cesarean scar. These tracts are thought to have formed due to damage of the decidua basalis during uterine surgery. Others suggest implantation of the gestational sac in a small dehiscence of a cesarean scar.[23] It is unclear if the risk of developing CSP increases with the number of previous CDs, the elapsed time between the current pregnancy and the prior CD, the size of the scar, or presence of a large scar niche.[16,22] Osborn and colleagues[18] report that 72% of CSPs occur in women with a history of 2 or more CDs. These researchers hypothesize that incomplete healing or increased fibrosis of the scar can be the cause of scar pregnancies. They believe that scar fibrosis after multiple CDs can lead to poor vascularity and impaired healing. This can result in small areas of dehiscence. Also, increased scar surface can act as an additional implantation site.

Ultrasound is the imaging modality of choice for initial diagnosis of CSP, with a reported sensitivity of 86% when using transvaginal techniques.[22] A combined transabdominal and transvaginal imaging approach should be used to reduce the risk of false-positive diagnoses. Through a full bladder on transabdominal imaging, a generalized view of the uterus, particularly the lower uterine segment, the bladder, and the adnexa, is obtained. Transvaginal ultrasound is then performed to evaluate the uterus, the lower uterine segment and its interface with the bladder, and the adnexa.[16]

The sonographic criteria for the diagnosis of CSP include the following: an empty endocervical and endometrial cavity, the presence of a gestational sac in the anterior lower uterine segment at the site of the cesarean scar, and thinning of the overlying myometrium between the gestational sac and the bladder. The myometrium will measure less than 5 mm in most cases, and as little as 2 mm in the rest.[18] A sagittal view reveals discontinuity of the anterior uterine wall, with bulging of the gestational sac through the gap. The adnexa should be carefully evaluated to ensure absence of an adnexal ectopic pregnancy. Doppler ultrasound also is a useful tool, and will demonstrate distinct peritrophoblastic vascularity surrounding the gestational sac. Pulsed Doppler ultrasound is helpful in the diagnosis of low-impedance, high-velocity arterial flow in the periphery of the gestational sac (**Fig. 4**).[22]

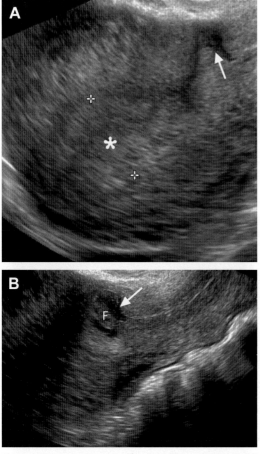

Fig. 4. Cesarean scar pregnancy with outward growth of the gestational sac. A woman presents with vaginal spotting at 7 weeks' gestation. (*A*) Long-axis transvaginal ultrasound image of the pelvis shows an empty uterine cavity containing some debris (between the first small caliper and the large *asterisk*), and fluid in the CD scar (*arrow*). (*B*) Further ultrasound imaging of the CD scar shows a gestational sac within the scar (*arrow*) containing a live fetus (F). This pregnancy was terminated by ultrasound-guided potassium chloride injection into the fetal pole.

Vial and colleagues[24] suggest 2 different types of CSPs. The first type is implanted on the scar and grows into the cervicoisthmic space and the uterine cavity, whereas the second type involves deep implantation into the scar with outward growth of the gestational sac. Therefore, there is a wide range of presentations of CSP with complete invagination of the sac into the scar to complete extension outside the scar. Pascual and colleagues[25] suggest that 3D gray-scale and power Doppler ultrasound is helpful for identifying subtle in diagnoses of subtle abnormalities of the uterine contour, as well as abnormal vascularity associated with the gestational sac (**Fig. 5**).

MRI is a useful tool for assessment of CSP, and is reserved as an adjunct to equivocal or complicated ultrasound examinations. Sagittal and axial T1-weighted and T2-weighted images can depict the gestational sac in the lower anterior myometrial scar.[18,22]

The main objectives in the management of CSP are prevention of related maternal complications and preservation of future fertility. Currently to our knowledge no standardized guidelines are available for the management of CSP. A few rare cases of successful pregnancies with expectant management have been reported in the literature.[26,27] Sinha and Mishra[28] reported a significant adverse outcome in cases of expectant management of cesarean scar pregnancies. The pregnancies in these few reported cases evolved into placenta accreta/increta, which led to uterine rupture, hysterectomy, and severe maternal morbidity.

Currently, the general recommendation in the literature for the management of CSP is early intervention by termination of pregnancy. Medical treatment of an unruptured CSP should be attempted in women who are hemodynamically stable.[29] Local injection of methotrexate into the gestational sac using transvaginal ultrasound guidance has shown a high success rate in the literature.[23] Some researchers report success with injection of potassium chloride into the gestational sac via a transvaginal approach.[30] Systemic methotrexate has a short half-life and possible decreased absorption into the CSP, as it is surrounded by fibrous scar tissue rather than normally vascularized myometrium. Therefore, some researchers consider this treatment method less favorable. Others argue that systemic methotrexate provides a noninvasive approach with an overall complication rate of 36%, and therefore should be considered a viable treatment for appropriately selected women.[31]

Other therapeutic methods described in the literature include a combination of medical treatments using different pharmacologic compounds, and a combination of medical and surgical treatments.[23] Uterine artery embolization with or without local methotrexate, and ultrasound-guided transvaginal saline infusion and aspiration of the gestational sac, also are described by researchers with some reported success.[30,32] Surgical therapeutic approaches include hysteroscopic evacuation of CSP with laparoscopic assistance, laparotomy and removal of the gestational sac with repair of the cesarean scar, suction curettage, and transvaginal resection of the gestational sac.[23,33–35]

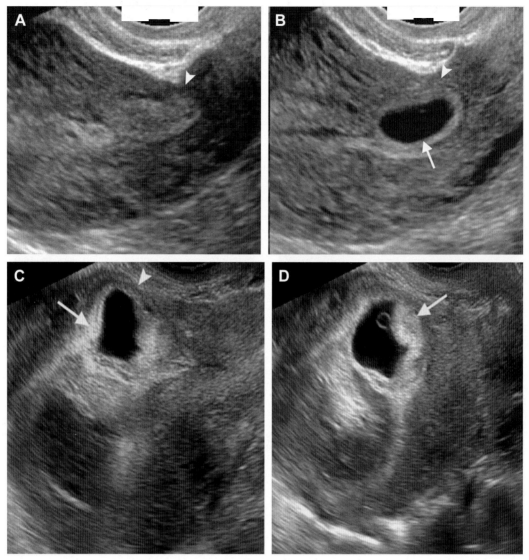

Fig. 5. Cesarean scar pregnancy with growth of the gestational sac into the cervicoisthmic space. A woman presents with vaginal spotting and lower pelvic pain at 6 weeks' gestation. (*A*) Long-axis gray-scale transvaginal ultrasound image of the lower uterine segment shows the decidual reaction from an implanted sac at the CD scar (*arrowhead*). (*B*) Long-axis gray-scale transvaginal ultrasound image obtained slightly lower shows the thin layer of myometrium (*arrowhead*) covering the gestational sac (*arrow*). (*C*) Transverse gray-scale ultrasound image at the same level shows the implanted gestational sac (*arrow*) at the CD scar (*arrowhead*). (*D*) Transverse gray-scale ultrasound image shows the thin layer of myometrium, which measured 3 mm (not shown). Note the formed placenta and yolk sac (*arrow*); however, a fetal pole was not yet seen. This pregnancy was highly desired, and the parents decided to carry it to term despite the significant risk of maternal morbidity. At 28 weeks' gestation, an MRI was performed, which showed uterine dehiscence and placenta percreta (not shown). Shortly after the MRI, the mother presented with premature rupture of membranes and severe fetal intrauterine growth restriction. The fetus was delivered at 29 weeks' gestation via a vertical hysterotomy. The mother lost 6 L of blood during fetal delivery, immediately after which uterine artery embolization and hysterectomy was performed. The mother received 4 units of blood transfusion, and both the mother and the fetus survived.

Dilatation and curettage is considered a less favorable treatment option, because it can increase the risk of bleeding, uterine rupture, or bladder damage.[16]

Pelvic Adhesions

Adhesions are fibrous bands that form between organs and/or the abdominal wall due to surgical tissue disruption and inflammation. General risk factors for adhesion formation include tissue ischemia/hypoxia, excessive organ manipulation, intraperitoneal hemorrhage, lysis of previous adhesions, and infection.[36]

CD is associated with an increased risk of adhesion development between the uterus and the surrounding tissues and organs. The reported incidence of adhesion formation after CD is 46% to 65%. This incidence and severity of adhesions increases with repeated CDs.[37] Nisenblat and colleagues[6] described dense adhesions as those resulting in fusion of the uterus to the anterior abdominal wall or the bladder. These investigators

reported a 0.2% incidence of dense adhesions in women with 1 CD versus a 51% incidence in women who have had 6 or more CDs.

Meticulous surgical technique with appropriate hemostasis, tissue manipulation, and minimization of tissue ischemia are important factors in prevention of adhesions.[38] Closure of the peritoneum after CD has been the subject of some debate in the literature. In a meta-analysis, Cheong and colleagues[39] reported an increased association of adhesion formation and nonclosure of the peritoneum after CD. Malvasi and colleagues[40] reported an increased risk of adhesions with closure of peritoneum after CD. Lyell,[37] on

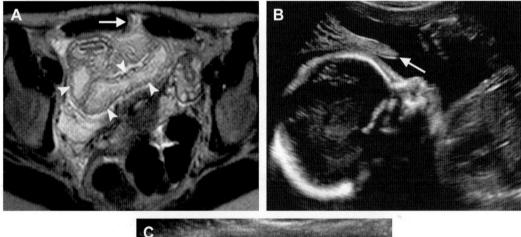

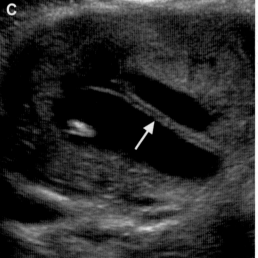

Fig. 6. Adhesions. (*A*) Intestinal obstruction due to adhesions. A woman with a history of 2 CDs presented with abdominal pain and vomiting. Axial T2-weighted MR enterography image with neutral enteric contrast shows mildly dilated bowel loops (*arrowheads*) tethered at the incision site of the anterior abdominal wall (*arrow*). Surgical evaluation revealed thick adhesions in the pelvis. (*B, C*) Thick uterine synechiae. Transverse gray-scale ultrasound images of a woman at 20 weeks' gestation with a history of multiple CDs were performed for fetal anatomic survey of the current pregnancy. Note the thick adhesions (*arrows*) in the uterine cavity. Fetal extremities floated between the adhesions without any fetal structural abnormalities (not shown).

the other hand, in a review of 173 women who had undergone CD, reported fewer dense adhesions in those with peritoneal closure after CD. Contrary to both groups, Kapustian and colleagues,[41] in a review of 533 women with closure and nonclosure of the peritoneum after CD, did not show a significant difference in adhesion rates between the 2 groups.

Adhesions in the pelvis are associated with several complications. These include bowel obstruction, decreased fertility, chronic pelvic pain, increased risk of bladder injury, and increased risk of perioperative bleeding (**Fig. 6**).[37,42,43] Tulandi and colleagues,[44] in a review of 1283 women who had undergone CD, found a statistically significant increase in the infant delivery time after each subsequent CD.

Scar Niche

A niche is a triangular or semicircular area at the site of the cesarean scar, which can act as a reservoir for fluid or blood.[22] In the literature it is also referred to by such terms as deficient cesarean scar, pouch, isthmocele, diverticulum, and cesarean scar defect. The niche prevalence ranges from a 24% to 70% detection rate by transvaginal ultrasound, and a 56% to 84% detection rate by sonohysterography. Risk factors include multiple CDs, trial of labor and vaginal delivery before CD, single-layer myometrial closure after CD, and retroflexion of the uterus.[45]

Abnormal uterine bleeding (postmenstrual bleeding, prolonged menstruation) is the most common symptom associated with scar niche. The underlying cause is likely poor myometrial contractility adjacent to the scar, or fibrotic changes at the site of the scar, which alter drainage of blood and fluid from the uterine cavity during menstruation.[46] The accumulated blood within the niche may act as a source of postmenstrual spotting. Additionally, the endometrium at the superior edge of the niche may act as a source of bleeding.[16] Bij de Vaate and colleagues[46] reported a prevalence of postmenstrual bleeding of 15% in women who did not have a niche versus 34% in those who had a detectible niche on a transvaginal ultrasound examination. Van der Voet and colleagues[47] also found an increased prevalence of niche in the cesarean scar in women who had less than 50% residual myometrium adjacent to the scar.

Various methods of niche detection are described in the literature. These include transvaginal ultrasound, sonohysterography, hysteroscopy, and hysterosalpingography.[45] On sonohysterography, the niche appears as a triangular or semicircular anechoic region within the cesarean scar, of variable size (**Fig. 7**).[48]

Several treatment methods for scar niche have been reported in the literature. These include administration of oral contraceptives, laparoscopic repair, laparoscopic-assisted vaginal repair, and hysteroscopic resection.[49]

Abdominal Wall Endometriosis

Endometriosis, defined as implantation of endometrial tissue outside the uterine cavity, is an uncommon but well-known complication of uterine procedures, including episiotomy, amniocentesis, and laparoscopic surgery. CD and hysterotomy are the most common surgeries associated with abdominal wall endometriosis (AWE). The cesarean scar is the most common site of AWE, with a reported incidence of approximately 0.03% to 0.4%.[50] The interval time between diagnosis of endometriosis and CD ranges from several months to years. Reports in the literature suggest an increased risk of CD-associated endometriosis, when the procedure is performed before the onset of spontaneous labor.[51]

The pathogenesis is believed to be due to implantation of endometrial tissue within the surgical incision. These cells incite a local inflammatory response and respond to hormonal stimulation. Symptoms are usually characterized by a palpable painful mass in the region of cesarean scar and cyclical pain associated with menses.[52] Endometriosis implants can be confined to the superficial layers of the anterior body wall, or may extend into deeper layers and

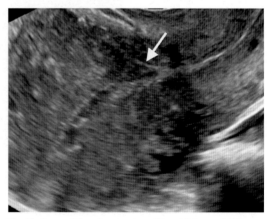

Fig. 7. Scar niche. A woman with a history of CD presented with lower abdominal pain and menorrhagia. Long-axis gray-scale ultrasound image of the uterus shows a niche at the level of the cesarean scar (*arrow*). No other pelvic abnormality was noted on the ultrasound examination.

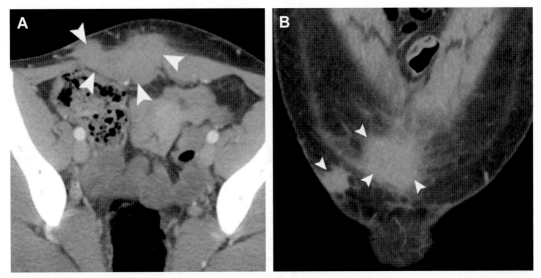

Fig. 8. Abdominal wall endometriosis. A woman with prior CDs presented with lower abdominal pain and a palpable mass on physical examination. (*A*) Axial and (*B*) coronal intravenous contrast-enhanced CT images of the pelvis show focal soft-tissue thickening (*arrowheads*) involving the subcutaneous fat and the right rectus muscle at the level of the CD scar. Pathologic evaluation revealed an endometriosis implant.

involve the rectus muscle. Rare utero-cutaneous fistulas also have been reported. Endometrial implants throughout the pelvic cavity are seen in 14% to 26% of patients.[53]

Scar endometriosis can be diagnosed by various imaging modalities; however, its appearance depends on the chronicity of the condition, phase of the menstrual cycle, size of the lesion, and the degree of associated inflammation and bleeding.[16,53]

Ultrasound is usually the first imaging modality in the assessment of such patients. On

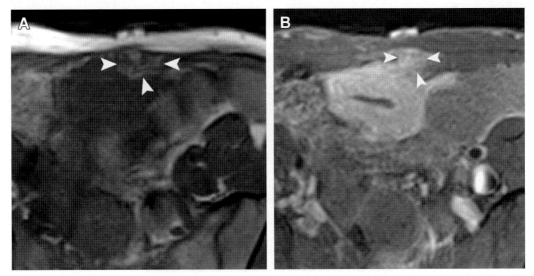

Fig. 9. Abdominal wall endometriosis. A woman presented with lower abdominal pain and a palpable nodule. (*A*) Axial T1-weighted MR image through the pelvis shows a focal soft-tissue nodule contiguous with the uterus at the level of a CD scar (*arrowheads*). Note the relatively high signal intensity within the nodule, compatible with the presence of blood products. (*B*) Axial fat-suppressed T1-weighted MR image with contrast through the pelvis shows an enhancing soft-tissue mass extending from the uterus at the level of the CD scar to the soft-tissue of the anterior abdominal wall (*arrowheads*). Pathologic examination revealed AWE.

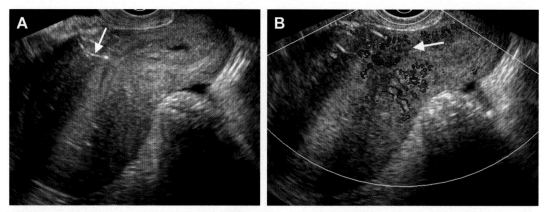

Fig. 10. Hypervascular granulation tissue. A woman with a history of multiple CDs presented with pain over an abdominal incision site. Long-axis (*A*) gray-scale and (*B*) Doppler ultrasound images of the uterus at the level of a cesarean scar (*arrows*) show abnormal increase in vascularity in that location. At surgery, significant adhesions were noted. Pathologic examination of the scar showed granulation tissue.

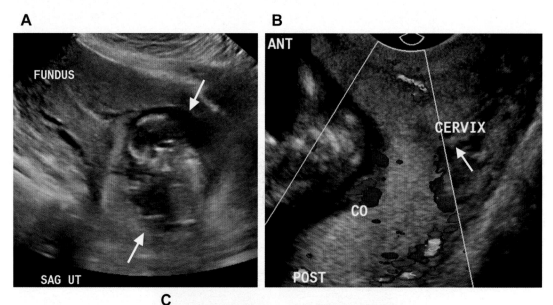

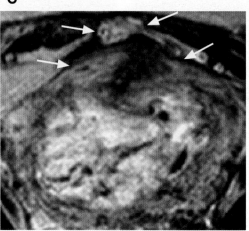

Fig. 11. Placenta percreta and complete previa, with a low-lying fetus in association with a CD scar. A woman presented at 13 weeks' gestation for fetal nuchal translucency measurement. (*A*) Long-axis gray-scale ultrasound image shows a fetus located in the lower uterine segment just above the cervix (*arrows*) with an empty uterine fundus. (*B*) Transverse Doppler image at the same level shows a complete placenta previa with the cord origin (CO) above the internal cervical os (*arrow*). The placenta has invaded the myometrium and the cervix. (*C*) Axial T2-weighted image through the lower uterus, from an MR examination performed shortly after the sonogram, shows invasion of a CD scar by the placenta, with extension of placental tissue beyond the myometrium (*arrows*).

ultrasound, scar endometriosis appears as a hypoechoic heterogeneous solid or partially cystic mass, which may have echogenic spots or septations representing fibrous components. The mass usually has irregular margins, and is vascular on color Doppler imaging. Focal pressure on the mass by the ultrasound probe can induce pain.[54] The appearance of scar endometriosis can be somewhat variable depending on the phase of the menstrual cycle in which it is imaged. Some scar endometriomas lesions may be associated with nodular thickening of their margins, some may contain cystic foci representing blood lacunae, and some may appear as punctate hypoechoic foci within the scar.[53] Picard and colleagues[55] suggest 3D ultrasound can be a useful tool in demonstrating the extent, margins, and configuration of AWE, and assists in surgical resection planning.

On CT, AWE may appear as a solid, soft-tissue mass with a variable enhancement pattern. Blood products may be present within the lesion, and feeding vessels can be seen in its periphery (**Fig. 8**).[53] On MRI, T1-weighted images may show hyperintense foci representing blood products, or the lesion may be isointense to muscle. AWE also may show heterogeneous signal intensity on T1-weighted and T2-weighted images due to presence of blood products of various ages. AWE can show enhancement after intravenous contrast administration (**Fig. 9**).[56]

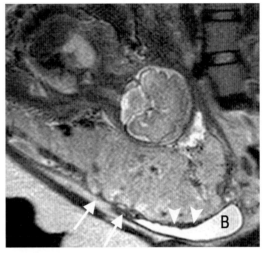

Fig. 13. Placenta previa and increta. A woman with a history of multiple CDs and an anterior placenta was screened with ultrasound for abnormal placentation, and was found to have suspicious findings. An MRI was requested for confirmation. Sagittal T2-weighted MR image of the lower uterine segment shows an anterior placenta, which is completely covering the internal cervical os (not shown). Note focal invasion of the placental tissue into the myometrium at the level of the CD scar (*arrows*), as well as the posterior bladder wall, with irregularity of the wall (*arrowheads*). B, bladder.

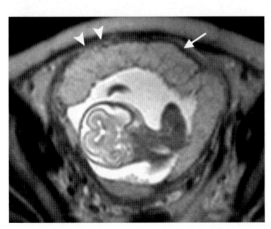

Fig. 12. Placenta accreta. A woman with a history of CDs and an anterior placenta during the current pregnancy was screened with ultrasound and was found to have suspicious findings for placenta accreta. An MRI was requested for confirmation. Axial T2-weighted, single-shot, fast-spin-echo image through the placenta at the level of the cesarean scar shows focal discontinuity (*arrowheads*) of the hypointense myometrium (*arrow*), which is highly consistent with placenta accreta.

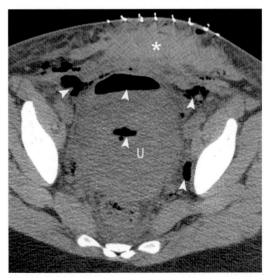

Fig. 14. Large abdominal wall hematoma after CD. A woman presented with a sudden bulge at the abdominal incision site and a drop in her hematocrit levels 2 days after CD. Axial noncontrast CT image at the level of the surgical incision in the pelvis shows a large hematoma in the subcutaneous fat (*asterisk*). Free gas in the pelvis and uterine cavity (*arrowheads*) is a normal postoperative finding. U, uterus.

The differential diagnosis for AWE includes abdominal wall lipoma, hernia, abscess, and tumors, including desmoid, fibrosis, lymphoma, sarcoma, and metastases.[16] Malignant transformation of AWE is rare, and is reported at a rate of approximately 0.9%. The most common tumor is clear cell carcinoma followed by endometrioid carcinoma.[57] The malignant transformation can occur any time between 3 and 39 years after the initial development of AWE, with an estimated average latency period of 17 years.[58]

Fine-needle aspiration and resection of the lesion with clear margins is the recommended treatment in the literature.[50] Other treatment options include chemotherapy and hormonal suppression. Wang and colleagues,[59] in a recent study, suggest ultrasound-guided high-intensity focused ultrasound as an effective and safe method of treatment of AWE.

Chronic Pelvic Pain

Chronic pelvic pain is defined as noncyclic pain in the lower abdomen, which is present for at least 6 months, occurs during the reproductive years, and affects daily activities.[60] The prevalence of chronic pain following CD is difficult to ascertain, as expression of pain is subjective and difficult to measure. Only a few studies in the literature have addressed this issue to our knowledge, with a reported incidence of 12.3% at 10 months after CD.[61] Kainu and colleagues[62] compared persistent pain after CD versus vaginal birth, and concluded that compared with vaginal delivery, chronic pain is more common 1 year after CD.

The type of incision used during CD can influence the risk of chronic pain development. A Pfannenstiel incision, which is most commonly used for CD, can result in neuroma formation, or entrapment of the iliohypogastric or ilioinguinal nerves, leading to development of chronic pelvic pain.[63] Repeated CDs can cause increasing fibrosis and subsequent increase in the risk of nerve entrapment.[64] The surgical technique may be an influencing factor as well. Surgical nonclosure of visceral and parietal peritoneum, length of the incision, and emergency CD are all associated with an increased likelihood of chronic pelvic pain (Fig. 10).[63,65]

Cesarean scar dehiscence and scar niche also can lead to chronic pelvic pain. Wang and colleagues[66] suggest that dysmenorrhea is associated with the width of the scar defect and repeated CDs, whereas postmenstrual bleeding and chronic pelvic pain are associated with the width of the defect only. Several reports in the

literature suggest resolution of symptoms after laparoscopic repair of the scar defect.[63,67]

Abdominal wall endometriosis and postoperative adhesions after CD can result in chronic pelvic pain as well. Adhesions are usually along the

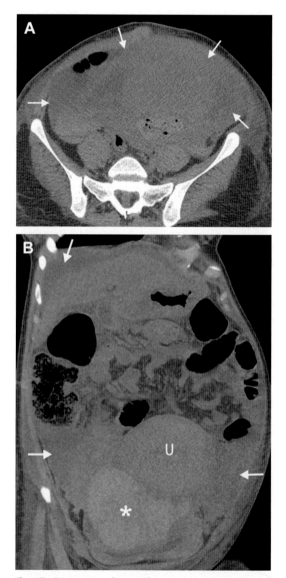

Fig. 15. Postpartum hemorrhage. A woman presented with sudden onset of abdominal pain and hemodynamic instability 3 days after vertical incision CD. (A) Axial and (B) coronal noncontrast CT images of the abdomen and pelvis show a large intraperitoneal and retroperitoneal hemorrhage (arrows), which extends from the pelvis into the upper abdomen. There also is a large blood clot in the cul-de-sac (asterisk). The patient was first managed conservatively; however, because of hemodynamic instability, she underwent subsequent successful angiography and uterine artery embolization. U, uterus.

anterior surface of the uterus at the interface between the abdominal wall and lower uterine segment. The likelihood of developing adhesions increases with multiple CDs. Adhesions also can lead to bowel obstruction, and prolonged surgical time in future CDs.[68] Seeding of the abdominal wall by endometrial cells from a CD or hysterectomy can result in AWE. These cells respond to hormonal stimulation, and cause an inflammatory response and pain in the adjacent tissue. The pain may be constant or may correlate with the menstrual cycle.[16]

Placentation Abnormalities

Multiple repeat CDs are associated with an increased risk of placenta previa as well as placentation abnormalities (accreta, increta, and percreta).[69] Placenta accreta is the mildest form of placentation abnormality, and is characterized by a defect in decidua basalis, allowing invasion of placental tissue into the myometrium. There is a fivefold increased risk of placenta previa and accreta with 2 or more CDs.[4,70] If the placenta implants on the cesarean scar, 20% to 40% of the time it is abnormally adherent, and can lead to uncontrollable postpartum bleeding and hysterectomy.[16]

Ultrasound is the initial imaging modality of choice for assessment of placentation abnormalities, as the cesarean scar and the implanted placenta are in the anterior pelvis. Both gray-scale and Doppler ultrasound are required for full evaluation of the placenta. On gray-scale ultrasound, the placenta is either low lying or is covering the internal cervical os. Gray-scale ultrasound findings of placenta accreta include loss of the subplacental hypoechoic clear space, large placental vascular spaces, bulging and/or interruption of the uterine wall and the uterus-bladder serosal surface, and extension of placental tissue beyond uterine serosal surface into the bladder or adjacent structures.[15] Comstock and colleagues[71] reported a sensitivity of 7% and a positive predictive value of 14% in diagnosis of placenta accreta, with loss of the subplacental clear space. These investigators suggested that presence of irregular linear vascular channels extending from the placenta into the myometrium increases the diagnostic capability, with a sensitivity of 50% and a positive predictive value of 88% (**Fig. 11**). Calì and colleagues[72] in a recent study suggested that 3D power Doppler technique plays a complementary role in the diagnosis of placentation abnormalities, by better depicting the associated

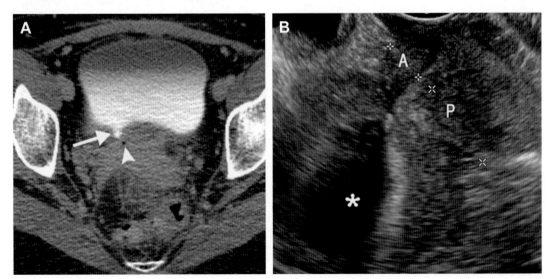

Fig. 16. Bladder and cervical injury. A woman with a recent CD presented with passage of air with urination and vaginal leaking. (*A*) An axial image through the pelvis from a CT cystogram shows tethering of the posterior bladder wall to the cervical region (*arrow*) and a small focus of air within the cervix (*arrowhead*). Surgical evaluation found that the cervix was sutured to the posterior bladder wall, resulting in a small fistula, which was repaired. (*B*) A pelvic ultrasound examination was performed for continued pelvic pain after surgical repair. Long-axis gray-scale image from the transvaginal ultrasound shows anterior cervical atrophy (small calipers) corresponding to the site of the surgical repair. There was fluid and debris within the uterine cavity (*asterisk*) due to cervical stenosis. A, anterior; P, posterior; large calipers demarcate posterior cervix.

irregular vascular channels. Shih and colleagues[73] suggested that criteria, including inseparable cotyledonal and intervillous circulations, intraplacental hypervascularity, and tortuous vascularity with irregular branching and multiple coherent vessels seen on the basal view, can all assist in the diagnosis of placentation abnormalities. They reported a specificity of 92% and a sensitivity of 97% when these criteria are used.

MRI has been used as an adjunct for diagnosis when ultrasound findings are inconclusive. On MRI, abnormal placentation is diagnosed by a heterogeneous placenta, which contains T2-hypointense intraplacental bands likely due to fibrin deposition. Bulging of the placenta or placenta-bladder margin, disorganized deep placental vessels, and invasion of the bladder or adjacent tissue are other possible findings (**Figs. 12 and 13**).[16]

In case of an undiagnosed placentation abnormality, the mother is at significant risk of severe uterine bleeding and placental retention. Also, subinvolution of the retained placenta can result in postpartum infection. Therefore,

delivery in such cases should be carefully planned. CD followed immediately by hysterectomy is the most definitive treatment; however, surgical intervention, and/or uterine artery embolization are other possible treatment considerations.[74]

Decreased Fertility

Several studies in the literature suggest decreased future maternal fertility after CD. Theoretically, uterine surgery can result in local vascular compromise and/or endometrial scarring, which can lead to subsequent decreased fertility. Pelvic adhesions also can result in decreased fertility because of tubal scarring and/or obstruction. Endometrial adhesions (synechiae) can interfere with implantation of fertilized eggs and resultant infertility.[2,44,75] Murphy and colleagues,[76] in a study of fertility in 4000 women,

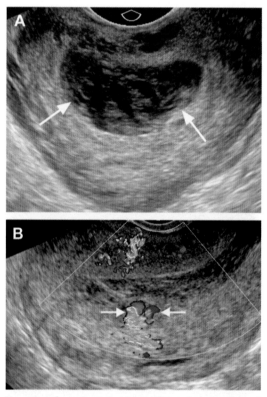

Fig. 18. Infected retained products of conception. A woman presented with fever and vaginal bleeding 2 weeks after CD. (*A*) Transvaginal transverse grayscale ultrasound image of the uterus shows heterogeneous material within the uterine cavity (*arrows*). (*B*) Long-axis Doppler ultrasound image of the uterus shows flow to the intrauterine contents (*arrows*). Surgical evacuation was performed. Pathologic examination revealed retained products of conception with evidence of associated infection.

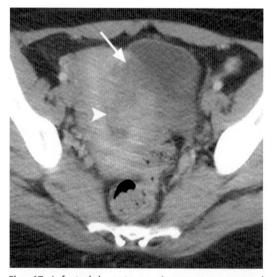

Fig. 17. Infected hematoma. A woman presented with abdominal pain and fever 2 weeks after CD. Axial contrast-enhanced CT image of the pelvis shows enhancing tissue within the endometrial cavity (*arrowhead*), which is contiguous with abnormal low density in the uterine wall. The uterine wall also appears disrupted (*arrow*). At surgery, hematoma and pus were present within the uterine cavity along with inflammatory changes in the uterine wall. The hematoma and pus were surgically evacuated, and the patient was treated with intravenous antibiotics.

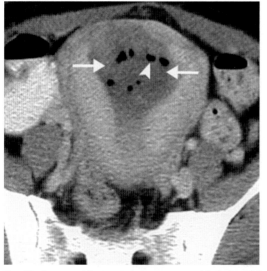

Fig. 19. Pyometritis. A woman presents with fever and pelvic pain 1 week after CD. Axial contrast-enhanced CT image of the pelvis shows fluid (*arrows*) and gas (*arrowhead*) filling the uterine cavity. On surgical evaluation, the uterine cavity was filled with pus.

found that those with a prior CD had a prolonged time from the time of pregnancy planning to the time of conception. This association was more prevalent in women with 2 or more pregnancies and a prior CD.

Multiple repeat CDs also are associated with an increased risk of hysterectomy. Marshall and colleagues,[4] in a recent review of the literature, found an increased incidence of hysterectomy of up to 8.9% in women with fewer than 5 CDs, and a 15-fold increased risk in those women with more than 5 CDs.

Other Complications

All CDs are associated with an increased risk of postpartum hemorrhage. This could be the result of uterine atony, placentation abnormalities, retained products of conception, acquired uterine arteriovenous malformation, excessive blood loss during delivery, lysis of adhesions, and uterine rupture (**Figs. 14** and **15**).[2,13,20]

Pelvic adhesions due to CD can lead to increased operative time and difficulty in delivery of the infant. They also can lead to operative complications, including bladder, ureter, and bowel injury. Incarcerated uterus is another rare complication in which the gravid uterus is trapped in the posterior pelvis (**Fig. 16**).[2,77]

With all CDs, there is an increased risk of postpartum febrile morbidity, which can result from postoperative endometritis, wound infection, infected postoperative pelvic fluid collections, postpartum appendicitis or pyelonephritis, and ovarian vein thrombophlebitis (**Figs. 17–21**).[13,78]

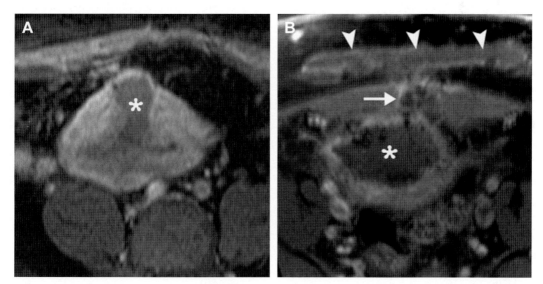

Fig. 20. Pyometritis, with uterine rupture and abscess. A woman presents with fever, severe abdominal pain, and an elevated white blood cell count 10 days after CD. (*A, B*) Axial T1-weighted fat-suppressed gadolinium-enhanced MR images of the pelvis show gas and fluid within the uterine cavity (*asterisk*) extending to the space anterior to the uterus (*arrow*), as well as into the subcutaneous fat at the level of cesarean scar (*arrowheads*). On surgical evaluation, this was shown to represent a ruptured uterine abscess.

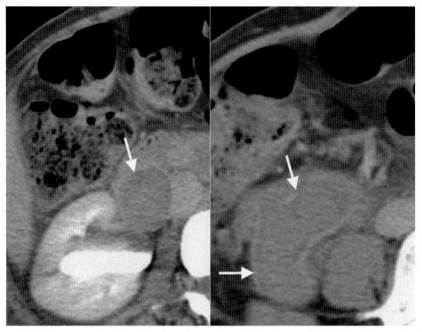

Fig. 21. Ovarian vein thrombophlebitis. A woman presents with flank pain and fever 7 days after CD. Delayed axial images from a contrast-enhanced CT examination of the abdomen and pelvis show a markedly dilated and acutely thrombosed right ovarian vein (*arrows*).

SUMMARY

The rate of CDs continues to rise, whereas the rate of vaginal delivery after cesarean birth continues to decline. Many women now tend to undergo multiple CDs, and therefore the associated chronic maternal morbidities are of growing concern. Accurate diagnosis of these conditions is crucial in maternal and fetal well-being. Many of these complications are diagnosed by imaging, and radiologists should be aware of the type and imaging appearances of these conditions.

REFERENCES

1. Martin JA, Hamilton BE, Osterman MJ, et al. Births: final data for 2012. National Vital Statistics Reports 2013;62(9):1–87.
2. Clark EA, Silver RM. Long-term maternal morbidity associated with repeat cesarean delivery. Am J Obstet Gynecol 2011;205(Suppl 6):S2–10.
3. Guise JM, Denman MA, Emeis C, et al. Vaginal birth after cesarean: new insights on maternal and neonatal outcomes. Obstet Gynecol 2010; 115(6):1267–78.
4. Marshall NE, Fu R, Guise JM. Impact of multiple cesarean deliveries on maternal morbidity: a systematic review. Am J Obstet Gynecol 2011;205(3):262. e1–8.
5. Silver RM, Landon MB, Rouse DJ, et al. Maternal morbidity associated with multiple repeat cesarean deliveries. Obstet Gynecol 2006;107(6): 1226–32.
6. Nisenblat V, Barak S, Griness OB, et al. Maternal complications associated with multiple cesarean deliveries. Obstet Gynecol 2006;108(1):21–6.
7. La Rosa MF, McCarthy S, Richter C, et al. Robotic repair of uterine dehiscence. JSLS 2013;17(1): 156–60.
8. American College of Obstetricians and Gynecologists. ACOG Practice bulletin no. 115: vaginal birth after previous cesarean delivery. Obstet Gynecol 2010;116:450–63.
9. Varner M. Cesarean scar imaging and prediction of subsequent obstetric complications. Clin Obstet Gynecol 2012;55(4):988–96.
10. Vikhareva Osser O, Valentin L. Clinical importance of appearance of cesarean hysterotomy scar at transvaginal ultrasonography in nonpregnant women. Obstet Gynecol 2011;117(3):525–32.
11. Gizzo S, Zambon A, Saccardi C, et al. Effective anatomical and functional status of the lower uterine segment at term: estimating the risk of uterine dehiscence by ultrasound. Fertil Steril 2013;99(2): 496–501.
12. Donnez O, Jadoul P, Squifflet J, et al. Laparoscopic repair of wide and deep uterine scar dehiscence after cesarean section. Fertil Steril 2008;89(4): 974–80.

13. Kamaya A, Ro K, Benedetti NJ, et al. Imaging and diagnosis of postpartum complications: sonography and other imaging modalities. Ultrasound Q 2009;25(3):151–62.

14. Yap OW, Kim ES, Laros RK. Maternal and neonatal outcomes after uterine rupture in labor. Am J Obstet Gynecol 2001;184(7):1576–81.

15. Di Salvo DN. Sonographic imaging of maternal complications of pregnancy. J Ultrasound Med 2003;22(1):69–89.

16. Rodgers SK, Kirby CL, Smith RJ, et al. Imaging after cesarean delivery: acute and chronic complications. Radiographics 2012;32(6):1693–712.

17. Maldjian C, Milestone B, Schnall M, et al. MR appearance of uterine dehiscence in the post-cesarean section patient. J Comput Assist Tomogr 1998;22(5):738–41.

18. Osborn DA, Williams TR, Craig BM. Cesarean scar pregnancy: sonographic and magnetic resonance imaging findings, complications, and treatment. J Ultrasound Med 2012;31(9):1449–56.

19. Seow KM, Huang LW, Lin YH, et al. Cesarean scar pregnancy: issues in management. Ultrasound Obstet Gynecol 2004;23(3):247–53.

20. Kim D, Moon NR, Lee SR, et al. Acquired uterine arteriovenous malformation in a cesarean scar pregnancy. Taiwan J Obstet Gynecol 2013;52(4):590–2.

21. Lin EP, Bhatt S, Dogra VS. Diagnostic clues to ectopic pregnancy. Radiographics 2008;28(6):1661–71.

22. Ash A, Smith A, Maxwell D. Caesarean scar pregnancy. BJOG 2007;114(3):253–63.

23. Litwicka K, Greco E. Caesarean scar pregnancy. Curr Opin Obstet Gynecol 2013;25(6):456–61.

24. Vial Y, Petignat P, Hohlfeld P. Pregnancy in a cesarean scar. Ultrasound Obstet Gynecol 2000;16(6):592–3.

25. Pascual MA, Hereter L, Graupera B, et al. Three-dimensional power Doppler ultrasound diagnosis and conservative treatment of ectopic pregnancy in a cesarean section scar. Fertil Steril 2007;88(3):706.e5–7.

26. Litwicka K, Greco E. Caesarean scar pregnancy. Curr Opin Obstet Gynecol 2011;23(6):415–21.

27. Nishida R, Yamada T, Yamada T, et al. Viable delivery after conservative management of a cesarean scar pregnancy. J Ultrasound Med 2013;32(9):1682–4.

28. Sinha P, Mishra M. Caesarean scar pregnancy: a precursor of placenta percreta/accreta. J Obstet Gynaecol 2012;32(7):621–3.

29. Timor-Tritsch IE, Monteagudo A. Unforeseen consequences of the increasing rate of cesarean deliveries: early placenta accreta and cesarean scar pregnancy. A review. Am J Obstet Gynecol 2012;207(1):14–29.

30. Ugurlucan FG, Bastu E, Dogan M, et al. Management of cesarean heterotopic pregnancy with transvaginal ultrasound–guided potassium chloride injection and gestational sac aspiration, and review of the literature. J Minim Invasive Gynecol 2012;19(5):671–3.

31. Bodur S, Gun I, Guido R. What is the role of primary methotrexate treatment in scar ectopic pregnancy? Am J Obstet Gynecol 2014;210:379–80.

32. Lui MW, Shek NW, Li RH, et al. Management of heterotopic cesarean scar pregnancy by repeated transvaginal ultrasonographic-guided aspiration with successful preservation of normal intrauterine pregnancy and complicated by arteriovenous malformation. Eur J Obstet Gynecol Reprod Biol 2014; 175:209–10.

33. Wang DB, Chen YH, Zhang ZF, et al. Evaluation of the transvaginal resection of low-segment cesarean scar ectopic pregnancies. Fertil Steril 2014; 101(2):602–6.

34. Demirel LC, Bodur H, Selam B, et al. Laparoscopic management of heterotopic cesarean scar pregnancy with preservation of intrauterine gestation and delivery at term: case report. Fertil Steril 2009;91(4):1293.e5–7.

35. Arslan M, Pata O, Dilek TU, et al. Treatment of viable cesarean scar ectopic pregnancy with suction curettage. Int J Gynaecol Obstet 2005;89(2):163–6.

36. El-Mowafi DM, Diamond MP. Are pelvic adhesions preventable? Surg Technol Int 2003;11:222–35.

37. Lyell DJ. Adhesions and perioperative complications of repeat cesarean delivery. Am J Obstet Gynecol 2011;205(Suppl 6):S11–8.

38. Bates GW, Shomento S. Adhesion prevention in patients with multiple cesarean deliveries. Am J Obstet Gynecol 2011;205(Suppl 6):S19–24.

39. Cheong YC, Premkumar G, Metwally M, et al. To close or not to close? A systematic review and a meta-analysis of peritoneal non-closure and adhesion formation after caesarean section. Eur J Obstet Gynecol Reprod Biol 2009;147(1):3–8.

40. Malvasi A, Tinelli A, Farine D, et al. Effects of visceral peritoneal closure on scar formation at cesarean delivery. Int J Gynaecol Obstet 2009; 105(2):131–5.

41. Kapustian V, Anteby EY, Gdalevich M, et al. Effect of closure versus nonclosure of peritoneum at cesarean section on adhesions: a prospective randomized study. Am J Obstet Gynecol 2012; 206(1):56.e1–4.

42. Andolf E, Thorsell M, Källén K. Cesarean delivery and risk for postoperative adhesions and intestinal obstruction: a nested case-control study of the Swedish medical birth registry. Am J Obstet Gynecol 2010;203(4):406.e1–6.

43. Gedikbasi A, Akyol A, Bingol B, et al. Multiple repeated cesarean deliveries: operative

complications in the fourth and fifth surgeries in urgent and elective cases. Taiwan J Obstet Gynecol 2010;49(4):425–31.

44. Tulandi T, Agdi M, Zarei A, et al. Adhesion development and morbidity after repeat cesarean delivery. Am J Obstet Gynecol 2009;201(1):56.e1–6.

45. Bij de Vaate AJ, van der Voet LF, Naji O, et al. The prevalence, potential risk factors for development and symptoms related to the presence of uterine niches following Cesarean section: a systematic review. Ultrasound Obstet Gynecol 2014;43:372–82.

46. Bij de Vaate AJ, Brölmann HA, van der Voet LF, et al. Ultrasound evaluation of the Cesarean scar: relation between a niche and postmenstrual spotting. Ultrasound Obstet Gynecol 2010;37(1):93–9.

47. Van der Voet LF, Bij de Vaate AM, Veersema S, et al. Long-term complications of caesarean section. The niche in the scar: a prospective cohort study on niche prevalence and its relation to abnormal uterine bleeding. BJOG 2013;121(2): 236–44.

48. Monteagudo A, Carreno C, Timor-Tritsch IE. Saline infusion sonohysterography in nonpregnant women with previous cesarean delivery: the "niche" in the scar. J Ultrasound Med 2001;20(10):1105–15.

49. Van der Voet LF, Vervoort AJ, Veersema S, et al. Minimally invasive therapy for gynaecological symptoms related to a niche in the caesarean scar: a systematic review. BJOG 2013;121(2): 145–56.

50. Ozel L, Sagiroglu J, Unal A, et al. Abdominal wall endometriosis in the cesarean section surgical scar: a potential diagnostic pitfall. J Obstet Gynaecol Res 2012;38(3):526–30.

51. Nominato NS, Prates LF, Lauar I, et al. Cesarean section greatly increases risk of scar endometriosis. Eur J Obstet Gynecol 2010;152(1):83–5.

52. Bektas H, Bilsel Y, Ersoz F, et al. Abdominal wall endometrioma; a 10-year experience and brief review of the literature. J Surg Res 2010;164(1):e77–81.

53. Gidwaney R, Badler RL, Yam BL, et al. Endometriosis of abdominal and pelvic wall scars: multimodality imaging findings, pathologic correlation, and radiologic mimics. Radiographics 2012;32(7): 2031–43.

54. Savelli L, Manuzzi L, Di Donato N, et al. Endometriosis of the abdominal wall: ultrasonographic and Doppler characteristics. Ultrasound Obstet Gynecol 2012;39(3):336–40.

55. Picard A, Varlet M, Guillibert F, et al. Three-dimensional sonographic diagnosis of abdominal wall endometriosis: a useful tool? Fertil Steril 2011; 95(1):289.e1–4.

56. Randriamarolahy A, Perrin H, Cucchi JM, et al. Endometriosis following cesarean section: ultrasonography and magnetic resonance imaging. Clin Imaging 2010;34(2):113–5.

57. Li X, Yang J, Cao D, et al. Clear-cell carcinoma of the abdominal wall after cesarean delivery. Obstet Gynecol 2012;120:445–8.

58. Da Ines D, Bourdel N, Charpy C, et al. Mixed endometrioid and serous carcinoma developing in abdominal wall endometriosis following Cesarean section. Acta Radiol 2011;52(5):587–90.

59. Wang W, Wang L, Wang J, et al. Ultrasound-guided high-intensity focused ultrasound treatment for abdominal wall endometriosis: preliminary results. Eur J Radiol 2011;79(1):56–9.

60. Almeida EC, Nogueira AA, Candido dos Reis FJ, et al. Cesarean section as a cause of chronic pelvic pain. Int J Gynaecol Obstet 2002;79(2):101–4.

61. Nikolajsen L, Sørensen HC, Jensen TS, et al. Chronic pain following caesarean section. Acta Anaesthesiol Scand 2004;48(1):111–6.

62. Kainu JP, Sarvela J, Tiippana E, et al. Persistent pain after caesarean section and vaginal birth: a cohort study. Int J Obstet Anesth 2010;19(1):4–9.

63. Silver RM. Delivery after previous cesarean: long-term maternal outcomes. Semin Perinatol 2010; 34(4):258–66.

64. Loos MJ, Scheltinga MR, Mulders LG, et al. The Pfannenstiel incision as a source of chronic pain. Obstet Gynecol 2008;111(4):839–46.

65. Rafique Z, Shibli KU, Russell IF, et al. A randomized controlled trial of the closure or non-closure of peritoneum at caesarean section: effect on post-operative pain. BJOG 2002;109(6):694–8.

66. Wang CB, Chiu WW, Lee CY, et al. Cesarean scar defect: correlation between cesarean section number, defect size, clinical symptoms and uterine position. Ultrasound Obstet Gynecol 2009;34(1):85–9.

67. Klemm P, Koehler C, Mangler M, et al. Laparoscopic and vaginal repair of uterine scar dehiscence following cesarean section as detected by ultrasound. J Perinat Med 2005;33(4):324–31.

68. Diamond MP. Postoperative adhesions: an underappreciated complication of cesarean deliveries. Am J Obstet Gynecol 2011;205(Suppl 6):S1.

69. Solheim KN, Esakoff TF, Little SE, et al. The effect of cesarean delivery rates on the future incidence of placenta previa, placenta accreta, and maternal mortality. J Matern Fetal Neonatal Med 2011; 24(11):1341–6.

70. Bowman Z, Eller A, Bardsley T, et al. Risk factors for placenta accreta: a large prospective cohort. Am J Perinatol 2013. [Epub ahead of print].

71. Comstock CH, Love JJ Jr, Bronsteen RA, et al. Sonographic detection of placenta accreta in the second and third trimesters of pregnancy. Am J Obstet Gynecol 2004;190(4):1135–40.

72. Calì G, Giambanco L, Puccio G, et al. Morbidly adherent placenta: evaluation of ultrasound diagnostic criteria and differentiation of placenta

accreta from percreta. Ultrasound Obstet Gynecol 2013;41(4):406–12.

73. Shih JC, Jaraquemada JM, Su YN, et al. Role of three-dimensional power Doppler in the antenatal diagnosis of placenta accreta: comparison with gray-scale and color Doppler techniques. Ultrasound Obstet Gynecol 2009;33(2):193–203.

74. Balayla J, Bondarenko HD. Placenta accreta and the risk of adverse maternal and neonatal outcomes. J Perinat Med 2013;41(2):141–9.

75. Myers EM, Hurst BS. Comprehensive management of severe Asherman syndrome and amenorrhea. Fertil Steril 2012;97(1):160–4.

76. Murphy DJ, Stirrat GM, Heron J, et al. The relationship between caesarean section and subfertility in a population-based sample of 14 541 pregnancies. Hum Reprod 2002;17(7):1914–7.

77. Gardner CS, Jaffe TA, Hertzberg BS, et al. The incarcerated uterus: a review of MRI and ultrasound imaging appearances. AJR Am J Roentgenol 2013;201(1):223–9.

78. Antonelli E, Morales MA, Dumps P, et al. Sonographic detection of fluid collections and postoperative morbidity following cesarean section and hysterectomy. Ultrasound Obstet Gynecol 2004; 23(4):388–92.

Index

Note: Page numbers of article titles are in **boldface** type.

Radiol Clin N Am 52 (2014) 1137–1143
http://dx.doi.org/10.1016/S0033-8389(14)00108-0
0033-8389/14/$ – see front matter © 2014 Elsevier Inc. All rights reserved.

Moving?

Make sure your subscription moves with you!

To notify us of your new address, find your **Clinics Account Number** (located on your mailing label above your name), and contact customer service at:

Email: journalscustomerservice-usa@elsevier.com

800-654-2452 (subscribers in the U.S. & Canada)
314-447-8871 (subscribers outside of the U.S. & Canada)

Fax number: 314-447-8029

Elsevier Health Sciences Division
Subscription Customer Service
3251 Riverport Lane
Maryland Heights, MO 63043

*To ensure uninterrupted delivery of your subscription, please notify us at least 4 weeks in advance of move.